AF856156

Botulinum Toxins in Clinical Aesthetic Practice

Third Edition

Volume One: Clinical Adaptations

Series in Cosmetic and Laser Therapy

Series Editors

Nicholas J. Gary P. Lask, and David J. Goldberg

Anthony V. Benedetto, *Botulinum Toxins in Clinical Aesthetic Practice, Third Edition: Two Volume Set*, ISBN 9781498716314

Robert Baran and Howard Maibach, *Textbook of Cosmetic Dermatology, Fifth Edition*, ISBN 9781482223934

Philippe Deprez, *Textbook of Chemical Peels, Second Edition: Superficial, Medium, and Deep Peels in Cosmetic Practice*, ISBN 9781482223934

Jenny Kim, Gary Lask, and Andrew Nelson, *Comprehensive Aesthetic Rejuvenation: A Regional Approach*, ISBN 9780415458948

David J. Goldberg and Alexander L. Berlin, *Disorders of Fat and Cellulite: Advances in Diagnosis and Treatment*, ISBN 9780415477000

Neil S. Sadick, Paul J. Carniol, Deborshi Roy, and Luitgard Wiest, *Illustrated Manual of Injectable Fillers: A Technical Guide to the Volumetric Approach to Whole Body Rejuvenation*, ISBN 9780415476447

Kenneth Beer, Mary P. Lupo, and Vic A. Narurkar, *Cosmetic Bootcamp Primer: Comprehensive Aesthetic Management*, ISBN 9781841846989

Anthony Benedetto, *Botulinum Toxins in Clinical Aesthetic Practice, Second Edition*, ISBN 9780415476362

Robert Baran and Howard I. Maibach, *Textbook of Cosmetic Dermatology, Fourth Edition*, ISBN 9781841847009

Neil Sadick, Diane Berson, Mary P. Lupo, and Zoe Diana Draelos, *Cosmeceutical Science in Clinical Practice*, ISBN 9780415471145

Paul Carniol and Gary Monheit, *Aesthetic Rejuvenation Challenges and Solutions: A Global Perspective*, ISBN 9780415475600

Avi Shai, Robert Baran, Howard I. Maibach, *Handbook of Cosmetic Skin Care, Second Edition*, ISBN 9780415467186

Benjamin Ascher, Marina Landau, and Bernard Rossi, *Injection Treatments in Cosmetic Surgery*, ISBN 9780415386517

David J. Goldberg, *Laser Hair Removal, Second Edition*, ISBN 9780415414128

Paul J. Carniol and Neil S. Sadick, *Clinical Procedures in Laser Skin Rejuvenation*, ISBN 9780415414135

C. William Hanke, Gerhard Sattler, and Boris Sommer, *Textbook of Liposuction*, ISBN 9781841845326

Botulinum Toxins in Clinical Aesthetic Practice

Third Edition

Volume One: Clinical Adaptations

Edited by

Anthony V. Benedetto

Clinical Professor of Dermatology
Perelman School of Medicine
University of Pennsylvania
and
Medical Director
Dermatologic SurgiCenter
Philadelphia, Pennsylvania

CRC Press
Taylor & Francis Group
Boca Raton London New York

CRC Press is an imprint of the
Taylor & Francis Group, an **informa** business

CRC Press
Taylor & Francis Group
6000 Broken Sound Parkway NW, Suite 300
Boca Raton, FL 33487-2742

© 2018 by Taylor & Francis Group, LLC
CRC Press is an imprint of Taylor & Francis Group, an Informa business

No claim to original U.S. Government works

Printed and bound in India by Replika Press Pvt. Ltd.

Printed on acid-free paper

International Standard Book Number-13: 978-1-138-30184-9 (Pack- Hardback and eBook)

This book contains information obtained from authentic and highly regarded sources. While all reasonable efforts have been made to publish reliable data and information, neither the author[s] nor the publisher can accept any legal responsibility or liability for any errors or omissions that may be made. The publishers wish to make clear that any views or opinions expressed in this book by individual editors, authors or contributors are personal to them and do not necessarily reflect the views/opinions of the publishers. The information or guidance contained in this book is intended for use by medical, scientific or health-care professionals and is provided strictly as a supplement to the medical or other professional's own judgement, their knowledge of the patient's medical history, relevant manufacturer's instructions and the appropriate best practice guidelines. Because of the rapid advances in medical science, any information or advice on dosages, procedures or diagnoses should be independently verified. The reader is strongly urged to consult the relevant national drug formulary and the drug companies' and device or material manufacturers' printed instructions, and their websites, before administering or utilizing any of the drugs, devices or materials mentioned in this book. This book does not indicate whether a particular treatment is appropriate or suitable for a particular individual. Ultimately it is the sole responsibility of the medical professional to make his or her own professional judgements, so as to advise and treat patients appropriately. The authors and publishers have also attempted to trace the copyright holders of all material reproduced in this publication and apologize to copyright holders if permission to publish in this form has not been obtained. If any copyright material has not been acknowledged please write and let us know so we may rectify in any future reprint.

Except as permitted under U.S. Copyright Law, no part of this book may be reprinted, reproduced, transmitted, or utilized in any form by any electronic, mechanical, or other means, now known or hereafter invented, including photocopying, microfilming, and recording, or in any information storage or retrieval system, without written permission from the publishers.

For permission to photocopy or use material electronically from this work, please access www.copyright.com (http://www.copyright.com/) or contact the Copyright Clearance Center, Inc. (CCC), 222 Rosewood Drive, Danvers, MA 01923, 978-750-8400. CCC is a not-for-profit organization that provides licenses and registration for a variety of users. For organizations that have been granted a photocopy license by the CCC, a separate system of payment has been arranged.

Trademark Notice: Product or corporate names may be trademarks or registered trademarks, and are used only for identification and explanation without intent to infringe.

Library of Congress Cataloging-in-Publication Data

Names: Benedetto, Anthony V., editor.
Title: Botulinum toxins in clinical aesthetic practice / edited by Anthony V. Benedetto.
Description: Third edition. | Boca Raton, FL : CRC Press/Taylor & Francis Group, 2018. | Includes bibliographical references and index.
Identifiers: LCCN 2017024412| ISBN 9781138301849 (v. 1 : pack- hardback and ebook : alk. paper) | ISBN 9781138304802 (v. 2 : pack- hardback and ebook : alk. paper) | ISBN 9780203729847 (v. 1 : ebook) | ISBN 9780203729755 (v. 2 : ebook)
Subjects: | MESH: Botulinum Toxins, Type A--therapeutic use | Dermatologic Agents--therapeutic use | Skin--drug effects | Cosmetic Techniques | Skin Diseases--drug therapy
Classification: LCC RL120.B66 | NLM QV 140 | DDC 615.9/5--dc23
LC record available at https://lccn.loc.gov/2017024412

Visit the Taylor & Francis Web site at
http://www.taylorandfrancis.com

and the CRC Press Web site at
http://www.crcpress.com

To Dianne, my loving wife of forty years, whose encouragement and support permitted me to accomplish that which seemed at times insurmountable and unattainable.

Contents

Preface

Because of the exponential developments in the clinical use of botulinum toxins (BoNTs), the need for a third edition quickly became a foregone conclusion. Maintaining the original mission of an instructional manual, this completely revamped and updated third edition attempts to record the phenomenal progress that has evolved in the use of BoNTs in clinical medicine over the past seven years. Updates of the literature, expanded indications, improved clinical photographs and illustrations, and newer and innovative ways to utilize the different BoNTs that are presently available worldwide are presented in this newly formatted third edition. It also has become strikingly obvious that BoNTs are injected in a variety of novel ways that differ from East to West. Therefore, a concerted effort has been made to include a profile of as many of the different BoNTs currently available around the world, including how they are utilized in a clinical aesthetic setting in both Western and Eastern cultures.

In the United States, glabellar and lateral canthal lines remain the only areas of the face that are approved by the FDA for the cosmetic use of onabotulinumtoxinA (OnaBTX-A) or BOTOX® Cosmetic. The other BoNTs available in the United States, abobotulinumtoxinA (AboBTX-A), incobotulinumtoxinA (IncoBTX-A), and rimabotulinumtoxinB (RimaBTX-B), have their own similar, but very specific, FDA indications. Consequently, except for glabellar and lateral canthal wrinkles, all the cosmetic injection techniques described in this third edition, as in the previous editions, apply to non-approved, off-label indications, which makes this book unlike most other textbooks in medicine.

It is sobering to realize that throughout human existence women and men have always sought ways to improve their appearance. To commence the in-depth and diverse discussions in this third edition on beautification and rejuvenation with BoNTs, Nina Jablonski, PhD, professor of anthropology at The Pennsylvania State University, and a world-renowned biological anthropologist and paleobiologist, provides us in her Prologue with a brief introduction to the evolutionary and anthropological perspectives on the importance of human facial attractiveness and expressivity. She cautions both patients and treating physicians in the over-use of face altering procedures that can effectively inhibit one's ability to express oneself accurately and in a completely natural manner.

Chapter 1 is written by Jean Carruthers, MD, to whom the world is indebted for her prescient identification of the cosmetic uses of the BoNTs. Dr. Jean Carruthers commences our venture through the fascinating evolving world of the BoNTs by presenting a historical account of the chronological events that led to the discovery, identification, isolation, and eventual synthesis of BoNTs for clinical use. Included is her seminal work in the development and advancement of the clinical uses of BoNT-A in ocular therapeutics, and her serendipitous discovery of its cosmetic properties. Jean describes the role she and her dermatologist husband, Dr. Alastair Carruthers, played in their provocatively sensitive introduction and promotion of the cosmetic uses of BoNT-A to the medical community.

Updates on the current advancements in the pharmacology and immunology of the different BoNTs are discussed by world-renowned scientists who are intimately involved in BoNT research and development. These include Chapter 2 by Mitchell F. Brin, MD, neurologist and one of the earliest clinical injectors of OnaBTX-A and now senior vice president of global drug development and chief scientific officer of BOTOX®, at Allergan Inc. (Irvine, CA). He presents an update on the pharmacology, immunology, recent developments, and future predictions on the use of BoNT-A. Chapter 3 by Juergen Frevert, PhD, head of botulinum toxin research at Merz Pharmaceuticals GmbH, (Potsdam, Germany), discusses the innovative pharmacology and immunology of a noncomplexed BoNT-A, and the advantages of its clinical uses.

Chapter 4 by the visionary dermatologist, Richard Glogau, MD, discusses the fascinating emerging science, development, and effective clinical uses of a new topically applied BoNT-A. Chapter 5 by Gary Monheit, MD, a dermatologist and leader in BoNT clinical research, and dermatologist James Highsmith, MD, elaborates on the recent advances of the different FDA approved BoNT-As and BoNT-B with updates on the pertinent literature and details on recent developments in their clinical use. Chapter 6 by Andy Pickett, PhD, Senior Program Leader & Scientific Expert, Neurotoxins for Galderma Aesthetic and Corrective, and Director and Founder of Toxin Science Limited, Wrexham, UK, identifies some of the different BoNTs used in clinical practice currently available in other parts of the world.

Chapter 7 by Alastair and Jean Carruthers, MD, presents updated and advanced clinical information on the adjunctive uses of the BoNTs in conjunction with injections of soft tissue fillers, and light- and energy-based devices for the aesthetic improvement of the face and body.

In Chapter 8, Arthur Swift, MD, an otorhinolaryngologist, Kent Remington, MD, a dermatologist, and Steve Fagien, MD, an ophthalmologist, add a new dimension to the aesthetic interpretation of how to use injectables when rejuvenating the face, change to including their explanation of facial proportions, geometrical Phi measurements, aesthetics, and beauty as they relate to the use of BoNTs.

For Chapter 9, dermatologists David Pariser, MD, and DeeAnna Glaser, MD, Secretary and President, respectively, of the International Hyperhidrosis Society, have comprehensively revised and updated the material on hyperhidrosis, discussing recent developments as well as new and different areas of treatment.

Chapter 10 by dermatologist Kevin C. Smith, MD, the master of novel injection techniques, along with dermatologists Irèn Kossintseva and Benjamin Barankin continues to enlighten us on unique ways to utilize BoNT-A for cosmetic and therapeutic purposes.

Chapter 11 by dermatologist and attorney David Goldberg, MD, JD, concludes the first volume with a revision and update of his chapter on the important medicolegal aspects of the cosmetic uses of BoNT.

Because of the ever-growing selection of the various BoNT products currently commercially available for clinical use in different parts of the world, the new Appendix 1 written by dermatologist Alica Sharova, MD, PhD, of Pirogov Russian National Research Medical University, Moscow, presents thought-provoking results of her metanalysis comparing consensus statements and recommendations for injecting different BoNT products in the United States, Russia, and different countries in Europe. She identifies and compares the fallacious recommendations of dose ratio equivalencies of the different available BoNTs injected, including number of injection points and dosaging for the different areas of the face and neck in males and females.

In the second volume, Sebastian Cotofana, PhD, a quintessential anatomist, has provided essential new material on functional facial anatomy in Chapter 12.

The nuclear Chapters 13, 14, and 15 on the cosmetic treatment of the face, neck, and chest with injections of BoNTs have been reorganized and expanded, assimilating many improved injection techniques by integrating updated information of recently published clinical and anatomical studies. All the anatomical figures and illustrations have been revised and enhanced throughout the text. The organization of these three chapters has remained the same. Each clinical topic is subdivided according to its facial and functional anatomy, and discussed in seven subheadings. The "Introduction" of each topic identifies the different anatomical changes acquired by men and women as they "age" and develop "wrinkles." Normal "Functional Anatomy" discusses the reasons these disconcerting changes and wrinkles occur so that a suitable plan of correction with a BoNT can be initiated. Functional anatomy is stressed and complemented by clinical photographs and detailed illustrations because the only way a physician injector can utilize any type of BoNT properly is to have an in-depth understanding of how to modify the normal and exaggerated movements of facial mimetic muscles and other potentially treatable muscles elsewhere in the body. When injections of a BoNT are appropriately performed, desirable and reproducible results without adverse sequelae are created. In the "Dilution" subheading, suggestions are given on how much diluent can be added to reconstitute a 100-unit vial of OnaBTX-A in order to arrive at various preferred concentrations per fluid volume dilutions when injecting certain muscles at different anatomical sites. The U.S. FDA-approved manufacturer's recommendation for the reconstitution of a 100-unit vial of OnaBTX-A is to add 2.5 mL of nonpreserved normal saline. This approved and recommended dilution is for injecting glabellar and lateral canthal frown lines only, since these areas on the face are the only approved indications for the cosmetic use of OnaBTX-A. However, when treating other areas of the face and body for cosmetic purposes, albeit in an off-label, unapproved manner, higher or lower dilutions of OnaBTX-A have proven to be more suitable and clinically more effective, depending on the muscles being treated. Options for "Dosing" are presented, with an emphasis placed on what to do and what not to do when injecting OnaBTX-A. Precise dosing and accurate injections of OnaBTX-A will diminish muscle movements of the face and body in a safe and reproducible way. Fastidious injection techniques are necessary to correct a particular aesthetic problem reliably, predictably, and for extended periods of time with any BoNT. "Outcomes" and results of different injection techniques are discussed to avoid "Complications" and adverse sequelae. Finally, how to inject a particular anatomical site and its projected results are summarized in the list of "Implications of Treatment".

Controversial and remarkable treatments for non-surgical breast augmentation for women and men are practiced by dermatologists Francisco Atamoros Perez and Olga Marcias Martinez and discussed in detail in Chapter 16. Their accumulated clinical evidence of the efficacy of BoNT-A injections of the pectoral area is clearly presented with an abundance of clinical illustrations.

Chapter 17, by a prominent and internationally well-known Korean dermatologist, Kyle Seo, MD, discusses the Asian perspective of the use of the different BoNTs currently available in his part of the world. Insight into the East and Southeast Asian cultural aesthetic needs and the Asian perception of aesthetics and beauty, is emphasized. He also presents a detailed description of the racial differences in the anatomy between Asians and Caucasians, which call for different indications and variations in appropriate dosing and injection points of BoNT-A treatments, necessary when treating Asian patients. He also provides some practical guidelines for the innovative use of BoNT-A in facial skin redraping and body muscle contouring injection techniques that are currently very popular in the East.

Many appendices supplying material for procedural reference conclude this second volume.

It is extremely fascinating and encouraging to understand that the cosmetic use of OnaBTX-A was initiated by the insight and convictions of two astute and courageous physicians, an ophthalmologist wife and her dermatologist husband. If it were not for the persistence of Jean and Alastair Carruthers in promoting their serendipitous observations, many other perceptive and insightful physicians would not have had the opportunity or the confidence to learn more about BoNT and its use in clinical aesthetic medicine. The challenge now being passed onto the reader is that with knowledge of how to inject a few drops of BoNT appropriately and safely, while treating patients with compassion and professionalism, additional innovative and ingenious uses of BoNT can be discovered, be they for cosmetic or therapeutic purposes.

We are all indebted to those physicians who have treated and continue to care for patients with BoNT for therapeutic and cosmetic purposes. Their commitment to the improvement of their patients' health and well-being through the advancement of sound and effective medical care is commendable and truly appreciated.

Finally, particular recognition and a special expression of gratitude is due to Kelly Heckler for her organizational skills and secretarial expertise that facilitated the completion of this book.

Anthony V. Benedetto, DO FACP
Philadelphia, PA

Acknowledgments

Many of the anatomical drawings not otherwise attributed (e.g., Figure 10.1) have base artwork from the Shutterstock archives and are reproduced with permission under licence; the annotations and overlays have been developed by the lead author of each chapter.

PROLOGUE An anthropological perspective on facial attractiveness and expressivity

Nina G. Jablonski

Humans are large-brained, long-lived primates that evolved in small, stable, and tightly knit social groups. In these groups, in the past and today, social cohesion has been essential for survival and communication has been essential for social cohesion. Communication in nonhuman primate and traditional human societies involves important vocal and tactile components, but is dominated by the exchange of visual information. The face is the primary portal from which this information emanates, and the "information content" of the face is vast. Gender is readily perceived by the relative masculinity or femininity of facial features, while color and texture of facial skin connote age and state of health, symmetry of facial features appears to indicate good health during all stages of development, and facial averageness connotes genetic heterozygosity.[1] Across cultures, the same features are also the primary source of judgements about attractiveness, with the universality of these preferences suggesting that, in the course of evolution, humans come to consider certain features attractive because they were displayed by healthy individuals.[2,3] Facial attractiveness is associated with many positive personal, professional and societal outcomes, especially for women.[4] In some cultures perceived Perceived facial attractiveness declines more in older women than in men, suggesting that there is probably greater selective pressure on older women to maintain high facial attractiveness.[5]

The static features of the face are only one aspect of the face's total information content, however. Facial expressions are as, or more important than the static attributes associated with attractiveness because they convey different kinds of information, about inner mood, intention and empathy. Humans and related species that live in complex social groups must be able to interpret the various meanings associated with facial appearance and the facial displays used in different emotional contexts.[6] The nonverbal information conveyed by postures and gestures (body language) is important in humans, but much of our capacity for nonverbal communication—especially in the expression of fear and anger witnessed by raising the hackles—has been lost as a result of loss of visible body hair in the human lineage.[7] Humans have thus become even more face-centric than our highly communicative nonhuman primate relatives.

The antiquity and importance of rich facial expressivity in humans must be considered in the contexts of cosmetic treatment of the face and facial beauty because practitioners and patients are confronted with a paradox when considering modification of the face. The quest for youthful looks and a face showing less visible evidence of age is at odds with the evolved, nuanced and robust communications functions of the human face. Over the life course, the habitual activities of the muscles of facial expression eventually produce lines and wrinkles in the skin, and the goal of much cosmetic intervention is the mitigation of these effects. But the very activities of human expression that lead to wrinkles are some of the most highly evolved of human signals and the most salient parts of the human communications repertoire. There is no easy or single solution to this paradox, but there is ample room for thoughtful exploration and discussion.

The importance of visual signals from the primate face is reflected in the number, size, and complex interconnections of the brain centers in the visual system, limbic system, and prefrontal cortex associated with the reception and interpretation of sensory information from faces.[8–10] The involvement of multiple homologous centers in the brains of macaque monkeys and humans implies the presence of these features in the last common ancestor of the monkey and human lineages, about 30 million years ago.[11] In nonhuman and human primates, the core areas involved in interpretation of static information from the face are the inferior occipital gyrus, fusiform gyrus, and the superior temporal sulcus. These areas in both hemispheres along with the amygdala, hippocampus, inferior frontal gyrus, and orbitofrontal cortex are recruited in the interpretation of facial expressions, and together comprise an extended system for facial processing.[10] The multiplicity and complex interconnectedness of the neural centers involved in the interpretation of both the invariant and changing modalities of facial input denote the preeminent importance of the face in the human social economy. Interpretation of invariant facial features is central to the recognition of identity, while interpretation of changeable aspects of the face is associated with speech and facial expression.

The primacy of the face and facial expression in human communication in humans is witnessed not only by the richness of the sensory systems associated with perception of facial information, but in the impressively complex motor systems that produce facial expressions.

The number and complexity of the intrinsic facial muscles in humans are far greater than in any other primate or mammal[12], a situation that makes for a wide range of facial expressions, from the most extreme and highly visible at a distance to the most subtle and nuanced perceptible only at close quarters. The muscles that produce these movements are described in great detail in the chapters that follow, but it warrants mention here that the muscles of facial expression that are most strongly conserved among mammals are those involved with the closure of the eyes and mouth, including the orbicularis oris and buccinator involved with chewing and swallowing. The muscles that are unique to humans, and highly structurally and functionally distinct, are the superficial perioral muscles, which are arrayed radially around the oral cavity and serve only mimetic function.[13] The most constant of these are the zygomaticus major, the levator labii superioris, the levator labii superioris alaquae nasi, the depressor anguli oris, and the depressor labii inferioris; the risorius and zygomaticus minor are the most individually variable. The wide range of subtle and finely graded facial expressions is made possible not only by the low innervation ratio of all the intrinsic facial muscles, but also by their polyneuronal innervation, that is, the high percentage of single muscle fibers innervated by multiple motor end-plates coming from different neurons.[13]

The fidelity and universality of the basic facial expressions of happiness, sadness, surprise, fear, disgust, and anger was first explored by Charles Darwin in *The Expression of the Emotions in Man and Animals* in 1872[14] and then placed on a sound empirical footing through the studies of Paul Ekman and colleagues.[15,16] It is widely recognized that, in addition to the six basic expressions, many more exist and are used regularly by humans. These compound expressions, as they have been described[17], include some of the most recognizable emotions: happily surprised, sadly surprised, sadly angry, fearfully disgusted, and appalled (Figure P.1).

The different basic and compound expressions use different facial muscles in different combinations, and to different extents. Among the muscles most commonly recruited in these expressions are those

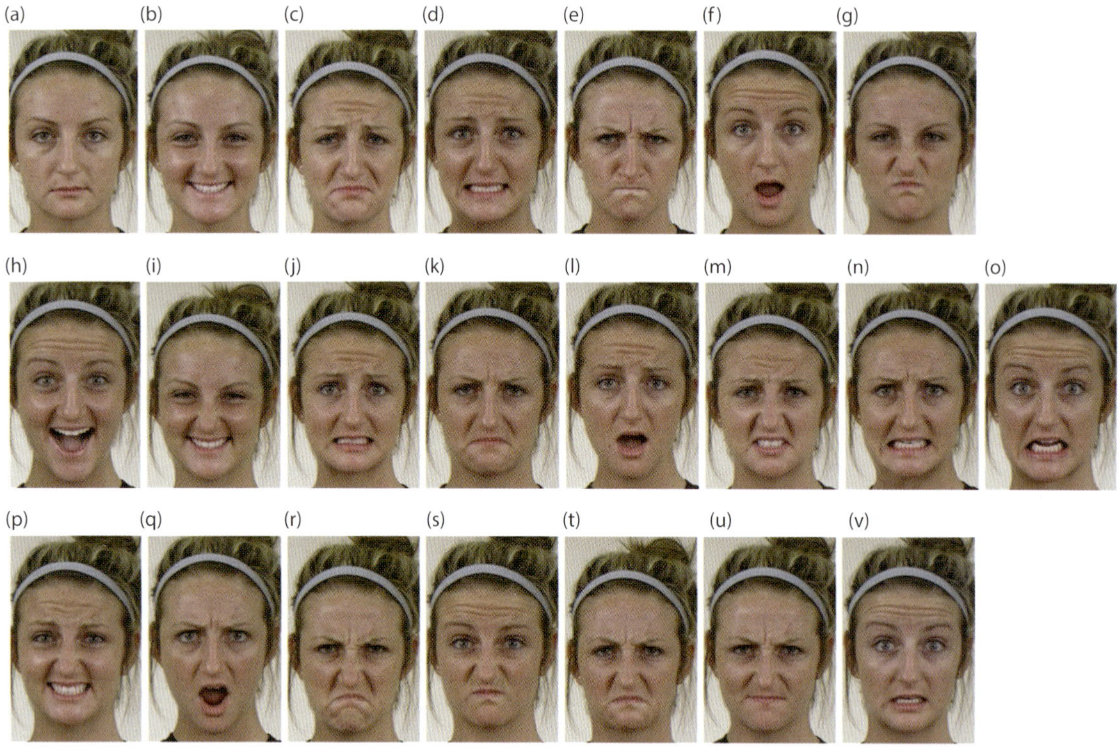

Figure P.1 Sample images illustrating basic and compound emotions, identified by Du and colleagues (2014). The images depict a neutral face (a), faces exhibiting the six basic emotions: (b) happy, (c) sad, (d) fearful, (e) angry, (f) surprised, and (g) disgusted; and 15 faces demonstrating compound emotions: (h) happily surprised, (i) happily disgusted, (j) sadly fearful, (k) sadly angry, (l) sadly surprised, (m) sadly disgusted, (n) fearfully angry, (o) fearfully surprised, (p) fearfully disgusted, (q) angrily surprised, (r) angrily disgusted, (s) disgustedly surprised, (t) appalled, (u) hatred, and (v) awed. (From Du S, Tao Y, and Martinez AM. *Proceedings of the National Academy of Sciences* 2014; 111(15): E1454–E1462, reproduced with permission of the authors and PNAS.)

most of the upper face commonly targeted in cosmetic procedures: the frontalis (especially the upper and middle fibers), the procerus, and the corrugator supercilii. Contraction of these muscles is required for expressions of recognition and concern, as well as in conveying sadness, anger and disgust.

The key questions, then, are what does treatment with botulinum neurotoxin (BoNT) do to human facial expressivity and mood, and does this matter? Facial expressions communicate emotions and mood, and are modified through social learning, primarily through imitation involving the intentional matching of the facial behaviors of others.[18] Because effective imitation of an emotional expression requires that the observer understand the relationship between production of the expression and the underlying emotional state that the expresser wants to convey, facial imitation involves empathy.[18] When an observer watches another person making an expression, covert activation of the facial muscles involved in producing the expressions occurs in the observer due to activation of neurons in the mirror neuron system.[19] Imitation of emotional facial expressions (such as anger, happiness, fear, and the other basic expressions) also involves activation of the insula and amygdala.[20] If an observer is prevented from making an expression (as when they are asked to hold a pencil firmly in their teeth), they become less able to detect the emotional expression of the observed face.[21,22] Failure to recognize emotion in others is also observed in people with Moebius syndrome, which impedes movement of the facial muscles.[23] Activation of the same cortical areas occurs when people are observing and imitating faces expressing emotion.[24] Thus, in emotion recognition, observation and action are linked together by the mirror neuron system.[25] The mental states and intentions of other people, thus, are embodied and not understood only through linguistic and mental processes.[25] In facial feedback, the motor action of forming an expression is sufficient to experience that expression.[26] The deliberate lowering of the eyebrows as in a frown, for instance, makes a person's mood more negative.[26]

It follows from this evidence that when the activity of facial muscles is partially blocked as the result of treatment with BoNT, there is a decrease in the strength of the emotional experience.[27] In the context of facial feedback theory, people treated with BoNT cannot express certain emotions as well, after treatment as before, and the loss of emotional experience is caused by the loss of feedback from making the expression.[26] The observation that emotions—including powerful negative emotions—are attenuated following treatment of specific facial muscles with BoNT has led to the adoption of BoNT injections as part of the armamentarium of techniques for treating clinical depression.[28] This is especially the case when BoNT injections are used in the upper face, to target fibers of the frontalis, procerus, and corrugator. Under these conditions, negative facial expressions are reduced to a greater extent than positive ones, yielded a net change in the valence of facial expressions and a reduction in the experience of negative emotions.[28–30] The role of positive social feedback and positive self-feedback (from looking in the mirror) probably also reduce depression.[28] A full discussion of the use of BoNT in the treatment of depression is beyond the scope of this prologue, but it is sufficient to state that BoNT is increasingly being used because of its psychoactive rather than its cosmetic effects. Regardless of the primary reasons for BoNT use, other impacts of partial facial immobilization have to be considered.

It has become increasingly common for people to choose to restrict the motion of their faces for cosmetic reasons for periods of many years, and for young adults to elect to start BoNT treatment before the appearance of facial lines. The unintended and long-term consequences of cosmetic BoNT injections have not been fully explored, and initial accounts have focused on the positive outcomes resulting from making people happier through reduction of the capacity to produce negative expressions. But mediation of facial affect with BoNT is a double-edged sword. There are many people today who cannot frown, and many who can't raise their eyebrows. Expressions of recognition, surprise, and concern for others are conveyed through contraction of the muscles of "negative affect," the frontalis and glabellar complex. Thus, BoNT reduces the ability to produce desirable expressions central to the demonstration of empathy as well as classic negative expressions of sadness, anger, and disgust. To what extent does this matter? Few systematic studies have been undertaken to explore the interpersonal and broader social ramifications of this phenomenon, but the preliminary indication is that chronic reduction of facial expressivity significantly impairs the abilities of treated individuals to interpret the emotions of others.[31] To these reports can be added the anecdotal accounts of people feeling uneasy around coworkers treated with BoNT whose expressions they cannot "read," as well the widely publicized on late-night television about a putative, frustrated child who couldn't interpret their parent's expressions: "I wish my teacher knew that I never can tell when Mommy's angry because her forehead doesn't move".[32] The importance of visible expressions of empathy or expressions of displeasure in the socialization of children cannot be overstated. A mother's scowl tells a child that something has gone wrong and that she is unhappy, and the establishment of this highly visible emotional vocabulary is an ancient and central part of human socialization.[33] A frown establishes a "current of connection," indicating that you understand another's distress.[34] As the visible repertoire of emotions develops and diversifies, a child's ability to immediately understand the actions of others develops and diversifies accordingly.[33] One of the cardinal characteristics of human beings is our ability to deal with sophisticated social environments, during which overt bodily behavior occurring in complex social interchanges is interpreted as an indication of our mental activity.[33] Although rarely discussed in the circles of cosmetic medicine, the reduction of the human capacity for empathy resulting from partial facial immobilization needs to be actively considered, discussed, and researched.

The paradox between the quests for lineless facial beauty and facial expressivity has not been resolved, and many important avenues of research about the consequences, especially, of long-term BoNT use require investigation. Thoughtful cosmetic practitioners will deal with this paradox and the related unknowns by being good scientists, and by undertaking attentive discussion of the costs and benefits of BoNT procedures with their patients. This is not an inconvenience, it's important. In connection with the use of BoNT on the face, the costs and risks are not only the medical ones enumerated in consent forms, but the more subtle ones of loss of efficacy of our highly evolved systems of visually based communication. Human beings are incessant communicators and ceaseless innovators. When we recognize that these two areas of human expertise are merged in cosmetic science, we can design new and nuanced interventions that will augment and not erase the best parts of our humanity.

REFERENCES

1. Little AC, Jones BC, and DeBruine LM. Facial attractiveness: Evolutionary based research. *Philos Trans R Soc Lond B Biol Sci* 2011; 366(1571): 1638–59.
2. Fink B, and Penton-Voak I. Evolutionary psychology of facial attractiveness. *Curr Dir Psychol Sci* 2002; 11(5): 154–8.
3. Bashour M. History and current concepts in the analysis of facial attractiveness. *Plast Reconstr Surg* 2006; 118(3): 741–56
4. Jackson LA. *Physical Appearance and Gender: Sociobiological and Sociocultural Perspectives SUNY Series in the Psychology of Women*. Albany, NY: State University of New York Press, 1992.
5. Maestripieri D, Klimczuk ACE, Traficonte DM, and Wilson MC. A greater decline in female facial attractiveness during middle age reflects women's loss of reproductive value. *Front Psychol* 2014; 5(179): 1–6.
6. Parr LA, Waller BM, and Fugate J. Emotional communication in primates: Implications for neurobiology. *Curr Opin Neurobiol* 2005; 15(6): 716–20.
7. Jablonski NG. *Skin: A Natural History*. Berkeley, CA: University of California Press, 2006.
8. Le Grand R, Mondloch CJ, Maurer D, and Brent HP. Early visual experience and face processing. *Nature* 2001; 410: 890.
9. de Haan M, Pascalis O, and Johnson MH. Specialization of neural mechanisms underlying face recognition in human infants. *J Cogn Neurosci* 2002; 14(2): 199–209.
10. Ishai A, Schmidt CF, and Boesiger P. Face perception is mediated by a distributed cortical network. *Brain Res Bull* 2005; 67(1–2): 87–93.
11. Steiper ME, Young NM, and Sukarna TY. Genomic data support the hominoid slowdown and an Early Oligocene estimate for the hominoid-cercopithecoid divergence. *Proc Natl Acad Sci* 2004; 101(49): 17021–26.
12. Huber E. Evolution of facial musculature and facial expression. *J Nerv Ment Dis* 1934; 79(1): 109.
13. Cattaneo L, and Pavesi G. The facial motor system. *Neurosci Biobehav Rev* 2014; 38: 135–59.
14. Darwin C. *The Expression of the Emotions in Man and Animals*. 3 ed. New York, New York: Oxford University Press, 1998.
15. Ekman P. *Emotions Revealed: Recognizing Faces and Feelings to Improve Communication and Emotional Life*. New York, New York: Time Books, 2003.
16. Eckman P, and Friesen WV. *Unmasking the Face: A Guide to Recognizing Emotions from Facial Clues*. Englewood Cliffs, NJ: Prentice-Hall, 1975.
17. Du S, Tao Y, and Martinez AM. Compound facial expressions of emotion. *Proc Natl Acad Sci* 2014; 111(15): E1454–62.
18. Braadbaart L, de Grauw H, Perrett DI, Waiter GD, and Williams JHG. The shared neural basis of empathy and facial imitation accuracy. *NeuroImage* 2014; 84: 367–75.
19. Dimberg U, Thunberg M, and Elmehed K. Unconscious facial reactions to emotional facial expressions. *Psychol Sci* 2000; 11(1): 86–9.
20. Pohl A, Anders S, Schulte-Rüther M, Mathiak K, and Kircher T. Positive facial affect – An fMRI study on the involvement of insula and amygdala. *PLOS ONE* 2013; 8(8): e69886.
21. Oberman LM, Winkielman P, and Ramachandran VS. Face to face: Blocking facial mimicry can selectively impair recognition of emotional expressions. *Soc Neurosci* 2007; 2(3–4): 167–78.
22. Niedenthal PM, Barsalou LW, Winkielman P, Krauth-Gruber S, and Ric F. Embodiment in attitudes, social perception, and emotion. *Pers Soc Psychol Rev* 2005; 9(3): 184–211.
23. Cole J. Empathy needs a face. *J Conscious Stud* 2001; 8(5–6): 51–68.
24. Leslie KR, Johnson-Frey SH, and Grafton ST. Functional imaging of face and hand imitation: Towards a motor theory of empathy. *NeuroImage* 2004; 21(2): 601–7.
25. Corradini A, and Antonietti A. Mirror neurons and their function in cognitively understood empathy. *Conscious Cogn* 2013; 22(3): 1152–61.

26. Lewis MB. Exploring the positive and negative implications of facial feedback. *Emotion* 2012; 12(4): 852–59.
27. Davis JI, Senghas A, Brandt F, and Ochsner KN. The effects of BOTOX injections on emotional experience. *Emotion* 2010; 10(3): 433–40.
28. Alam M, Barrett KC, Hodapp RM, and Arndt KA. Botulinum toxin and the facial feedback hypothesis: Can looking better make you feel happier? *J Am Acad Dermatol* 2008; 58(6): 1061–72.
29. Finzi E. *The Face of Emotion: How Botox Affects Our Moods and Relationships*. New York: Palgrave Macmillan, 2013.
30. Hennenlotter A, Dresel C, Castrop F, Ceballos-Baumann AO, Wohlschläger AM, and Haslinger B. The link between facial feedback and neural activity within central circuitries of emotion—New insights from botulinum toxin–induced denervation of frown muscles. *Cereb Cortex* 2009; 19(3): 537–42.
31. Neal DT, and Chartrand TL. Embodied emotion perception amplifying and dampening facial feedback modulates emotion perception accuracy. *Soc Psychol Pers Sci* 2011; 2(6): 673–78.
32. Real Time with Bill Maher. 2015. *I Wish My Teacher Knew ...* April 25, 2015 [cited August 5, 2015]. Available from http://www.real-time-with-bill-maher-blog.com/index/2015/4/25/i-wish-my-teacher-knew.
33. Sinigaglia C, and Sparaci L. Emotions in action through the looking glass. *J Anal Psychol* 2010; 55(1): 3–29.
34. Crapanzano A. 2012. Frozen in Time. *Marie Claire*, December, 150–6.

1 Botulinum toxin and its development in clinical medicine

Jean Carruthers and Alastair Carruthers

INTRODUCTION

In the aftermath of the Napoleonic wars (1799–1815) in Europe in the early nineteenth century, Dr. Justinus Kerner, an astute German physician and poet, noted that there seemed to be a substance in sausages that was causing people to die of a mysterious paralytic disease. Dr. Kerner postulated that this substance could possibly be helpful in treating overactive muscle conditions. Subsequent characterization of this substance and research led San Francisco ophthalmologist Dr. Alan Scott to consider using botulinum toxin type A (BoNT-A) as an alternative to surgery in the treatment of strabismus. In 1982, Ophthalmologist/Dermatologist Dr. Jean Carruthers had the opportunity to undertake a Fellowship with Dr. Scott and subsequently with Dr. Joseph Tsui and other Vancouver neurologists and published the first study of treating patients with dystonias with BoNT-A. Drs. Jean and her husband Alastair Carruthers then treated the first cosmetic patient, thus beginning a new era in the use of biologic substances considered to be deadly poisons as safe clinical modalities in the cosmetic as well as in the medical world.

SAUSAGE POISONING AND *CLOSTRIDIUM BOTULINUM*

At the end of the eighteenth century, the number of cases of fatal food poisoning throughout the southwest German region of Württemberg increased, likely due to widespread poverty after the devastating Napoleonic Wars (1795–1813) and subsequent unsanitary food production in rural areas.[1] In 1793, after 13 people fell ill and after 6 died during an outbreak in the small village of Wildbad in Württemberg, medical officers in the region scrambled to understand and identify the cause. By 1811, the Department of Internal Affairs of the Kingdom of Württemberg had pinpointed prussic acid in undercooked blood sausages as the culprit. In 1820, the district medical officer and poet, Justinus Kerner (1786–1862) published his first monograph on sausage poisoning, with a complete clinical description and summary of 76 case histories.[2] In a quest to extract and isolate the unknown toxic substance he called "fat poison" or "fatty acid," Kerner began to experiment on animals and himself in the pharmacist's laboratory, eventually publishing the first complete monograph containing the clinical evaluation and summary of 155 cases and accurate descriptions of all gastrointestinal, autonomic, and neuromuscular symptoms and signs of botulism.[3] From his experimentation, Kerner deduced that his fat poison acted by an interruption of the peripheral and autonomic nervous signal transmission, leaving the sensory signal transmission intact. In the final paragraph of his monograph, Kerner discussed the potential use of the toxin for the treatment of a variety of disorders characterized by "sympathetic overactivity" (e.g., St. Vitus' dance or Sydenham's chorea, a disorder characterized by jerky, uncontrollable movements, either of the face or of the arms and legs) and hypersecretion of bodily fluid, as well as for treating ulcers, delusions, rabies, plague, tuberculosis, and yellow fever. Sausage poisoning was eventually named botulism, after the Latin word *botulus*, meaning sausage.

In December 1895, 34 people in the small Belgian village of Ellezelles fell ill with symptoms of mydriasis, diplopia, dysphagia, dysarthria, and increasing muscle paralysis after eating pickled and smoked ham.[4] After examining the ham and conducting autopsies on the 3 patients who died, microbiologist Emile Pierre Van Ermengem (1851–1922) of the University of Ghent isolated an anaerobic microorganism that he called *Bacillus botulinus*—later renamed *Clostridium botulinum*.[5]

In 1904, an outbreak of food poisoning in Darmstadt, Germany involving canned white beans, led to the discovery of two serologically distinct strains of *C. botulinum*; these were eventually classified alphabetically as types A and B by Georgina Burke at Stanford University in 1919.[6] Over the next decades, cases of botulism became more frequent with the increased popularity of canned food products, and additional strains—types C, D, E, F, and G—were identified.[7]

CLINICAL DEVELOPMENT OF BOTULINUM TOXIN

With the advent of war, the potential uses of botulinum toxins took on a more sinister edge. In 1928, Herman Sommer and colleagues at the University of California, San Francisco isolated pure botulinum toxin type A (BoNT-A) as a stable acid precipitate.[8] As World War II approached, the United States government—along with multiple countries engaged in biowarfare programs—began intensive research into biological weapons, assembling bacteriologists and physicians in a laboratory at Camp Detrick (later named Fort Detrick) in Maryland to investigate dangerous and infectious bacteria and toxins.[7] In 1946, Carl Lamanna and colleagues developed concentration and crystallization techniques for the toxin that were subsequently used by Edward J. Schantz, a young U.S. army officer stationed at Fort Detrick, to produce the first batch of BoNT-A which was the basis for the later clinical product.[9,10] In 1972, President Richard Nixon signed the Biological and Toxic Weapons Convention, effectively putting an end to all investigations on biological agents for use in war, and Fort Detrick was closed. Schantz took his research to the University of Wisconsin, where he produced a large amount (150 mg) of BoNTA (batch 79–11) that remained in clinical use in the United States until December 1997.[11]

In the late 1960s and early 1970s, Alan Scott (Figure 1.1), an ophthalmologic surgeon at the Smith-Kettlewell Eye Research Foundation in San Francisco, began to experiment with BoNTA, supplied by Schantz, as a potential non-surgical treatment of strabismus.[12] Scott published his first primate studies in 1973,[13] and human studies with BoNT-A (then named Oculinum®) began in 1977. When he injected the toxin using a newly developed practical electromyographic (EMG) device (Figure 1.2)—a Teflon-coated needle used as an electrode that produced an auditory signal when the tip of the needle came close to motor endplates when the muscle was activated, allowing for precise placement of material[14]—strabismus could be treated relatively easily without invasive surgery for the first time. The publication of his landmark paper in 1980 showing that the toxin could correct gaze misalignment in humans[15] revolutionized the treatment of strabismus and subsequently of many other muscular disorders.

In 1989, the Food and Drug Administration (FDA) approved Oculinum®—subsequently acquired and renamed BOTOX® by Allergan Inc. (Irvine, CA)—for the nonsurgical correction of strabismus, blepharospasm, hemifacial spasm, and Meige's syndrome in adults, and clinical use expanded to include the treatment of cervical dystonia and spasmodic torticollis.[16,17]

THE BIRTH OF BOTOX® COSMETIC

By the late 1980s, nearly 10,000 patients had received multiple injections of BoNT-A for the treatment of benign essential blepharospasm with no evidence of antibody formation or systemic complications over 6 years of continued use,[18] and Scott's work planted

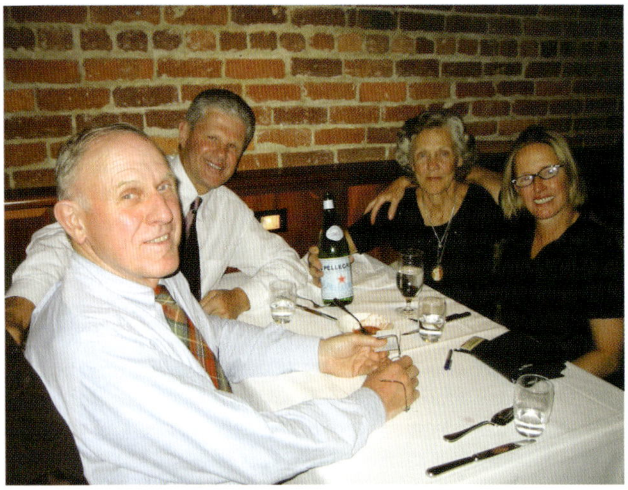

Figure 1.1 Alan B. Scott, MD, San Francisco ophthalmologist and strabismologist who was the first to use BoNT-A therapeutically and to recognize its many potential uses.

the seeds for its future cosmetic applications. In Vancouver, British Columbia, Jean Carruthers noticed a remarkable and unexpected effect in the brow of a patient treated for blepharospasm: a noticeable reduction in the appearance of glabellar furrows, giving her a more serene, untroubled expression. Jean discussed the observation with her dermatologist spouse, Alistair, who was attempting to soften the forehead wrinkles of his patients using soft-tissue augmenting agents available in the late 1980s, including collagen, silicone, or autologous fat, none of which worked particularly well—or with minimal risk—in the glabella. The timing for a non-invasive and easy injectable treatment that carried little risk of complication could not have been more perfect. The Baby Boomers—those 80 million babies born between 1946 and 1964—had all grown up and were clamoring to fix the lines, folds, and wrinkles that made them look older than they felt.[19]

After a conversation with Alan Scott, who confirmed he had treated a few patients for cosmetic purposes in 1985, we injected a small amount of BoNT-A between the brows of our then-assistant—now known as "patient zero"—and awaited the results. Seventeen more patients followed, aged 34–51, who would become part of the first published report on the efficacy of BoNT-A for glabellar rhytides (Figure 1.3).[20] The study attracted a flurry of interest and similar

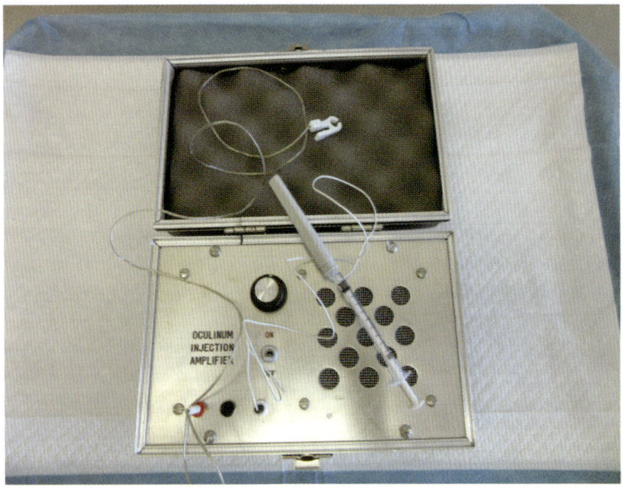

Figure 1.2 Early studies with BoNT-A used with EMG guidance.

trials showing remarkable effects indicating that BoNT-A was indeed a novel and promising treatment for unsightly facial rhytides.[21–23] Between 1992 and 1997, the popularity of cosmetic off-label use grew so rapidly that Allergan's supply temporarily ran out.[24]

By 2002, investigators had established an excellent safety profile for therapeutic doses of the toxin, and numerous open-label studies totaling more than 800 subjects demonstrated the safe and effective use of BoNT-A for improvements in the appearance of hyperfunctional facial rhytides.[25] In the United States, the FDA had approved BoNT-A for strabismus, blepharospasm, hemifacial spasm, and cervical dystonia. Additional approvals had been granted in the United Kingdom for axillary hyperhidrosis, and in Canada for axillary hyperhidrosis, focal muscle spasticity, and for the cosmetic treatment of glabellar wrinkles. In April 2002, on the heels of two large, double-blind, placebo-controlled, randomized, multicenter clinical trials,[26,27] the FDA approved BoNT-A for the non-surgical reduction of glabellar furrows, and the world of facial rejuvenation changed dramatically.

In the 1980s and 1990s, the concept of using botulinum toxin as a therapeutic agent seemed to be at best folly and at worst dangerous. Those of us who had had considerable experience in its use knew that the key to safety, as with any other drug, was the dosage administered. The difficulty was that the units of measurements were in billionths (nanograms) of a gram and the measurement needed to be biologic with "Mouse units."[28] Dr. Ross Kennedy and I performed a prospective randomized clinical trial of patients with misaligned eyes who had no ability to use the eyes together (fusion). We compared BoNT-A to adjustable suture surgery and found the BoNT-A superior in this group of patients. It showed that this modality was safe in this group and yet would not replace traditional surgery for other groups. The periocular safety was also studied in our 1995 paper[29] showing that the production of eyelid ptosis was the specific location of the injecting needle and thus could, with good technique, largely be avoided. In 1995 we used BoNT-A to treat congenital motor nystagmus ("shaking eyes") with a substantial improvement in vision.[30]

The cosmetic uses of BoNT-A spread from its initial use for glabellar frown lines[31] to realizing that we could shape the face in different ways such as being able predictably to elevate the whole eyebrow[32] and to titrate the widening of the eyelid fissure.[33] In 2000 we published on the combined use of BoNT-A with ablative CO_2 laser resurfacing.[34] We started to treat headache pain because our patients were so positive about the effects, even when this was felt not to work with current neurology theories.[35]

By 2003 we had started to use BoNT-A in the mid- and lower face and neck[36] and also were using combination treatments with hyaluronic acid fillers for deep resting glabellar rhytides.[37] With Bob Weiss, Vic Narukar, and Tim Flynn we explored the combination with Intense Pulsed Light (IPL)[38] and in 2004 we showed that injecting BoNT-A with IPL full face caused a 15% improvement in pigment reduction.[39]

By now there was a need to study dose ranging and we looked at men[40] and women[41] and showed that men have much larger dose requirements than women do.

In 2005, we published our first long-term safety review.[42] We started to study Patient Reported Outcomes (PROs) in 2007[43] and we all now realized that this was the hugely important yardstick for the evaluation of cosmetic treatments. The next step was the development of validated rating scales to aid the precision of both patient and investigator ratings.[44–46]

In the early days, fillers were felt to belong only in the lower face and neuromodulators in the upper. With Gary Monheit we did a three-arm prospective randomized study of the separate and combined use of fillers and neuromodulators in the perioral region.[47]

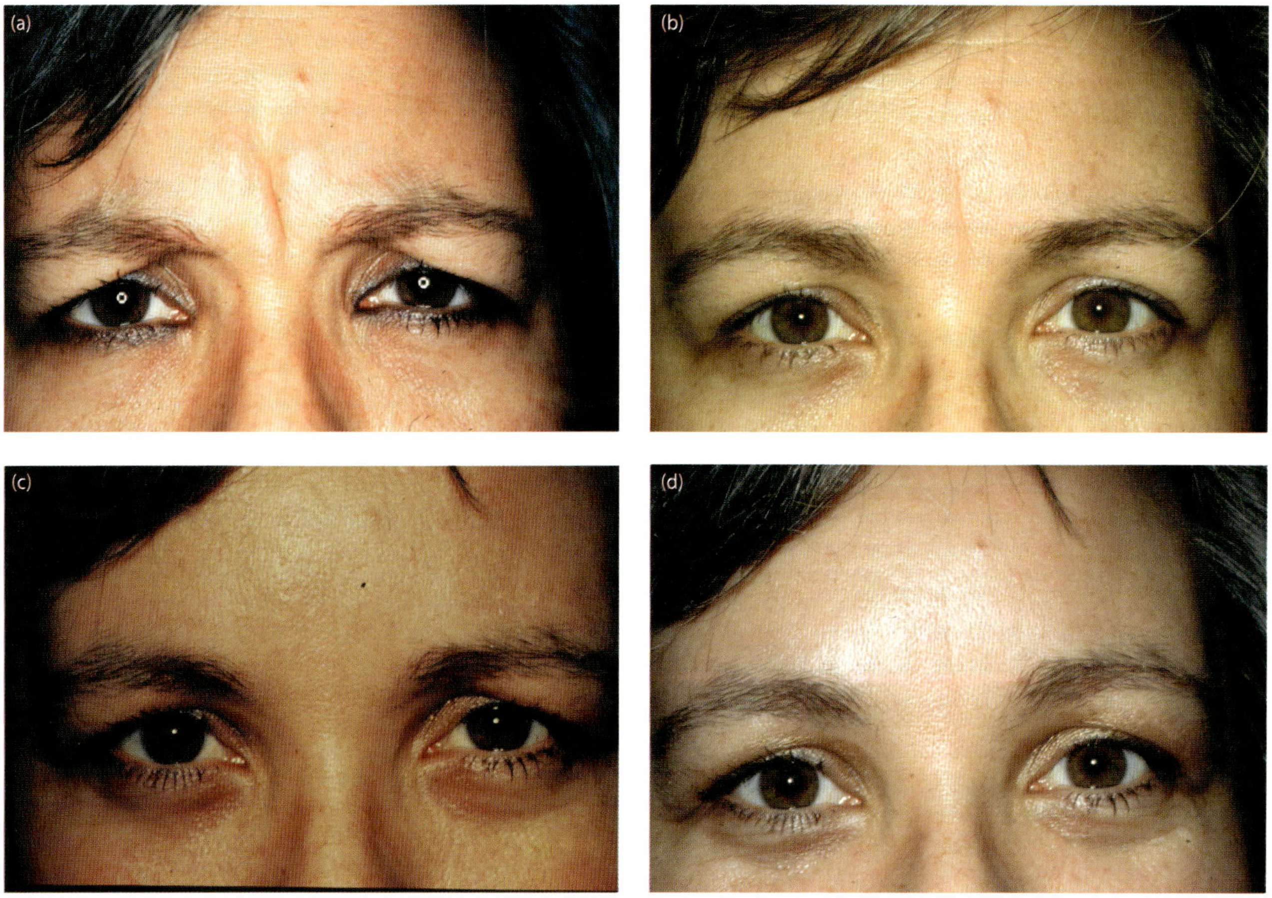

Figure 1.3 Patient zero—BoNT-A for the treatment of glabellar rhytides (a) pre-operative, frowning; (b) pre-operative, resting; (c) post-operative, attempting to frown; (d) post-operative, resting. (From Jean DA et al. *J Dermatol Surg Oncol* 1992; 18: 17, with permission.)

The combination was the clear winner.[47] In October 2012, Jean gave a TEDx talk "How a Feared Poison Became a World Class Multipurpose Drug."

Also in 2012, Jean and Alastair were awarded the prestigious Eugene Van Scott Award from the American Academy of Dermatology. Our presentation was titled "You want to Inject What?"—a phrase some of our many early patients had used when we were discussing treatment options in the early days.[19]

The worldwide popularity of the aesthetic use of BoNT-A has allowed many authors from many countries the opportunity to work together to pool concepts and new ideas for combined uses of botulinum toxins with other treatment modalities.[48,49]

Finally, derivative structures in the molecular structure of BoNT-A as in daxibotulinumtoxinA (DaxiBTX-A) has allowed a second generation of BoNT-A neuromodulators to take their first steps on the cosmetic and therapeutic stage.[50] Also most interesting, a new presentation of a short-acting neuromodulator BoNT-E is currently undergoing clinical trials.

SUMMARY

Thirty years ago, the idea of using a fatal, toxic agent to treat medical disorders and cosmetic rhytides was met with frank disbelief.[19] Today, BoNT-A has become one of the most versatile pharmaceuticals across diverse areas of medicine, with multiple formulations available globally for a broad range of therapeutic and cosmetic applications. Now the treatment of choice for smoothing hyperkinetic lines and shaping the face, alone or in combination with other rejuvenating procedures, and used for a variety of movement, pain, autonomic nervous system, and gastrointestinal and genitourinary disorders, among others, BoNT-A has firmly planted itself in clinical history, thanks to the dedication and sometimes dogged determination of medical innovators.

REFERENCES

1. Erbguth FJ. Historical notes on botulism, Clostridium Botulinum, Botulinum Toxin, and the idea of the therapeutic use of the toxin. *Mov Disord* 2004; 19: S3.
2. Kerner J. *New Observations on the in Wurttemberg Incipient Fatal Poisoning by the Consumption of Smoked Sausages*. Tübingen: Osiander; 1820.
3. Kerner J. *The Fat or the Fatty Acid and its Effects on the Animal Organism: An Inquiry for the Investigation of the Spoiled Sausages Toxic Substance*. Stuttgart, Tübingen: Cotta; 1822.
4. Erbguth FJ. Historical notes on botulism, Clostridium Botulinum, Botulinum Toxin, and the idea of the therapeutic use of the toxin. *Mov Disord* 2004; 19: S6.
5. Van Ermengem EP. A new anaerobic bacillus and its relation to botulism. *Rev Infect Dis* 1979; 1: 701.
6. Burke GS. The occurrence of bacillus botulinus in nature. *J Bacteriol* 1919; 4: 541.
7. Erbguth FJ. From poison to remedy: The Chequered history of botulinum toxin. *J Neural Transm* 2008; 115: 562.
8. Snipe PT, Sommer H. Studies on botulinus toxin. 3. Acid preparation of botulinus toxin. *J Infect Dis* 1928; 43: 152.
9. Lamanna C, Eklund HW, McElroy OE. Botulinum toxin (type A); including a study of shaking with chloroform as a step in the isolation procedure. *J Bacteriol* 1946; 52: 1–13.

10. Schantz EJ, Johnson EA. Botulinum toxin: The story of its development for the treatment of human disease. *Perspect Biol Med* 1997; 40: 317.
11. Ting PT, Freiman A. The story of clostridium botulinum: From food poisoning to botox. *Clin Med* 2004; 4: 260.
12. Erbguth FJ. From poison to remedy: The Chequered history of botulinum toxin. *J Neural Transm* 2008; 115: 563.
13. Scott FJ et al. Pharmacologic weakening of extraocular muscles. *Invest Ophthalmol* 1973; 12: 924.
14. Jampolsky A. What can electromyography do for the ophthalmologist? *Invest Ophthalmol* 1970; 8: 570.
15. Scott AB. Botulinum toxin injection into extraocular muscles as an alternative to strabismus surgery. *Ophthalmol* 1980; 87: 1044.
16. Tsui J et al. A pilot study on the use of botulinum toxin in spasmodic torticollis. *Can J Neurol Sci* 1985; 12: 314.
17. Carruthers J, Stubbs HA. Botulinum toxin for benign essential blepharospasm, hemifacial spasm and age-related lower eyelid ectropion. *Can J Neurol Sci* 1987; 14: 42.
18. Tsui J et al. Production of circulating antibodies to botulinum a toxin in patients receiving repeated injections for dystonia. *Ann Neurol* 1988; 23: 181.
19. Carruthers A, Carruthers J. You want to inject what? *Dermatol Surg* 2015; 41: S2–8.
20. Carruthers JDA, Carruthers A. Treatment of glabellar frown lines with C. Botulinum-A exotoxin. *J Dermatol Surg Oncol* 1992; 18: 17.
21. Blitzer A et al. Botulinum toxin for the treatment of hyperfunctional lines of the face. *JAMA Otolaryngol Head Neck Surg* 1993; 119: 1018.
22. Keen M et al. Botulinum toxin A for hyperkinetic facial lines: Results of a double-blind, placebo-controlled study. *Plast Reconstr Surg* 1994; 94: 94.
23. Lowe NJ et al. Botulinum A exotoxin for glabellar folds: A double-blind, vehicle-controlled study with an electromyographic injection technique. *J Am Acad Dermatol* 1996; 35: 569.
24. Kuczynski A. *Drought over, Botox is Back. New York Times*; 1997.
25. Carruthers A, Carruthers J. History of cosmetic botulinum toxin. In: *Botulinum Toxin, Carruthers A, Carruthers J*, (ed). New York: Elsevier; 2013, 16.
26. Carruthers JA et al. A multicenter, double-blind, randomized, placebo-controlled study of the efficacy and safety of botulinum toxin type A in the treatment of glabellar lines. *J Am Acad Dermatol* 2002; 46: 840.
27. Carruthers JD et al. Double-blind, placebo-controlled study of the safety and efficacy of botulinum toxin type A for patients with glabellar lines. *Plast Reconstr Surg* 2003; 112: 1089.
28. Carruthers JDA, Kennedy RA, Bagaric D. Botulinum versus adjustable suture surgery in the treatment of horizontal misalignment in adult patients lacking fusion. *JAMA Ophthalmol* 1990; 108(10): 1432–5.
29. Carruthers JDA, Carruthers JA, Bagaric D. Can ptosis Incidence be reduced after lid injections of botulinum A exotoxin for blepharospasm and hemifacial spasm. *Can J Ophthalmol* 1995; 30: 147.
30. Carruthers JDA. The treatment of congenital nystagmus with Botox. *J Pediatr Ophthalmol Strabismus* 1995; 32(5): 306–8.
31. Carruthers JDA, Carruthers JA. Treatment of glabellar frown lines with C. botulinum-A exotoxin. *J Dermatol Surg Oncol* 1992; 18(1): 17–21.
32. Huilgol SC, Carruthers A, Carruthers JDA. Raising eyebrows with botulinum toxin. *Dermatol Surg* 1999; 25(5): 373–6.
33. Flynn TC, Carruthers A, Carruthers JDA. The use of the Ultra-Fine II short needles 0.3 cc insulin syringe for botulinum toxin injections. *J Am Acad Dermatol* 2002; 46(6): 931–3.
34. Carruthers JDA, Carruthers JA, Zelichowska A. The power of combined therapies: BOTOX and ablative facial laser resurfacing. *Am J Cosmetic Surg* 2000; 17(3): 129–31.
35. Carruthers A, Langtry JAA, Carruthers JDA, Robinson G. Improvement of tension-type headache when treating wrinkles with botulinum toxin A injections. *Headache* 1999; 39: 662–5.
36. Carruthers A, Carruthers JDA. Aesthetic use of botulinum A exotoxin in the mid and lower face and neck. *Derm Surg* 2003; 29(5): 468–76.
37. Carruthers JDA, Carruthers A, Maberley D. Deep resting glabellar rhytides respond to BTX-A and Hylan B. *Derm Surg* 2003; 29(5): 539–4.
38. Carruthers JDA, Weiss R, Narurkar V, Corcoran T. Intense pulsed light and botulinum toxin type A for the aging face. *J Cosmet Dermatol* 2003; 16(S5): 1–16.
39. Carruthers JDA, Carruthers A. The effect of full-face broad and light treatments alone and in combination with bilateral crow's feet BTX-A chemodenervation. *Dermatol Surg* 2004; 30(3): 355–66.
40. Carruthers JA, Carruthers JDA. Dose-ranging study of botulinum toxin type A in the treatment of glabellar rhytides in females. *Dermatol Surg* 2005; 31(4): 414–22.
41. Carruthers JA, Carruthers JDA. A prospective, double-blind, randomized, parallel group, dose-ranging study of botulinum toxin type A in men with glabellar rhytides. *Dermatol Surg* 2005; 31(10): 1297–303.
42. Carruthers JDA, Carruthers A. Long term safety review of subjects treated with botulinum toxin type A (BoNT/A) for cosmetic use. P03. Toxins 2005. *Neurotox Res* 2006; 9(203): 225.
43. Carruthers JA, Carruthers JDA. Patient reported outcomes with botulinum neurotoxin type A. *J Cosmet Laser Ther* 2007; 9(suppl 1): 32–27.
44. Fagien S, Carruthers JDA. A comprehensive review of patient-reported satisfaction with botulinum toxin type A for aesthetic procedures. *Plast Reconstr Surg* 2008; 122(6): 1915–25.
45. Carruthers JA, Carruthers JDA. A validated facial grading scale—the future of facial ageing measurement tools? *J Cosmet Laser Ther* 2010; 12(5): 235–41.
46. Carruthers JA, Carruthers JDA. A single-center dose-comparison study of botulinum neurotoxin type A in females with upper facial rhytids: Assessing patients' perception of treatment outcomes. *J Drugs Dermatol.* 2009; 8(10): 924–9.
47. Carruthers JDA, Carruthers A, Monheit GD, Davis PG. Multicenter, randomized, parallel-group study of onabotulinumtoxinA and hyaluronic acid dermal fillers (24-mg/ml smooth, cohesive gel) alone and in combination for lower facial rejuvenation: Satisfaction and patient-reported outcomes. *Dermatol Surg* 2010; 36(Suppl 4): 2135–45.
48. Carruthers JDA, Burgess C, Day D et al. Consensus recommendations for combined aesthetic interventions in the face using botulinum toxin, fillers, and microfocused ultrasound with visualization. *Dermatol Surg* 2016; 00: 1–12.
49. Carruthers J, Carruthers A. A multimodal approach to rejuvenation of the lower face. *Dermatol Surg* 2016; 00: 1–5.
50. Carruthers J, Solish N, Humphrey S et al. Injectable DaxibotulinumtoxinA for the treatment of glabellar lines A, phase 2, randomized, dose-ranging, double-blind, multicenter comparison with OnabotulinumtoxinA and placebo. *Dermatol Surg* 2017. doi: 10.1097/DSS.0000000000001206 (online).

BIBLIOGRAPHY

American Society of Plastic Surgeons. 2015. *2014 Plastic Surgery Statistics Report*. http://www.plasticsurgery.org.

Blitzer, A, Brin M, Keen MS, Aviv JE. Botulinum toxin for the treatment of hyperfunctional lines of the face. *Arch Otolaryngol Head Neck Surg* 1993; 119: 1018–22.

Burke, GS. The occurrence of bacillus botulinus in nature. *J Bacteriology* 1919; 4: 541–53.

Carruthers A, Carruthers J. You want to inject what? *Dermatol Surg* 2045; 41: S2–8.

Carruthers A, Carruthers J. History of cosmetic botulinum toxin. In: *Botulinum Toxin*. Carruthers A, Carruthers J, (ed). New York: Elsevier; 2013, 13–7.

Carruthers, JD, Lowe NJ, Menter MA, Gibson J, Eadie N. Double-blind, placebo-controlled study of the safety and efficacy of botulinum toxin type A for Patients with glabellar lines. *Plast Reconstr Surg* 2003; 112: 1089–98.

Carruthers JA, Lowe NJ, Menter MA, Gibson J, Nordquist M, Mordaunt J, Walker P, Eadie N. A multicenter, double-blind, randomized, placebo-controlled study of the efficacy and safety of botulinum toxin type A in the treatment of glabellar lines. *J Am Acad Dermatol* 2002; 46: 840–9.

Carruthers JDA, Carruthers A. Treatment of glabellar frown lines with C. Botulinum-A exotoxin. *Journal of Dermatologic Surgery and Oncology* 1992; 18: 17–21.

Carruthers J, Stubbs HA. Botulinum toxin for benign essential blepharospasm, hemifacial spasm and age-related lower eyelid ectropion. *Can J Neurol Sci* 1987; 14: 42–5.

Erbguth FJ. From poison to remedy: The Chequered History of botulinum toxin. *J Neural Transm* 2008; 115: 559–5.

Erbguth FJ. Historical notes on botulism, Clostridium Botulinum, botulinum toxin, and the idea of the therapeutic use of the toxin. *Movement Disorders* 2004; 19: S2–6.

Jampolsky A. What can electromyography do for the ophthalmologist? *Invest Ophthalmol* 1970; 8: 570–99.

Keen M, Blitzer A, Aviv J, Binder A, Prystowsky J, Smith H, Brin M. Botulinum toxin A for hyperkinetic facial lines: Results of a double-blind, placebo-controlled study. *Plast Reconstr Surg* 1994; 94(1994): 94–9.

Kerner J. *New Observations on the in Wurttemberg Incipient Fatal Poisoning by the Consumption of Smoked Sausages*. Tübingen: Osiander; 1820.

Kerner J. *The Fat or the Fatty Acid and its Effects on the Animal Organism: an Inquiry for the Investigation of the Spoiled Sausages Toxic Substance*. Stuttgart, Tübingen: Cotta; 1822.

Kuczynski A. Drought over, Botox is back. *New York Times*; 1997. http://www.nytimes.com/1997/12/14/style/pulse-drought-over-botox-is-back.html.

Lamanna C, Eklund HW, McElroy OE. Botulinum toxin (Type A); Including a study of shaking with chloroform as a step in the isolation procedure. *J Bacteriol* 1946; 52: 1–13.

Lowe NJ, Maxwell A, Harper H. Botulinum A exotoxin for glabellar folds: A double-blind, vehicle-controlled study with an electromyographic injection technique. *J Am Acad Dermatol* 1996; 35: 569–72.

Schantz EJ, Johnson EA. Botulinum toxin: The story of its development for the treatment of human disease. *Perspect Biol Med* 1997; 40:317–27.

Scott AB. Botulinum toxin injection into extraocular muscles as an alternative to strabismus surgery. *Ophthalmol* 1980; 87: 1044–99.

Scott AB, Rosenbaum A, Collins CC. Pharmacologic weakening of extraocular muscles. *Invest Ophthalmol* 1973; 12: 924–7.

Snipe PT, Sommer H. Studies on botulinus toxin. 3. Acid preparation of botulinus toxin. *J Infect Dis* 1928; 43: 152–60.

Ting PT, Freiman A. The story of clostridium botulinum: From food poisoning to botox. *Clin Med* 2004; 4: 258–61.

Tsui J, Wong NLM, Wong E, Calne DB. Production of circulating antibodies to Botulinum A toxin in patients receiving repeated injections for dystonia. *Ann Neurol* 1988; 23: 181.

Tsui JK, Eisen A, Mak E, Carruthers J, Scott A, Calne DB. A pilot study on the use of botulinum toxin in spasmodic torticollis. *Can J Neurol Sci* 1985; 12: 314–16.

Van Ermengem EP. A new anaerobic bacillus and its relation to botulism. *Review of Infectious Diseases* 1979; 1: 701–19.

2 Botulinum toxins: Pharmacology, immunology, and current developments

Mitchell F. Brin

INTRODUCTION

Like digitalis, atropine, and ziconotide, botulinum toxins (BoNTs) are natural substances that have become useful medicines. As proteins synthesized by living organisms (clostridial bacteria), BoNTs are biological products as opposed to conventional, synthetic drugs. For clinical use, BoNTs are isolated, purified, and formulated into specific products in a complex series of steps strictly regulated by governmental agencies in most countries where the products are approved. The manufacturing method determines not only the purity of the final product, but also the reproducibility of unit activity—the dosage measurement for BoNTs. The final formulations of the products are also critical because they can affect product stability, efficacy, safety, and immunogenicity.

SYNTHESIS AND STRUCTURE

BoNTs are produced as multimeric protein complexes consisting of the ~150 kDa neurotoxin and associated hemagglutinin and non-hemagglutinin proteins. These neurotoxin associated proteins (NAPs) stabilize and protect the ~150 kDa neurotoxin from degradation in the gastrointestinal tract.[1,2] The NAPs also exert biologically relevant *in vivo* activity, as demonstrated by the distinct pharmacodynamic curves in mice following intraperitoneal and intravenous injection of the ~150 kDa versus 900 kDa molecule.[3] Interactions between BoNT proteins and NAPs are influenced by the microenvironment, including pH,[4] but are more difficult to study following therapeutic administration in humans. During the manufacturing of BoNTA for clinical use, proprietary procedures are used to determine which, if any, of the NAPs are retained in the final product.

Different bacterial strains synthesize complexes that vary in size and protein composition, as well as neurotoxin serotype.[5] Seven different BoNT serotypes are recognized: A, B, C1, D, E, F, and G. Serotypes A through F form the 300 kDa complex; serotypes A, B, C1, and D form the 500–700 kDa complex; and only type A forms the 900 kDa complex.[6,7] Type G forms the 500 kDa complex.[8] Some clostridial strains are mosaics, containing genes encoding parts of one serotype and parts of another; the newly identified botulinum toxin may be a new serotype H or may be a mosaic of types A and F.[9,10] Mosaic toxins have previously been described for types C1 and D,[11] and for types F and A.[12] Toxin variants within the serotypes (e.g., A1, A2, etc.) have also been identified, with reported differentiating preclinical *in vivo* profiles.[13,14]

The active BoNT protein in all serotypes is synthesized as a single chain of approximately 150 kDa that must be nicked or cleaved by proteases in order to be active (Figure 2.1).[15] Cleavage results in a di-chain molecule consisting of an approximately 100-kDa heavy chain and an approximately 50-kDa light chain, linked by a disulfide bond.[5] The protein comprises four domains consisting of the ~50 kDa light chain and three domains of the heavy chain: the ~50 kDa H_N membrane translocation domain, the ~25 kDa H_{CN} domain, and the ~25 kDa H_{CC} binding domain.[17]

PHARMACOLOGY

General Mechanism of Action

BoNTs exert their activity through a multistep process: binding to nerve terminals, internalization, translocation of the light chain across endosomal membrane, and inhibition of vesicular neurotransmitter release. This chapter focuses on recent developments in the mechanism of action; several comprehensive reviews are available for additional information.[17,18]

Binding

The binding of BoNTs to nerve cell membranes is characterized by a series of protein-lipid and protein-protein interactions with cellular membrane components that facilitate its internalization. Binding has been explained via a multireceptor model, in which the co-receptor comprises a ganglioside and protein component. BoNTs interact with gangliosides that are highly concentrated on presynaptic terminals.[19–22] Gangliosides are believed to mediate the initial low affinity contact between the BoNT and the neuronal membrane.[22,23] Ganglioside binding increases the local concentration of BoNT at the membrane surface, permitting it to diffuse in the plane of the membrane and bind its high affinity protein receptor (Figures 2.1 and 2.2).[22]

Botulinum neurotoxin A (BoNT-A) binding to gangliosides is mediated not only by the H_{CC} domain,[18] but also by parts of the H_N domain (amino acid residues H_N729-845).[25] A conserved ganglioside binding site motif has been identified in the H_C domain in all serotypes examined thus far except type D,[26] but affinities for various gangliosides differ between and within serotypes (e.g., A1, A2, etc.) produced by different clostridial strains.[27–29] Whether the H_{CN} domain has a function is unknown, but it may be involved in binding phosphatidylinositol phosphate (PIP).[18]

Synaptic vesicle protein 2 (SV2) is a protein receptor for BoNT types A, C1, D, E, and F and is localized to synaptic vesicles.[26,30–32] During exocytosis, portions of SV2 proteins are exposed to the cytoplasm, providing an exposed surface to which BoNTs can bind.[30,31] SV2 has at least three isoforms (SV2A, SV2B, and SV2C) that bind several BoNT serotypes with varying affinities (Table 2.1).

Synaptotagmins I and II are protein receptors for BoNT types B and G.[33,34] Synaptotagmins are localized to synaptic vesicle membranes where they sense calcium and trigger vesicle fusion.[35] Binding of types B and G to these proteins leads to their internalization into neurons.[34,36]

The C terminal domain of BoNTA shows homology with fibroblast growth factors (FGFs) and FGF receptor-3 (FGFR3) has been identified as an additional protein receptor for BoNTA in neuroblastoma cells, although the significance of this binding *in vivo* is not yet known.[37]

Internalization and translocation

After binding to gangliosides and protein co-receptors, BoNTs are internalized via receptor-mediated endocytosis into an endosome/vesicle. The light chain is translocated across the vesicle membrane in a series of steps still under study; recent evidence supports the following mechanism (Figure 2.3).[38,39] ATPase pumps in the vesicle membrane concentrate protons into lumen, decreasing intravesicular pH. The acidic environment of the endosome causes a conformational change in the neurotoxin-receptor complex that promotes insertion of the heavy chain into the endosomal membrane. The H_N domain of the heavy chain forms a channel and the H_C domain is needed for the light chain to unfold so that it can move through the channel into the cytosol.[38] The disulfide bond between the heavy and light chains is necessary for translocation across the synaptic vesicle membrane, but is ultimately reduced for the light chain to separate and interact with SNAP-25 (see the following).

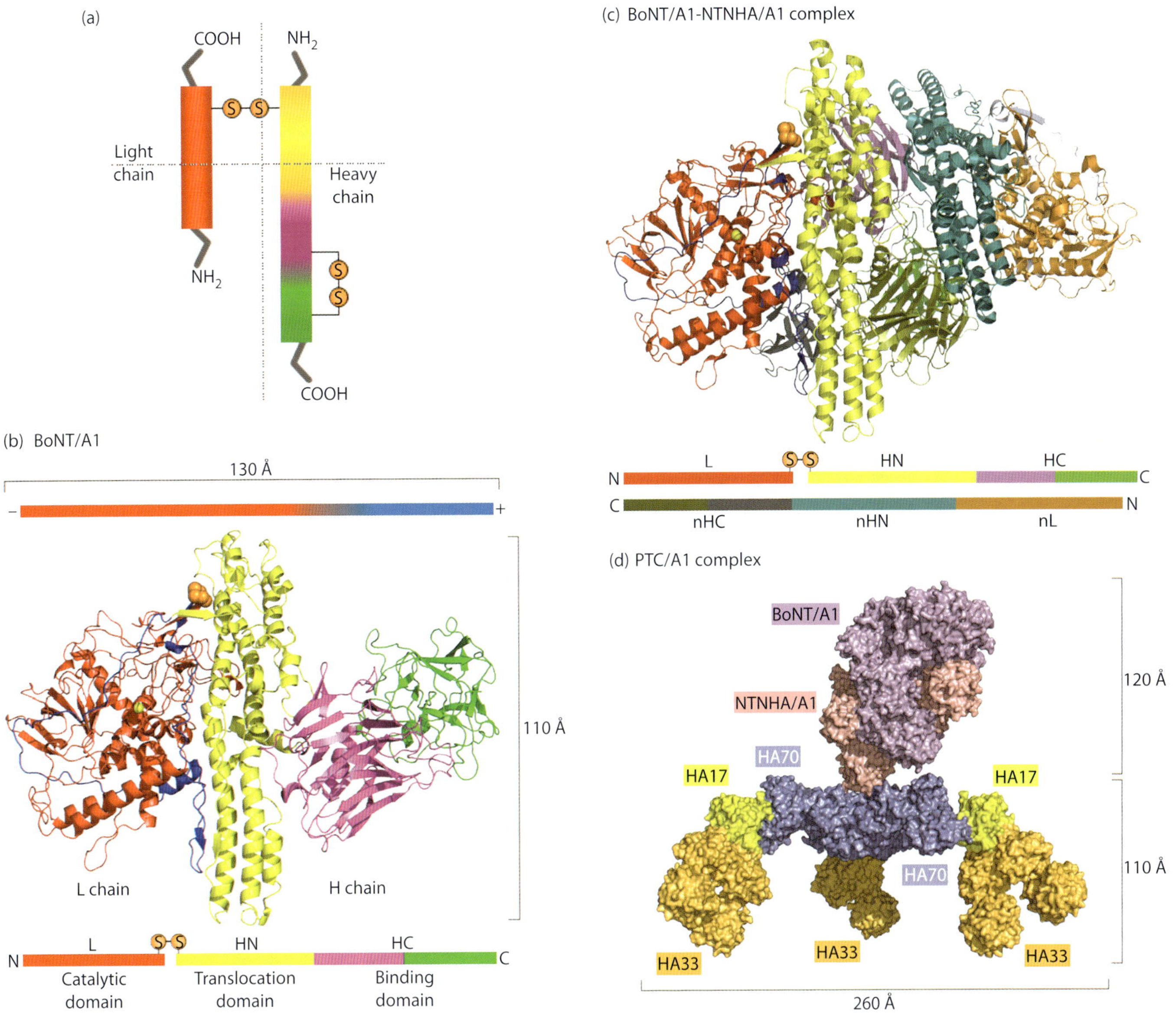

Figure 2.1 Schematic drawing showing structure of BoNT activated di-chain protein ~100-kDaa and ~50-kDaa chains (a) and diagrams of crystal structure of botulinum toxin A1 (BoNT-A1)[16] (b–d). The four individual protein domains interact with cellular membrane components in a series of protein-lipid and protein-protein interactions that facilitate the internalization of BoNT. These include the following: the H_C domain binds specifically to nerve terminals, with the H_{CC}, domain binding gangliosides and the H_{CN} domain possibly binding phosphatidylinositol phosphate (PIP),[18] the H_N domain forms a pore in the endosome that translocates the L chain into the nerve terminal cytosol, and the L chain is a metalloprotease that cleaves one or more SNARE (soluble N-ethylmaleimide-sensitive factor attachment protein receptor) proteins that mediate vesicular neurotransmitter release. A peptide belt (dark blue) surrounds the L domain and the inter-chain disulfide bond (orange), links the L chain to the H_N domain. (Figures b–d are reprinted from Rossetto O et al. *Nat Rev Microbiol* 12(8): 535–49. By permission from Macmillan Publishers Ltd., copyright 2014.)

Enzymatic Activity

Inside the cytosol, the light chain cleaves one or more of the SNARE (soluble N-ethylmaleimide-sensitive factor attachment protein receptor) proteins necessary for vesicle docking and fusion (Figure 2.4). Each serotype cleaves a specific peptide bond on one or more of the SNARE proteins in a zinc-dependent process.[43]

BoNT types A and E cleave SNAP-25 at different sites, and the effects of type E are much shorter. Evidence indicates that the type A light chain and its cleavage product ($SNAP\text{-}25_{197}$) localize to the plasma membrane, whereas the type E light chain is distributed throughout the cell cytoplasm.[44] The localization of type A light chain to the plasma membrane is decreased following mutation of the dileucine motif. Mutation of the dileucine motif of type A also leads to rapid recovery of neuromuscular function in rats.[45] More recently, mutation of the two leucines has been found to prevent interactions between the light chain and septins—intracellular structural proteins found clustered with the light chain at the plasma membrane (Figure 2.5).[46] The dileucine mutation also increases degradation of the type A light chain, as does interference with light chain-septin clustering. In contrast, the type E light chain does not interact with septins. These data indicate that the clustering of the type A light chain with septins at the plasma membrane via interactions with the dileucine motif is critical for its stability; these characteristics importantly contribute to the duration of action of BoNTA in clinical use.[44,46] Type A is the only botulinum neurotoxin serotype that contains a dileucine motif at the C terminus of the light chain.[44]

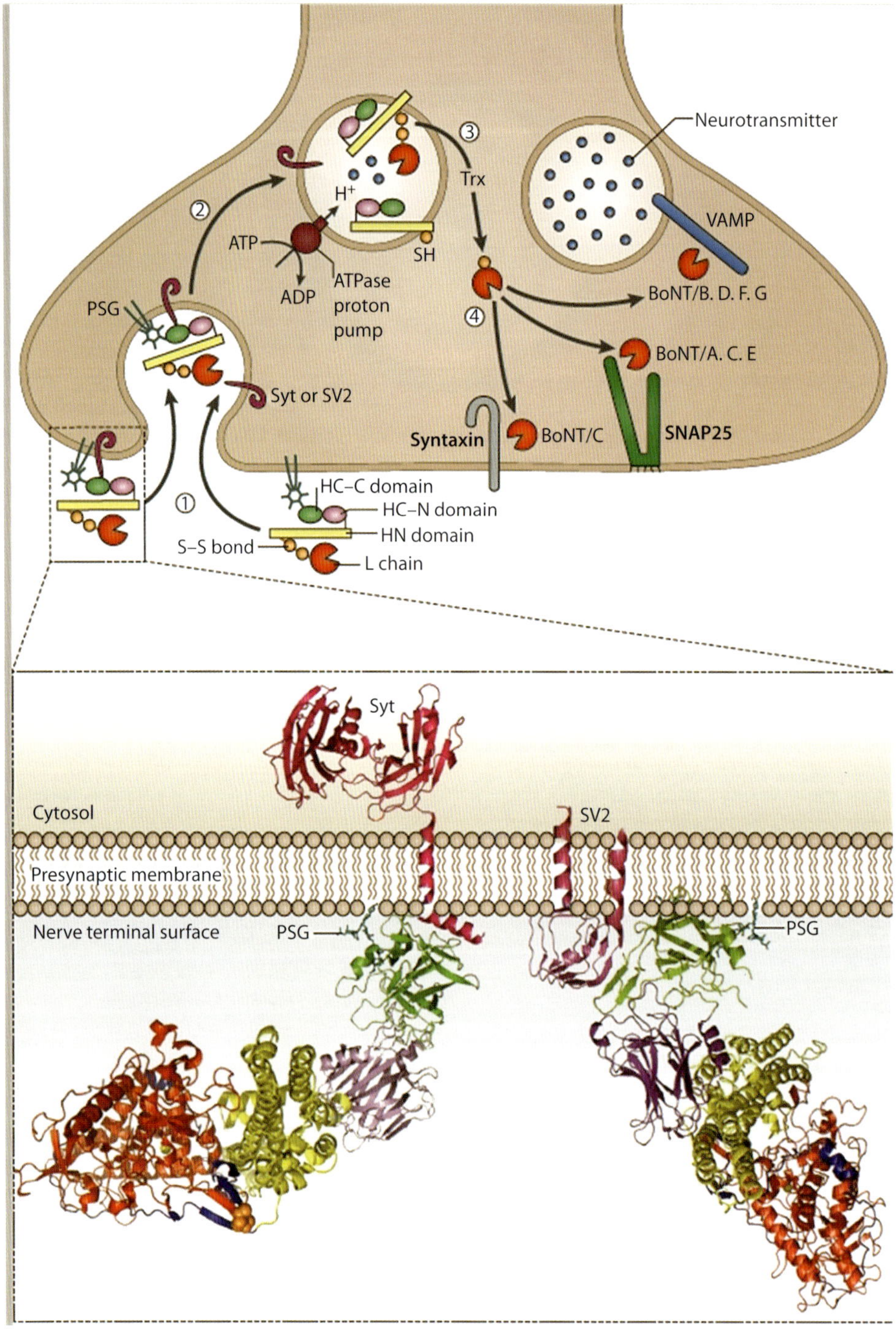

Figure 2.2 Binding and trafficking of BoNTs inside nerve terminals. The carboxy-terminal end of the HC domain (the HC-C domain) binds to a polysialoganglioside (PSG) present on the presynaptic membrane, followed by binding to a protein (either synaptotagmin [Syt] or SV2) located inside the exocytosed synaptic vesicle or on the presynaptic membrane (Step 1). The crystal structure of botulinum toxin B (BoNT-B) bound to Syt and PSG is shown on the lower left-hand side and the crystal structure of BoNT-A bound to PSG and to SV2 is shown on the lower right-hand side. BoNT is then endocytosed inside synaptic vesicles (Step 2), exploiting the vesicular ATPase proton pump that drives neurotransmitter reuptake. As the vesicle is acidified, BoNT becomes protonated, which results in translocation of the L chain across the synaptic vesicle membrane (Step 3) into the cytosol. Translocation can also occur across the endosomal membrane following the fusion of a synaptic vesicle with an endosome (which seems to occur in cultured neurons).[24] The L chain is released from the HN domain following cleavage of the inter-chain disulfide bond (S–S; shown in orange). The L-chain metalloproteases of BoNT-B, BoNT-D, BoNT-F, and BoNT-G cleave VAMP, the L-chain metalloproteases of BoNT-A and BoNT-E cleave SNAP25, and the L-chain metalloprotease of BoNT-C cleaves both SNAP25 and syntaxin (Step 4), all of which inhibit neurotransmitter release. (Reprinted from Rossetto O et al. *Nat Rev Microbiol* 12(8): 535–49. By permission from Macmillan Publishers Ltd., copyright 2014.)

In vitro, under the experimental conditions studied, BoNTA binding and internalization occur within minutes and proteolysis of SNAP-25 can be detected within half an hour.[47] Although traditionally called a neurotoxin because of its potential to cause generalized muscle weakness, BoNTA is not cytotoxic.[48,49]

Clinical Pharmacology

Mechanistically, the universal process of SNARE-mediated synaptic vesicle trafficking is the ultimate pharmacological target for BoNTs in neurons that are capable of binding and internalizing the toxin.[50]

Table 2.1 Receptors for BoNT Serotypes

Serotype	Cell membrane binding	Protein receptor
A	GT1b, GD1a	FGFR3 > SV2C > SV2A > SV2B;
B	GT1b, GD1a	Synaptotagmin II > Synaptotagmin I
C1	GD1b, GT1b	SV2
D	GT1b, GD1b, GD2	SV2B > SV2C > SV2A
E	GD1a	SV2A > SV2B
F	GD1a	SV2
G	GT1b	Synaptotagmin I ~ Synaptotagmin II

Source: Adapted from Lam KH et al. *Prog Biophys Mol Biol* 2015; 117(2–3): 225–31.)

Note: FGFR3 = fibroblast growth factor receptor 3, SV2 = secretory vesicle 2; >indicates comparative *in vitro* affinity.

Pharmacology in Neuromuscular Conditions: Extrafusal and Intrafusal Muscle Fibers

In the extrafusal motor nerve terminal, denervation leads to the increased production of growth factors, such as insulin-like growth factor-1 (IGF-1), and effects on related signaling pathways[51] that stimulate sprout development. Sprouts appear at motor-nerve terminals and nodes of Ranvier within 2 days of BoNTA injection into mammalian soleus muscles that persist and become more complex for at least 50 days.[52] Sprouts may establish functional synaptic contacts,[52] but the role of these sprouts in functional recovery of the neurons is not firmly established. Using a sensitive measure, Rogozhin and colleagues found that quantal neurotransmitter release could be detected in the vicinity of sprouts and the original terminals at about the same time, and the original terminals accounted for more than 80% of total acetylcholine release, suggesting that the spouts are relatively ineffectual.[53,54]

As exocytosis is restored, the original terminals recover and the sprouts regress.[55] After reinnervation is complete, the target tissue is fully functional[52] and there is no clinical indication that post-botulinum reinnervation produces functionally substandard synapses. However, in rats, acetylcholine release recovers more slowly after multiple than single injections.[53]

The SNARE-mediated mechanism inhibiting acetylcholine release occurs not only at alpha motor neurons, which innervate extrafusal muscle fibers, but also at gamma motor neurons, which innervate intrafusal muscle fibers. Intrafusal fibers make up muscle spindles (Figure 2.6)—the proprioceptive organs that are sensitive to stretch and are important in setting the resting tone and reflex sensitivity of muscle. Inhibition of gamma motor neurons decreases activation of muscle spindles, which effectively changes the sensory afferent system by reducing the Ia afferent traffic. However, this mechanism likely does not occur in facial muscles as they are reported to lack muscle spindles.[56,57]

Preclinical and clinical studies indicate that BoNT-A affects afferent pathways via inhibition of neural input to intrafusal fibers.[58–62] Thus, the overall effect of BoNT-A therapy may be a combination of a direct effect on the primary nerve-end organ communication (i.e., the alpha motor neuron innervating muscle) coupled with an indirect effect on the overall system (i.e., via afferent effects associated with toxin-induced chemodenervation of the gamma motor neuron).

The most common BoNT products in clinical use are onabotulinumtoxinA (Allergan), abobotulinumtoxinA (Ipsen), incobotulinumtoxinA (Merz), and rimabotulinumtoxinB (Solstice). BoNTs are most often injected into overactive skeletal muscles that vary depending on the condition to be treated and the patient's individual presentation. The clinical onset of action following intramuscular injection is generally reported to be within 3–7 days, with a peak effect in approximately 2–4 weeks. However, when injected into small muscles for the treatment of glabellar lines, the onset of clinical effects have been reported within 24 hours.[63,64] The duration of beneficial effects of each treatment is approximately 3–5 months following intramuscular injection,[65] although some differences have been noted.[66] The duration of BoNT-B is somewhat shorter than that of type A, and has been reported as 6–12 weeks in the management of facial lines.[67] Most patients respond to BoNT-A for many years without decrements in safety, responsiveness, or quality of life, and without increased doses.[68,69]

Pharmacology in Dermal Conditions

Eccrine sweat glands are widely distributed over the body, with areas around the sweat coil and duct densely vascularized and innervated by sympathetic postganglionic terminals.[70] Unlike most sympathetic neurons, those that innervate eccrine sweat glands are cholinergic; they also co-release neuropeptides such as calcitonin gene related peptide (CGRP) and vasoactive intestinal polypeptide (VIP).[71] Apocrine sweat glands are distributed only in hairy areas such as axillary, mammary, perineal, and genital regions, where they respond to both epinephrine and norepinephrine, although whether they are activated via sympathetic innervation, circulating levels of these neurotransmitters, or local intradermal release is not yet known. Apocrine sweat

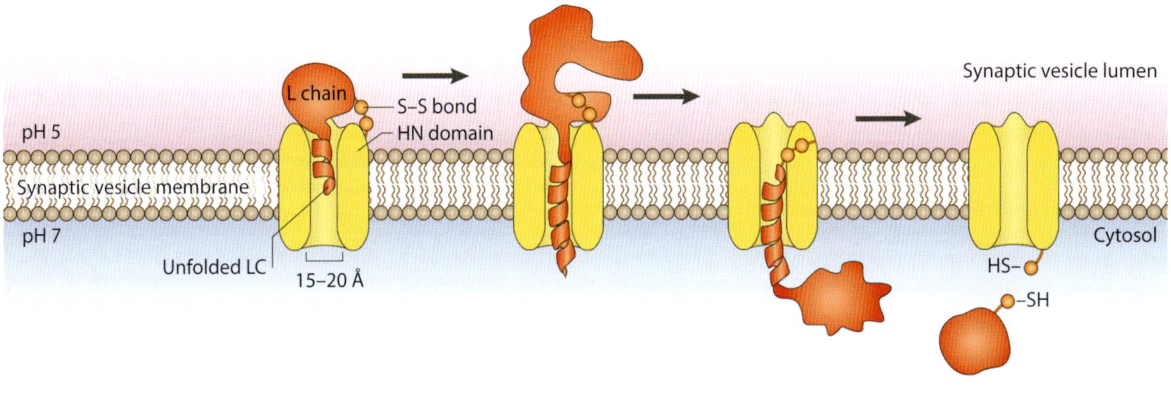

Figure 2.3 Model for the molecular events that occur during L-chain translocation across the synaptic vesicle membrane. Acidification of the synaptic vesicle lumen via action of the ATPase proton pump causes a conformational change in the HN domain, which enables it to penetrate the lipid bilayer. This leads to the formation of a channel that chaperones the partially unfolded L chain across the membrane. The inter-chain disulfide bond (S–S bond) is proposed to cross the membrane at a late stage during translocation, and its reduction on the cytosolic side of the synaptic vesicle membrane releases the L chain into the cytosol. (Reprinted by permission from Rossetto O et al. *Nat Rev Microbiol* 12(8): 535–49, Macmillan Publishers Ltd., copyright 2014.)

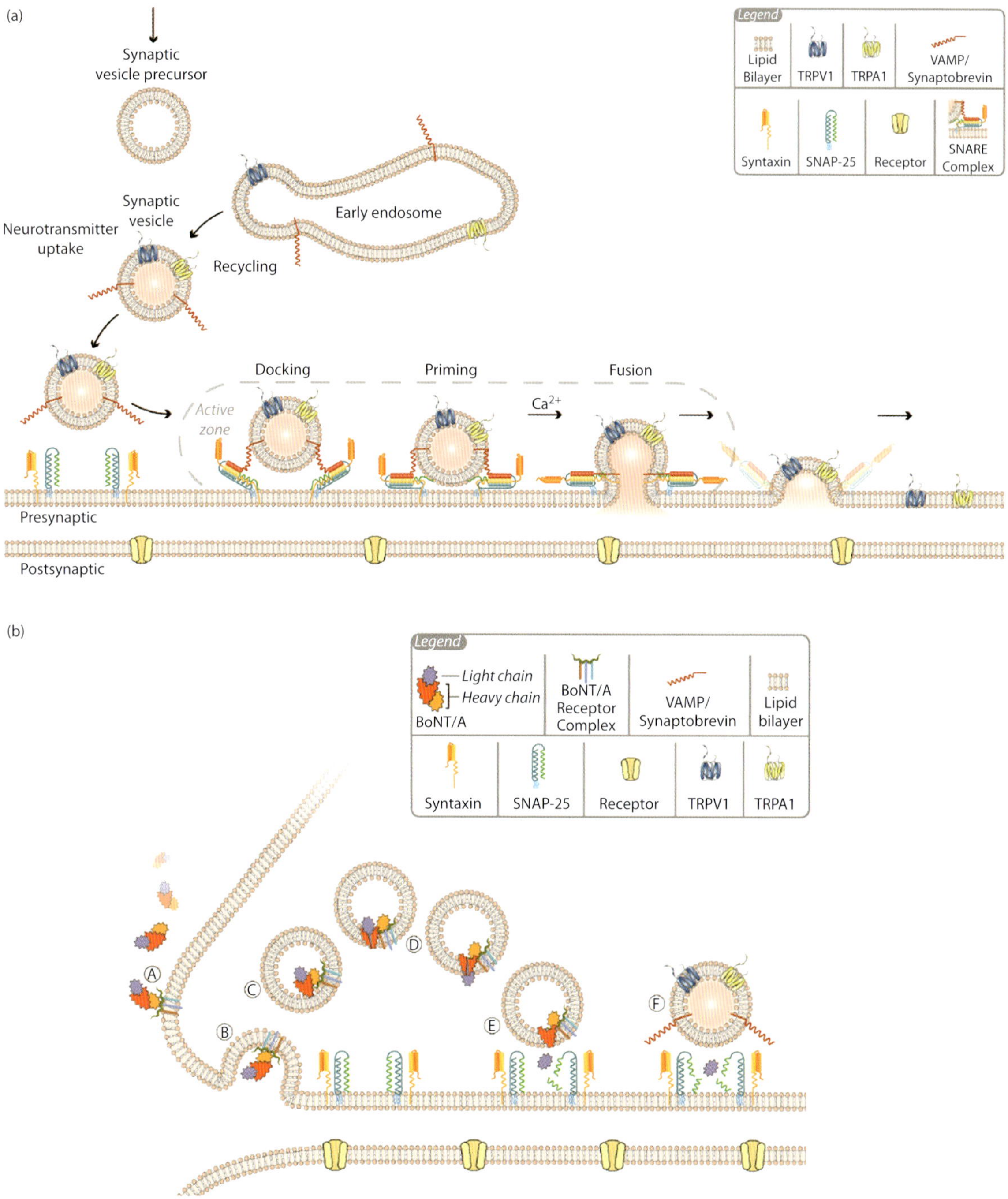

Figure 2.4 BoNT-A mechanism of action: Synaptic vesicle delivery of luminal *content* neurotransmitters and lipid bilayer *cargo* ion channels and receptors. (a) Synaptic vesicle (SC) delivery of luminal contents such as neurotransmitters and lipid bilayer cargo[108] including ion channels and receptors. SVs form a reserve pool at the nerve terminal and may be filled with neurotransmitters. Most SVs are decorated with multiple proteins:[40] membrane-associated protein receptors, transient receptor potential cation channel vanilloid subfamily, member 1 (TRPV1), and transient receptor potential cation channel ankyrin subfamily, member 1 (TRPA1) are depicted. SVs dock adjacent to the nerve terminal and inner membrane active zone and undergo an adenosine triphosphate (ATP)-dependent priming step that enables response to the Ca^{2+} signal that triggers fusion, exocytosis, and consequent delivery of not only SV contents into the extracellular space, but also lipid membrane and associated protein cargo into the cell surface. Successful fusion requires an interaction between the vesicle-associated membrane protein (VAMP)/synaptobrevin with the internal membrane surface proteins synaptosomal-associated protein of molecular weight 25 kDaa (SNAP-25) and syntaxin, which together form the SNARE (soluble NSF [N-ethylmaleimide-sensitive factor] attachment protein receptor) complex; other associated proteins (e.g., Munc18, Rab) are involved but not depicted.[41] The SV membrane may fully fuse into the terminal membrane (full collapse fusion), thus delivering the protein receptors (e.g., TRPV1 or TRPA1) into the cell surface. Excess terminal recycling through one of the endocytosis pathways[42] is not depicted. OnaBTX-A cleaves SNAP-25, impairing SV fusion and the regulated delivery of receptors TRPV1 or TRPA1 to the terminal membrane, thus downregulating receptor activity. An SV with both luminal contents and vesicular lipid bilayer cargo is diagrammed for illustration purposes. (b) OnaBTX-A mechanism of action. (A) OnaBTX-A heavy chain binds to an acceptor complex comprised of three components: ganglioside GT1b, synaptic vesicle glycoprotein 2 (SV2), and fibroblast growth factor receptor 3 (FGFR3); (B) internalization into an endosome that (C) acidifies; (D) conformational change that enables the light chain to traverse the endosomal wall; (E) cytosolic light chain specifically cleaves SNAP-25 (synaptosomal-associated protein of molecular weight 25 kDaa), one of the SNARE attachment protein receptors required for SV membrane docking; (F) SNARE disruption prevents SV fusion with the terminal membrane. This prevents SV content delivery of neurotransmitters to the synaptic cleft in addition to SV cargo delivery and cell surface expression of relevant peripheral nerve receptors and ion channels. (Figures courtesy of Maria Rivero [Allergan, Inc., Irvine, CA]. [a] Modified from Burstein R et al. *Cephalalgia* 2014; 34(11): 853–69; [b] reprinted from Whitcup SM et al. *Ann N Y Acad Sci* 2014; 1329: 67–80 via a Creative Commons License.)

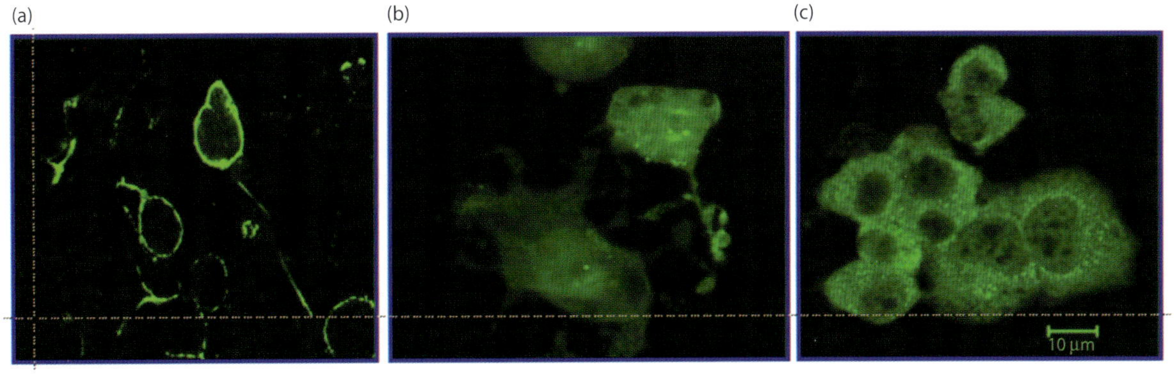

Figure 2.5 Subcellular localization of light chain in differentiated rat pheochromocytoma cells (PC12). Green fluorescent protein-light chain type A (GFP-LCA) localized in a punctate manner in specific areas at the plasma membrane of the cell body and neurites, with no fluorescence in the cytoplasm of cells (a). In contrast, the GFP-LCE (b) localizes in a punctate manner in the cell cytoplasm and the GFP-LCB (c) is dispersed throughout the cell including the nucleus.

glands have also been described in hairy regions where they respond to acetylcholine, norepinephrine, and epinephrine.[70]

Sebaceous glands in the skin are also sensitive to acetylcholine, but they are not directly innervated by autonomic fibers (although nerve fibers are evident in their vicinity).[72] *In vitro*, acetylcholine stimulates sebum production in human sebaceous glands by acting on nicotinic cholinergic receptors, and specifically nicotinic acetylcholine receptors alpha-7 (nAchRα7), which are present *in vitro* and *in vivo*.[73] Notably, acetylcholine is released from non-neuronal sebaceous cells in an autocrine fashion and may not be SNARE mediated; the non-neuronal actions of acetylcholine in skin have been reviewed.[74] Non-neuronal acetylcholine release in human skin is partially mediated via organic cation transporters.[75,76]

Hyperhidrosis

The sympathetic, cholinergic innervation of eccrine sweat glands provides the basis for BoNT-A use in focal hyperhidrosis, in which the medication is injected intradermally. The onset of action of BoNT-A

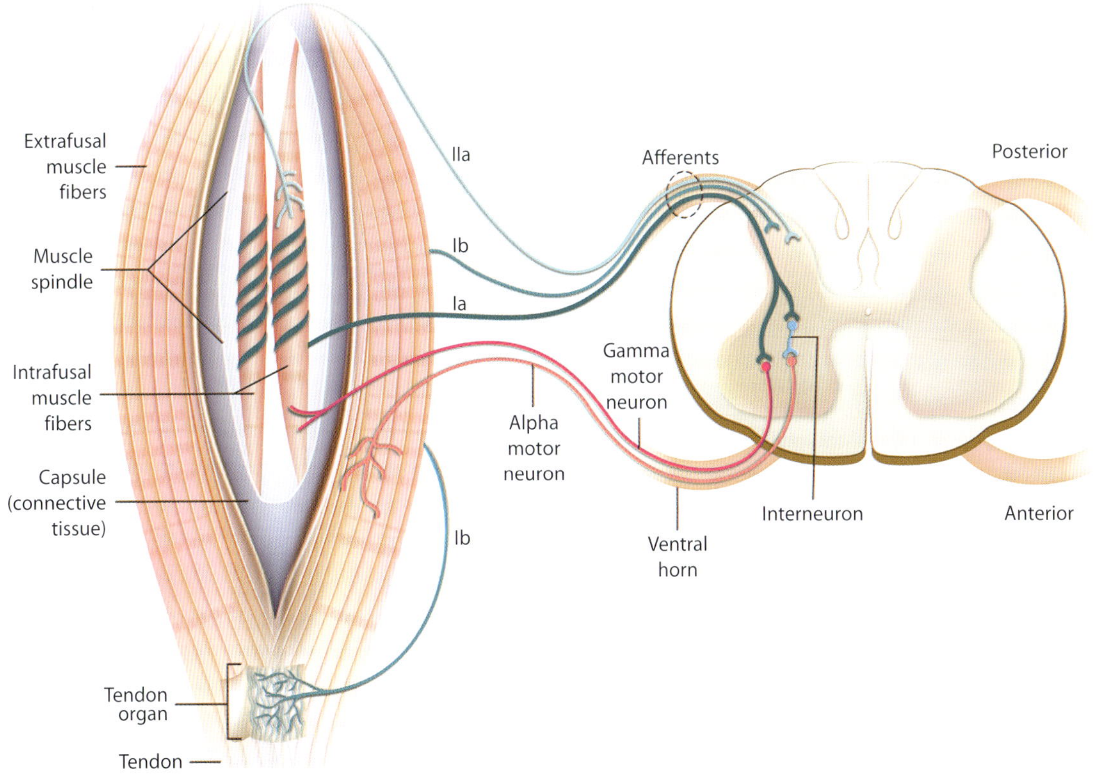

Figure 2.6 Motor and sensory innervation of muscle. Acetylcholine is released from alpha and gamma motor neurons that originate in the spinal cord (right). Alpha motor neurons innervate extrafusal muscle fibers and gamma motor neurons innervate intrafusal fibers of the muscle spindle (left). Activation of gamma motor neurons keeps the muscle spindle taut and sensitive to stretch. Group Ia and Group IIa afferent fibers convey information about muscle length; Group Ia fibers also convey information about the rate of length change. By inhibiting acetylcholine release from gamma motor neurons, BoNTA may affect muscle spindle activity and, consequently, sensory information conveyed back to the spinal cord. Golgi tendon organs sense muscle tension and are innervated by Group Ib afferents. (Figure courtesy of Maria Rivero [Allergan, Inc., Irvine, CA]).

in various forms of focal hyperhidrosis is within 1 week,[77] and benefits last approximately 7 months with OnaBTX-A, although 22%–28% of patients may experience benefits for at least a year.[78,79]

Preliminary studies in other dermal conditions

Serendipitous observations by investigators treating migraine and facial tics suggest that BoNT-A may also have beneficial effects on sebaceous cysts[80] and acne.[81] Several subsequent studies designed to evaluate the effects of OnaBTX-A or BoNT-A (Medytox) on sebum production support this effect.[73,82]

Several case reports and small, open studies have documented beneficial effects of OnaBTX-A and AboBTX-A in rosacea.[83–85] Beneficial effects of OnaBTX-A and AboBTX-A have also been reported in patients with psoriasis and with AboBTX-A in an animal model of psoriasis.[86–88]

BoNT-A has also been studied in cutaneous scarring following speculation that it may reduce the muscle tension that leads to scar production during wound healing.[89] Several small, randomized studies have found that OnaBTX-A injections improve the appearance of scars associated with facial wounds.[90,91] Subsequent case reports have also noted improvement in scarring and pain associated with keloids following BoNT-A.[92,93] A randomized study documented greater improvements in keloid volume and subjective symptoms such as pain following intralesional BoNT-A than corticosteroids.[94]

Studies on fibroblasts isolated from human scar tissue have found that BoNT-A inhibits the growth of fibroblasts and fibroblast differentiation into myofibroblasts, as well as decreases production of the scar-inducing protein, transforming growth factor-beta 1 (TGF-β1).[95,96] In a preclinical scar model, BoNT-A reduced collagen deposition and scarring.[97] In tissue from human keloid scars, BoNT-A has been found to alter expression of multiple scar-related proteins, including vascular endothelial growth factor (VEGF), platelet derived growth factor (PDGF), TGF-β1, and matrix metalloprotease-1 (MMP-1).[98] However, other preclinical work indicates that BoNT-A decreases collagen I production in human dermal fibroblasts.[99] Other researchers have found that BoNT-A significantly antagonizes premature senescence of human dermal fibroblasts *in vitro* induced by ultraviolet radiation, raising the potential of antiphotoaging effects.[100]

Pharmacology in Overactive Bladder/Neurogenic Detrusor Overactivity

Micturition comprises both motor and sensory components. Release of acetylcholine and ATP from parasympathetic nerves mediates the elimination of urine, with acetylcholine dominating under normal conditions and ATP dominating under pathological conditions.[101,102] Sensory mechanisms in the bladder likely mediate the sensation of urgency in overactive bladder. Bladder afferent neurons express numerous receptors, including transient receptor potential vanilloid 1 (TRPV1) that respond to heat, acidic pH, voltage, and endovanilloids,[103] tyrosine kinase receptor A that respond to nerve growth factor, and purinergic receptors (e.g., P2X3) that respond to ATP.[104,105]

The effects of BoNT-A on acetylcholine release from motor terminals are well documented, and growing evidence indicates that BoNT-A has several different sensory actions in the bladder.[105] For example, in preclinical studies, BoNT-A inhibits ATP release from cultured urothelial cells, which may stimulate purinergic receptors on bladder afferents.[106] The effects of BoNT-A have also been studied in a model of spinal cord injury, in which animals show an increase in resting ATP release, an increase in hypoosmotic-evoked ATP release, and a decrease in hypoosmotic-evoked NO release from the urothelium. Although BoNT-A does not affect the increase in resting ATP release, it significantly inhibits the hypoosmotic-evoked urothelial ATP release.[107] BoNT-A also restores the hypoosmotic-evoked inhibition of NO release in these animals. The authors suggest that changes in the ratio of ATP-mediated excitation and NO-mediated inhibition promote hyperactivity in the bladder that can be largely reversed by BoNT-A. Finally, peripheral administration of BoNT-A cleaves SNAP-25 and prevents the SNARE-mediated vesicle-fusion process, which consequently impairs transfer of the vesicular lipid bilayer cargo,[108] TRPV1 and P2X3, to neural membranes.[109,110]

Clinical evidence from patients with neurogenic detrusor overactivity indicates that BoNT-A normalizes disease-associated pathology. Patients with neurogenic detrusor overactivity exhibit increased levels of TRPV1 and P2X3 receptors in the suburothelial bladder.[111,112] The expression of P2X3 and TRPV1 in urinary bladder epithelial cells of these patients decreases significantly (without any loss of fiber density) 4 weeks after BoNT-A treatment, and improvements in patients' sensation of urgency and urodynamic physiology parameters are correlated with the temporal change in P2X3 immunoreactivity.[105] Urinary NGF levels, normalized to creatinine, are significantly higher than controls for untreated patients with either neurogenic or idiopathic detrusor overactivity, and clinical response to OnaBTX-A is associated with the reduction of these levels in both patient populations.[113]

In the treatment of overactive bladder, OnaBTX-A is injected into the smooth detrusor muscle of the urinary bladder and in the Phase 3 program for idiopathic overactive bladder,[114–116] the duration of effect was approximately 7–8 months, with consistent benefits observed following multiple injections up to 3.5 years.[117] Similarly, in the Phase 3 program for neurogenic detrusor overactivity, the duration of effect (time to retreatment) was approximately 8–10 months,[118,119] with consistent benefits observed following multiple injections up to 4 years.[120,121]

Pharmacology in Chronic Migraine

Chronic migraine is characterized by dysfunction in the trigeminovascular pathway, including central and peripheral sensitization involving peripheral release of proinflammatory mediators such as substance P, glutamate, and CGRP.[122,123] Activation of the peripheral pathway via meningeal nociceptors may involve a variety of receptors including TRP channels, P2X3 receptors that are sensitive to ATP, dopaminergic receptors (D1 and D2), and serotonergic 5HT1b/1d receptors.[123]

BoNT-A inhibits the release of substance P from cultured dorsal root ganglion neurons.[124] and the stimulated but not basal release of CGRP from cultured trigeminal ganglia neurons.[125] Moreover, in preclinical studies, BoNT-A reduces mechanical pain in peripheral trigeminovascular neurons in a manner consistent with inhibition or reduction of surface expression of mechano-sensitive ion channels.[123,126] Thus, OnaBTX-A may exert its prophylactic effects in chronic migraine through a dual mechanism that includes inhibition of SNARE-mediated vesicular release of inflammatory neurochemicals and peptides from the peripheral terminals of nociceptive primary afferent neurons, in addition to inhibition/downregulation of relevant peripheral nerve receptors and ion channels in a pathologic state.

For the treatment of chronic migraine, OnaBTX-A is injected into the craniofacial-cervical region as a prophylactic therapy. Beneficial effects are observed by week 4, and injection may be repeated every 12 weeks.[127] The Phase 3 data demonstrated the safety and efficacy of repeated OnaBTX-A injections for up to 56 weeks[128] and medical records of patients receiving OnaBTX-A for up to 9 treatment cycles (~2 years) demonstrated extended efficacy in a real-world setting via reduced headache days.

Overall, at least three lines of evidence indicate that BoNT-A regulates neurotransmitter release and receptor levels in pathological or stimulated states but not in the normal or basal states in conditions with a sensory component: (1) BoNT-A inhibits stimulated but not basal CGRP release from trigeminal cells, of potential relevance to migraine;[125] (2) BoNT-A normalizes the alterations in urothelial ATP and NO release induced by chronic spinal cord injury;[107] and (3) in the pathologic state of neurogenic detrusor overactivity, BoNT-A normalizes the concentration of TRPV1 and P2X3 in the bladder.[105] The latter observation (3) is consistent with the proposed dual regulation of surface expression/insertion of TRPs through the constitutive pathway, in which TRP channels reach the plasma membrane via exocytosis from the trans-Golgi or early endosomes, and the regulated vesicular pathway, in which receptors are transported as cargo in the lipid bilayer of neurotransmitter or neuropeptide vesicles that dock and fuse with the membrane in a SNARE-dependent process.[103] In this model, BoNT-A inhibits the SNARE-regulated mechanism of receptor insertion but not the constitutive expression of these sensory receptors.

Lack of Retrograde Transport at Relevant Preclinical Doses

Historically, a major distinction between tetanus toxin and BoNT has been that the former undergoes retrograde transport and transcytosis across neurons to exert effects in the central nervous system, whereas the latter does not.[129] It is notable that clinical tetanus results in a spastic paralysis and botulinum toxin results in peripheral muscle relaxation. However, over the past decade, several groups have reported the retrograde transport of BoNT-A under experimental conditions that appear to contradict this distinction.[130–132]

Studies reporting retrograde transport and transcytosis used high locally administered doses of BoNT, in marked contrast to the comparatively low doses used clinically. For example, the study by Antonucci and colleagues used a high dose laboratory preparation of BoNT-A injected into a single site of the rat whisker pad (135 pg),[130] which is approximately 450 pg/kg. By way of comparison, patients treated with OnaBTX-A for facial indications typically receive approximately 20 units (or 3 pg/kg) administered into multiple muscles, which, per kilogram, is approximately 150-fold lower than the dose used by the Antonucci and colleagues.[133]

Dose response studies by Dolly and colleagues help clarify the retrograde transport conversation. Using a model of compartmented cultures of rat sympathetic neurons, these investigators applied picomolar (pM) concentrations of BoNT-A to neurites and measured transport to cell bodies as percent total SNAP-25 in the cleaved form.[134] Results showed that BoNT-A acted locally except at high doses; for example, addition of 10 pM BoNT-A to neurites led to approximately one-third of total SNAP-25 cleaved in the neurites but virtually no cleaved SNAP-25 in the cell body compartment. The authors note that this amount of BoNT-A is equivalent to 75 mouse LD_{50} units and exceeds the maximum recommended clinical dose of 50 units per injection site for BoNT-A complex by 50%. At doses of 10^4 pM, which are 1000 times higher than the ~10 pM doses used clinically, BoNT-A applied to distal neurites did induce SNAP-25 cleavage in the central compartment, (indicating some retrograde transmission), but did not block synaptic transmission at cell bodies and therefore had no functional effect. No transcytosis was observed in these studies.

A recent study provided additional insights using a highly selective antibody for the BoNT-A-cleaved substrate ($SNAP25_{197}$) combined with 3-dimensional imaging.[135] In this study, $SNAP25_{197}$ was confined to motor neurons following injection of a low dose into the rat hindlimb; at a higher saturating dose, sporadic staining was observed in distal muscles and associated spinal cord regions, consistent with systemic spread of toxin, but was confined to the motor neuron and there was no evidence for transcytosis.

DIFFERENCES BETWEEN BoNT PRODUCTS

The clinical pharmacology of BoNTs is influenced by the bacterial strain, methods of isolation and purification, serotype, formulation, and procedures used to determine biological activity (see Reference 66 for review). These factors vary for each commercially available BoNT product and can affect its clinical profile.

Units of Biological Activity

Differences in unit potency and the noninterchangeability of units among BoNT products result from differences in the assays used to determine biological activity of bulk drug substance. Each manufacturer uses a unique, product-specific method and reference standard for testing.

Biological assays involving animals are sensitive to variations in animal strain, age, sex, diet, temperature, caging, season, and even the liquid used to dilute the product.[136] Notably, manufacturers of the main BoNT-A products use different diluents for LD_{50} unit testing: Allergan uses saline (the diluent also used for clinical reconstitution),[137] and Ipsen uses gelatin phosphate buffer.[138] Merz adds human serum albumin (HSA) as a stabilizer to their undisclosed diluent,[139] and stabilizers have been shown to enhance the activity of BoNT-A products at low concentrations in preclinical tests.[140]

Difference in LD_{50} assays mean that units are not interchangeable even for products labeled as containing the same number of units per vial. In a comparison of two BoNT-A products, both labeled at 100 units, one of the products (incobotulinumtoxinA) was found to contain substantially fewer units per vial when compared against an Allergan reference standard for OnaBTX-A.[137,141] When these two BoNT-A products were compared in the Merz LD_{50} assay, in which the products are diluted with a solution containing added HSA as a stabilizer and compared against the Merz reference standard, the potency was comparable.[139] These findings confirm that the potencies of the two BoNT-A products are differentially affected by the diluent and stabilizers, indicating that assay conditions markedly influence potency measurements reflecting underlying product differences.

Historically, the mouse-defined LD_{50} has been the global standard for BoNT-A potency testing used by all manufacturers, but the trend is toward less animal use in biological assays. Allergan has implemented a cell-based potency assay optimized for OnaBTX-A that meets the stringent approval requirements of global regulatory agencies for replacement of an animal LD_{50} test.[142] This rigorous, cross-validated assay does not change OnaBTX-A product or potency, and significantly reduces the use of animals for testing.

Current Regulatory Approvals of BoNT-A Products

Most regulatory agencies worldwide require that manufacturers meet strict guidelines governing the manufacture and clinical development of pharmaceutical products. These guidelines promote quality, purity, consistent biological activity, and lack of contamination. An official product approval for a specific disease or condition (i.e., "indication") is granted only after rigorous clinical trials demonstrate efficacy and safety. These studies provide important efficacy, safety, dosing, and injection site information specific to the individual product. The licensed indications for BoNT products differ based on whether the manufacturers have conducted the necessary studies as required by the regulatory agencies (Table 2.2). Approved indications for each product vary by country; practitioners should consult local labeling materials for details.

Table 2.2 Approved Indications[a] for the Main BoNT Products Available in the United States (US) and European Union (EU)[b]

Indication[a]	OnaBTX-A	AboBTX-A	IncoBTX-A
Therapeutic			
Strabismus	US	–	–
Blepharospasm	US, EU	EU	US, EU
Hemifacial spasm	EU	EU	–
Cervical dystonia	US, EU	US, EU	US, EU
Primary axillary hyperhidrosis	US, EU	–	–
Focal upper-limb spasticity	US, EU	US, EU	EU
Focal lower-limb spasticity	US, EU	EU	–
Juvenile cerebral palsy (dynamic equinus foot deformity)	EU	US, EU	–
Chronic migraine	US, EU	–	–
Neurogenic detrusor overactivity	US, EU	–	–
Overactive bladder	US, EU	–	–
Aesthetic			
Glabellar lines	US, EU	US, EU	US, EU
Crow's feet lines	US, EU	–	EU
Forehead lines	US	–	EU

[a]Approved indications, precise indication wording, and associated limitations vary from country to country. Consult local labeling for details.
[b]Majority of EU5 countries (France, Germany, Italy, Spain, United Kingdom).

Unlicensed Products

The noninterchangeability of BoNTs has become even more prominent with the unscrupulous use of counterfeit and unlicensed products. One study evaluated a BoNT-A product CNBTX-A (Nanfeng) that was previously available in China but was not approved there or in any other country.[143] The label on each vial indicated 55 units, however, the product was not accompanied by a package insert or dosing recommendations. Testing against an Allergan reference standard showed that a vial of CNBTX-A contained 243 units of biological activity.[143] Serious consequences could have resulted if clinicians had obtained this nonapproved product and applied it to patients based on doses of an approved product. In another instance, a highly concentrated laboratory preparation of BoNT, labeled for laboratory use only, was illegally administered to four individuals in a Florida clinic for cosmetic purposes.[144] All of the individuals exposed to this laboratory preparation experienced progressive muscle weakness and were hospitalized.[144]

The dangers of using unlicensed BoNT preparations are unambiguous: clinicians risk patient safety and incur professional liability.[145,146] It is critical that clinicians verify the BoNT product they are using and use it at doses recommended by the manufacturer and documented in the published clinical literature.

IMMUNOLOGY

Under certain circumstances (e.g., dose and frequency), BoNTs can elicit immune responses that neutralize the protein's activity. Only antibodies directed against the 150-kDa neurotoxin are neutralizing.[147] Antibodies may occasionally be formed against the nontoxin proteins in the BoNT complex, but these do not appear to affect clinical responsiveness.[147] Others have argued that the NAPs may serve as immune adjuvants,[148] but the low rates of neutralizing antibody formation with OnaBTX-A and AboBTX-A[149–151] suggest that such hypothetical effects are not established.

Within the BoNT-A molecule, antibodies directed against certain peptides within amino acid residues 449–1296 of the heavy chain are neutralizing.[152] Nearly all of the regions overlap or coincide with the regions on the protein that bind to synaptosomes *in vitro*.[152] Similar results have been found for BoNT-B.[153] The pattern of antibody recognition varies among patients with neutralizing antibodies, such that not all patients develop antibodies to the same portion of the BoNT molecule,[152] underscoring the potential role of individual genetic factors in neutralizing antibody development.[154]

In recent clinical studies, the rates of neutralizing antibody formation are low for the main three BoNT-A products:[155] 0% with OnaBTX-A (observed at study conclusion) in glabellar lines and 1.2% in cervical dystonia,[149,150] 0% with AboBTX-A in glabellar lines and less than 3% in cervical dystonia[151] and 1.1% with IncoBTX-A in their overall development program.[156,157] Clinical trials have not directly compared neutralizing antibody rates between different BoNT products, but the aforementioned numbers suggest that studies would not find meaningful differences. Moreover, some patients with neutralizing antibodies continue to respond to BoNT injections.[158]

SUMMARY AND CONCLUSIONS

BoNTs continue to stimulate both basic and clinical research. In the past few years, advances in understanding BoNT binding and internalization mechanisms have been reported, with increasingly detailed information on protein domains and their interactions with protein and lipid components at the plasma membrane. Mechanisms of action beyond the inhibition of acetylcholine release from neurons are also an active area of research, as evidenced by the effects of OnaBTX-A on afferent/sensory mechanisms that are consistent with the treatment of chronic migraine and lower urinary tract disorders.

Clinical studies have evaluated BoNT-A for many dermal conditions beyond hyperhidrosis and hyperfunctional facial lines in aesthetics. Initial reports from these small studies indicate that BoNT-A may reduce dermal sebum production/secretion and scar formation and improve the appearance of keloids. As research and development of BoNTs advance, it seems likely that additional applications will be identified for these important, but noninterchangeable, therapeutic proteins.

ACKNOWLEDGMENTS

The author acknowledges the assistance of Mary Ann Chapman, PhD in the preparation of this chapter, and reviews by Conor Gallagher, PhD; Birgitte Jacky, PhD; and Edward Hsia, PhD.

REFERENCES

1. Sharma SK, Singh BR. Hemagglutinin binding mediated protection of botulinum neurotoxin from proteolysis. *J Nat Toxins* 1998; 7(3): 239–53.
2. Sharma SK, Singh BR. Enhancement of the endopeptidase activity of purified botulinum neurotoxins A and E by an isolated component of the native neurotoxin associated proteins. *Biochemistry* 2004; 43(16): 4791–8.
3. Lamanna C, Spero L, Schantz EJ. Dependence of time to death on molecular size of botulinum toxin. *Infect Immun* 1970; 1(4): 423–4.
4. Matsui T, Gu S, Lam KH, Carter LG, Rummel A, Mathews II, Jin R. Structural basis of the pH-dependent assembly of a botulinum neurotoxin complex. *J Mol Biol* 2014; 426(22): 3773–82.
5. Sakaguchi G, Kozaki S, Ohishi I. Structure and function of botulinum toxins. In J. E. AIouf (ed). *Bacterial Protein Toxins*, London: Academic Press; 1984, 435–43.
6. Sakaguchi G, Ohishi I, Kozai S. Purification and oral toxicities of Clostridium botulinum progenitor toxins. In: Lewis GEJ (ed). *Biomedical Aspects of Botulism*. New York: Academic Press; 1981, 21–34.
7. Inoue K, Fujinaga Y, Watanabe T, Ohyama T, Takeshi K, Moriishi K, Nakajima H, Inoue K, Oguma K. Molecular composition of Clostridium botulinum type A progenitor toxins. *Infect Immun* 1996; 64(5): 1589–94.
8. Terilli RR, Moura H, Woolfitt AR, Rees J, Schieltz DM, Barr JR. A historical and proteomic analysis of botulinum neurotoxin type/G. *BMC Microbiol* 2011; 11: 232.
9. Maslanka SE, Luquez C, Dykes JK et al. A novel botulinum neurotoxin, previously reported as serotype H, has a hybrid-like structure with regions of similarity to the structures of serotypes A and F and is neutralized with serotype A antitoxin. *J Infect Dis* 2016; 213: 379–85.
10. Yao G, Lam KH, Perry K, Weisemann J, Rummel A, Jin R. Crystal structure of the receptor-binding domain of botulinum neurotoxin type HA, also known as type FA or H. *Toxins (Basel)*. 2017; 9(3). pii: E93. doi: 10.3390/toxins9030093.
11. Moriishi K, Koura M, Abe N, Fujii N, Fujinaga Y, Inoue K, Ogumad K. Mosaic structures of neurotoxins produced from Clostridium botulinum types C and D organisms. *Biochim Biophys Acta* 1996; 1307(2): 123–6.
12. Gonzalez-Escalona N, Thirunavukkarasu N, Singh A, Toro M, Brown EW, Zink D, Rummel A, Sharma SK. Draft genome sequence of bivalent clostridium botulinum strain IBCA10-7060, Encoding botulinum neurotoxin B and a New FA mosaic type. *Genome Announc* 2014; 2(6). pii: e01275-14. doi: 10.1128/genomeA.01275-14.
13. Whitemarsh, RC, Tepp WH, Bradshaw M, Lin G, Pier CL, Scherf JM, Johnson EA, Pellett S. Characterization of botulinum neurotoxin A subtypes 1 through 5 by investigation of activities in mice, in neuronal cell cultures, and in vitro. *Infect Immun* 2013; 81(10): 3894–902.
14. Aktories K. Clostridium botulinum C2 toxin and C. botulinum C3 ADP-ribosyltransferase. In: Herken H, Hucho F (eds). *Selective Neurotoxicity*. Berlin: Springer-Verlag; 1994, 841–54.
15. DasGupta BR. Activation of Clostridium botulinum type B toxin by an endogenous enzyme. *J Bacteriol* 1971; 108(3): 1051–7.
16. Lacy DB, Tepp W, Cohen AC, DasGupta BR, Stevens RC. Crystal structure of botulinum neurotoxin type A and implications for toxicity. *Nat Struct Biol* 1998; 5(10): 898–902.
17. Pantano S, Montecucco C. The blockade of the neurotransmitter release apparatus by botulinum neurotoxins. *Cell Mol Life Sci* 2014; 71(5): 793–811.
18. Montal M. Botulinum neurotoxin: A marvel of protein design. *Annu Rev Biochem* 2010; 79: 591–617.
19. Eidels L, Proia RL, Hart DA. Membrane receptors for bacterial toxins. *Microbiol Rev* 1983; 47(4): 596–620.
20. Yowler BC, Schengrund CL. Botulinum neurotoxin A changes conformation upon binding to ganglioside GT1b. *Biochemistry* 2004; 43(30): 9725–31.
21. Yowler BC, Kensinger RD, Schengrund CL. Botulinum neurotoxin A activity is dependent upon the presence of specific gangliosides in neuroblastoma cells expressing synaptotagmin I. *J Biol Chem* 2002; 277(36): 32815–9.
22. Stenmark P, Dupuy J, Imamura A, Kiso M, Stevens RC. Crystal structure of botulinum neurotoxin type A in complex with the cell surface co-receptor GT1b-insight into the toxin-neuron interaction. *PLoS Pathog* 2008; 4(8): e1000129.
23. Montecucco C, Rossetto O, Schiavo G. Presynaptic receptor arrays for clostridial neurotoxins. *Trends Microbiol* 2004; 12(10): 442–6.
24. Harper CB, Martin S, Nguyen TH et al. Dynamin inhibition blocks botulinum neurotoxin type A endocytosis in neurons and delays botulism. *J Biol Chem* 2011; 286(41): 35966–76.
25. Ayyar BV, Aoki KR, Atassi MZ. The C-terminal heavy-chain domain of botulinum neurotoxin A is not the only site that binds neurons, as the N-terminal heavy-chain domain also plays a very active role in toxin-cell binding and interactions. *Infect Immun* 2015; 83(4): 1465–76.
26. Rummel A, Hafner K, Mahrhold S, Darashchonak N, Holt M, Jahn R, Beermann S, Karnath T, Bigalke H, Binz T. Botulinum neurotoxins C, E and F bind gangliosides via a conserved binding site prior to stimulation-dependent uptake with botulinum neurotoxin F utilising the three isoforms of SV2 as second receptor. *J Neurochem* 2009; 110(6): 1942–54.
27. Strotmeier J, Gu S, Jutzi S et al. The biological activity of botulinum neurotoxin type C is dependent upon novel types of ganglioside binding sites. *Mol Microbiol* 2011; 81(1): 143–56.
28. Kroken AR, Karalewitz AP, Fu Z, Kim JJ, Barbieri JT. Novel ganglioside-mediated entry of botulinum neurotoxin serotype D into neurons. *J Biol Chem* 2011; 286(30): 26828–37.
29. Kull S, Schulz KM, Weisemann J et al. Isolation and functional characterization of the novel Clostridium botulinum neurotoxin A8 subtype. *PLoS One* 2015; 10(2): e0116381.
30. Mahrhold S, Rummel A, Bigalke H, Davletov B, Binz T. The synaptic vesicle protein 2C mediates the uptake of botulinum neurotoxin A into phrenic nerves. *FEBS Lett* 2006; 580(8): 2011–4.
31. Dong M, Yeh F, Tepp WH, Dean C, Johnson EA, Janz R, Chapman ER. SV2 is the protein receptor for botulinum neurotoxin A. *Science* 2006; 312(5773): 592–6.
32. Lam KH, Yao G, Jin R. Diverse binding modes, same goal: The receptor recognition mechanism of botulinum neurotoxin. *Prog Biophys Mol Biol* 2015; 117(2–3): 225–31.
33. Dong M, Tepp WH, Liu H, Johnson EA, Chapman ER. Mechanism of botulinum neurotoxin B and G entry into hippocampal neurons. *J Cell Biol* 2007; 179(7): 1511–22.
34. Jin R, Rummel A, Binz T, Brunger AT. Botulinum neurotoxin B recognizes its protein receptor with high affinity and specificity. *Nature* 2006; 444(7122): 1092–5.
35. Fernandez-Chacon, R, Konigstorfer A, Gerber SH, Garcia J, Matos MF, Stevens CF, Brose N, Rizo J, Rosenmund C, Sudhof TC. Synaptotagmin I functions as a calcium regulator of release probability. *Nature* 2001; 410(6824): 41–9.
36. Dong M, Richards DA, Goodnough MC, Tepp WH, Johnson EA, Chapman ER. Synaptotagmins I and II mediate entry of botulinum neurotoxin B into cells. *J Cell Biol* 2003; 162(7): 1293–303.

37. Jacky BP, Garay PE, Dupuy J et al. Identification of fibroblast growth factor receptor 3 (FGFR3) as a protein receptor for botulinum neurotoxin serotype A (BoNT/A). *PLoS Pathog* 2013; 9(5): e1003369.
38. Fischer A, Montal M. Molecular dissection of botulinum neurotoxin reveals interdomain chaperone function. *Toxicon* 2013; 75: 101–7.
39. Rossetto O, Pirazzini M, Montecucco C. Botulinum neurotoxins: Genetic, structural and mechanistic insights. *Nat Rev Microbiol* 2014; 12(8): 535–49.
40. Takamori S, Holt M, Stenius K et al. Molecular anatomy of a trafficking organelle. *Cell* 2006; 127(4): 831–46.
41. Jahn R, Fasshauer D. Molecular machines governing exocytosis of synaptic vesicles. *Nature* 2012; 490(7419): 201–7.
42. Sudhof TC. The synaptic vesicle cycle. *Annu Rev Neurosci* 2004; 27: 509–47.
43. Pellizzari R, Rossetto O, Schiavo G, Montecucco C. Tetanus and botulinum neurotoxins: Mechanism of action and therapeutic uses. *Philos Trans R Soc Lond B Biol Sci* 1999; 354(1381): 259–68.
44. Fernandez-Salas E, Steward LE, Ho H, Garay PE, Sun SW, Gilmore MA, Ordas JV, Wang J, Francis J, Aoki KR. Plasma membrane localization signals in the light chain of botulinum neurotoxin. *Proc Natl Acad Sci USA* 2004; 101(9): 3208–13.
45. Wang J, Zurawski TH, Meng J, Lawrence G, Olango WM, Finn DP, Wheeler L, Dolly JO. A dileucine in the protease of botulinum toxin A underlies its long-lived neuroparalysis: Transfer of longevity to a novel potential therapeutic. *J Biol Chem* 2011; 286(8): 6375–85.
46. Vagin O, Tokhtaeva E, Garay PE et al. Recruitment of septin cytoskeletal proteins by botulinum toxin A protease determines its remarkable stability. *J Cell Sci* 2014; 127(Pt 15): 3294–308.
47. Simpson LL. Kinetic studies on the interaction between botulinum toxin type A and the cholinergic neuromuscular junction. *J Pharmacol Exp Ther* 1980; 212(1): 16–21.
48. Kurokawa Y, Oguma K, Yokosawa N, Syuto B, Fukatsu R, Yamashita I. Binding and cytotoxic effects of Clostridium botulinum type A, C1 and E toxins in primary neuron cultures from foetal mouse brains. *J Gen Microbiol* 1987; 133(9): 2647–57.
49. Pamphlett R. Axonal sprouting after botulinum toxin does not elicit a histological axon reaction. *J Neurol Sci* 1988; 87(2–3): 175–85.
50. Popoff MR, Poulain B. Bacterial toxins and the nervous system: Neurotoxins and multipotential toxins interacting with neuronal cells. *Toxins (Basel)* 2010; 2(4): 683–737.
51. Shen J, Ma J, Lee C, Smith BP, Smith TL, Tan KH, Koman LA. How muscles recover from paresis and atrophy after intramuscular injection of botulinum toxin A: Study in juvenile rats. *J Orthop Res* 2006; 24(5): 1128–35.
52. Meunier FA, Herreros J, Schiavo F. Molecular mechanism of action of botulinal neurotoxins and the synaptic remodeling they induce in vivo at the skeletal neuromuscular junction. In: *Neurotoxicology Handbook*, Massar EJ (eds) Totwa, NJ: Humana Press; 2001, 1, 307–49.
53. Rogozhin AA, Pang KK, Bukharaeva E, Young C, Slater CR. Recovery of mouse neuromuscular junctions from single and repeated injections of botulinum neurotoxin A. *J Physiol* 2008; 586(13): 3163–82.
54. Ko CP. Do nerve terminal sprouts contribute to functional recovery from botulinum neurotoxin A? *J Physiol* 2008; 586(13): 3021.
55. de Paiva A, Meunier FA, Molgo J, Aoki KR, Dolly JO. Functional repair of motor endplates after botulinum neurotoxin type A poisoning: Biphasic switch of synaptic activity between nerve sprouts and their parent terminals. *Proc Natl Acad Sci USA* 1999; 96(6): 3200–5.
56. Goodmurphy CW, Ovalle WK. Morphological study of two human facial muscles: Orbicularis oculi and corrugator supercilii. *Clin Anat* 1999; 12(1): 1–11.
57. Urban PP, Bohl J, Abrao L, Stofft E. Facial muscles lack muscle spindles [abstract]. *Klin Neurophysiol* 2004; 35: 297.
58. Filippi GM, Errico P, Santarelli R, Bagolini B, Manni E. Botulinum A toxin effects on rat jaw muscle spindles. *Acta Otolaryngol* 1993; 113(3): 400–4.
59. Rosales RL, Arimura K, Takenaga S, Osame M. Extrafusal and intrafusal muscle effects in experimental botulinum toxin-A injection. *Muscle Nerve* 1996; 19(4): 488–96.
60. Phadke CP, On AY, Kirazli Y, Ismail F, Boulias C. Intrafusal effects of botulinum toxin injections for spasticity: Revisiting a previous paper. *Neurosci Lett* 2013; 541: 20–3.
61. Trompetto C, Bove M, Avanzino L, Francavilla G, Berardelli A, Abbruzzese G. Intrafusal effects of botulinum toxin in post-stroke upper limb spasticity. *Eur J Neurol* 2008; 15(4): 367–70.
62. Trompetto C, Curra A, Buccolieri A, Suppa A, Abbruzzese G, Berardelli A. Botulinum toxin changes intrafusal feedback in dystonia: A study with the tonic vibration reflex. *Mov Disord* 2006; 21(6): 777–82.
63. Beer KR, Boyd C, Patel RK, Bowen B, James SP, Brin MF. Rapid onset of response and patient-reported outcomes after onabotulinumtoxinA treatment of moderate-to-severe glabellar lines. *J Drugs Dermatol* 2011; 10(1): 39–44.
64. Blitzer A, Binder WJ, Aviv JE, Keen MS, Brin MF. The management of hyperfunctional facial lines with botulinum toxin. A collaborative study of 210 injection sites in 162 patients. *Arch Otolaryngol Head Neck Surg* 1997; 123(4): 389–92.
65. Brashear A, Watts MW, Marchetti A, Magar R, Lau H, Wang L. Duration of effect of botulinum toxin type A in adult patients with cervical dystonia: A retrospective chart review. *Clin Ther* 2000; 22(12): 1516–24.
66. Brin MF, James C, Maltman J. Botulinum toxin type A products are not interchangeable: A review of the evidence. *Biologics* 2014; 8: 227–41.
67. Lowe NJ, Yamauchi PS, Lask GP, Patnaik R, Moore D. Botulinum toxins types A and B for brow furrows: Preliminary experiences with type B toxin dosing. *J Cosmet Laser Ther* 2002; 4(1): 15–8.
68. Hsiung GY, Das SK, Ranawaya R, Lafontaine AL, Suchowersky O. Long-term efficacy of botulinum toxin A in treatment of various movement disorders over a 10-year period. *Mov Disord* 2002; 17(6): 1288–93.
69. Defazio G, Abbruzzese G, Girlanda P et al. Botulinum toxin A treatment for primary hemifacial spasm: A 10-year multicenter study. *Arch Neurol* 2002; 59(3): 418–20.
70. Wilke K, Martin A, Terstegen L, Biel SS. Neurobiology of skin appendages: Eccrine, apocrine, and apoeccrine sweat glands. In: Granstein, RD, Luger, TA (eds). *Neuroimmunology of the Skin*. Berlin: Springer-Verlag; 2009, 167–75.
71. Lindh B, Hokfelt T. Structural and functional aspects of acetylcholine peptide coexistence in the autonomic nervous system. *Prog Brain Res* 1990; 84: 175–91.
72. Plewig G, Kligman AM. Sebaceous glands. In: *Acne and Rosacea*. Berlin: Springer; 2000, 57–81.
73. Li ZJ, Park SB, Sohn KC, Lee Y, Seo YJ, Kim CD, Kim YS, Lee JH, Im M. Regulation of lipid production by acetylcholine signalling in human sebaceous glands. *J Dermatol Sci* 2013; 72(2): 116–22.
74. Kurzen H, Wessler I, Kirkpatrick CJ, Kawashima K, Grando SA. The non-neuronal cholinergic system of human skin. *Horm Metab Res* 2007; 39(2): 125–35.

75. Schlereth T, Birklein F, an Haack K, Schiffmann S, Kilbinger H, Kirkpatrick CJ, Wessler I. In vivo release of non-neuronal acetylcholine from the human skin as measured by dermal microdialysis: Effect of botulinum toxin. *Br J Pharmacol* 2006; 147(2): 183–7.
76. Wessler I, Kirkpatrick CJ. Acetylcholine beyond neurons: The non-neuronal cholinergic system in humans. *Br J Pharmacol* 2008; 154(8): 1558–71.
77. Lowe NJ, Yamauchi PS, Lask GP, Patnaik R, Iyer S. Efficacy and safety of botulinum toxin type A in the treatment of palmar hyperhidrosis: A double-blind, randomized, placebo-controlled study. *Dermatol Surg* 2002; 28(9): 822–7.
78. Naumann M, Lowe NJ, Kumar CR, Hamm H. Botulinum toxin type A is a safe and effective treatment for axillary hyperhidrosis over 16 months: A prospective study. *Arch Dermatol* 2003; 139(6): 731–6.
79. Lowe NJ, Glaser DA, Eadie N, Daggett S, Kowalski JW, Lai PY, G. North American Botox in Primary Axillary Hyperhidrosis Clinical Study. Botulinum toxin type A in the treatment of primary axillary hyperhidrosis: A 52-week multicenter double-blind, randomized, placebo-controlled study of efficacy and safety. *J Am Acad Dermatol* 2007; 56(4): 604–11.
80. Turner IM, Agrillo T. Migraine, botulinum toxin type-A, and the disappearing sebaceous cyst. *Headache* 2005; 45(2): 166–7.
81. Diamond A, Jankovic J. Botulinum toxin in dermatology - beyond wrinkles and sweat. *J Cosmet Dermatol* 2006; 5(2): 169.
82. Min P, Xi W, Grassetti L et al. Sebum production alteration after botulinum toxin type A injections for the treatment of forehead rhytides: A prospective randomized double-blind dose-comparative clinical investigation. *Aesthet Surg J* 2015; 35(5): 600–10.
83. Park KY, Hyun MY, Jeong SY, Kim BJ, Kim MN, Hong CK. Botulinum toxin for the treatment of refractory erythema and flushing of rosacea. *Dermatology* 2015; 230(4): 299–301.
84. Bloom BS, Payongayong L, Mourin A, Goldberg DJ. Impact of intradermal abobotulinumtoxinA on facial erythema of rosacea. *Dermatol Surg* 2015; 41:(Suppl 1): S9–16.
85. Dayan SH, Pritzker RN, Arkins JP. A new treatment regimen for rosacea: OnabotulinumtoxinA. *J Drugs Dermatol* 2012; 11(12): e76–9.
86. Gilbert E, Ward NL. Efficacy of botulinum neurotoxin type A for treating recalcitrant plaque psoriasis. *J Drugs Dermatol* 2014; 13(11): 1407–8.
87. Zanchi M, Favot F, Bizzarini M, Piai M, Donini M, Sedona P. Botulinum toxin type-A for the treatment of inverse psoriasis. *J Eur Acad Dermatol Venereol* 2008; 22(4): 431–6.
88. Ward NL, Kavlick KD, Diaconu D, Dawes SM, Michaels KA, Gilbert E. Botulinum neurotoxin A decreases infiltrating cutaneous lymphocytes and improves acanthosis in the KC-Tie2 mouse model. *J Invest Dermatol* 2012; 132(7): 1927–30.
89. Gassner HG, Sherris DA, Otley CC. Treatment of facial wounds with botulinum toxin A improves cosmetic outcome in primates. *Plast Reconstr Surg* 2000; 105(6): 1948–53; discussion 54-5.
90. Gassner HG, Brissett AE, Otley CC, Boahene DK, Boggust AJ, Weaver AL, Sherris DA. Botulinum toxin to improve facial wound healing: A prospective, blinded, placebo-controlled study. *Mayo Clin Proc* 2006; 81(8): 1023–8.
91. Ziade M, Domergue S, Batifol D, Jreige R, Sebbane M, Goudot P, Yachouh J. Use of botulinum toxin type A to improve treatment of facial wounds: A prospective randomised study. *J Plast Reconstr Aesthet Surg* 2013; 66(2): 209–14.
92. Uyesugi B, Lippincott B, Dave S. Treatment of a painful keloid with botulinum toxin type A. *Am J Phys Med Rehabil* 2010; 89(2): 153–5.
93. Robinson AJ, Khadim MF, Khan K. Keloid scars and treatment with Botulinum Toxin Type A: The Belfast experience. *J Plast Reconstr Aesthet Surg* 2013; 66(3): 439–40.
94. Shaarawy E, Hegazy RA, Abdel Hay RM. Intralesional botulinum toxin type A equally effective and better tolerated than intralesional steroid in the treatment of keloids: A randomized controlled trial. *J Cosmet Dermatol* 2015; 14(2): 161–6.
95. Xiao Z, Zhang F, Lin W, Zhang M, Liu Y. Effect of botulinum toxin type A on transforming growth factor beta1 in fibroblasts derived from hypertrophic scar: A preliminary report. *Aesthetic Plast Surg* 2010; 34(4): 424–7.
96. Jeong HS, Lee BH, Sung HM, Park SY, Ahn DK, Jung MS, Suh IS. Effect of botulinum toxin type A on differentiation of fibroblasts derived from scar tissue. *Plast Reconstr Surg* 2015; 136(2): 171e–8e.
97. Xiao Z, Qu G. Effects of botulinum toxin type A on collagen deposition in hypertrophic scars. *Molecules* 2012; 17(2): 2169–77.
98. Xiaoxue W, Xi C, Zhibo X. Effects of botulinum toxin type A on expression of genes in keloid fibroblasts. *Aesthet Surg J* 2014; 34(1): 154–9.
99. Oh SH, Lee Y, Seo YJ, Lee JH, Yang JD, Chung HY, Cho BC. The potential effect of botulinum toxin type A on human dermal fibroblasts: An in vitro study. *Dermatol Surg* 2012; 38(10): 1689–94.
100. Permatasari F, Hu YY, Zhang JA, Zhou BR, Luo D. Anti-photoaging potential of Botulinum Toxin Type A in UVB-induced premature senescence of human dermal fibroblasts in vitro through decreasing senescence-related proteins. *J Photochem Photobiol B* 2014; 133: 115–23.
101. Nausch B, Heppner TJ, Nelson MT. Nerve-released acetylcholine contracts urinary bladder smooth muscle by inducing action potentials independently of IP3-mediated calcium release. *Am J Physiol Regul Integr Comp Physiol* 2010; 299(3): R878–88.
102. Dolly JO, Lawrence GW. Chapter 3: Molecular basis for the therapeutic effectiveness of botulinum neurotoxin type A. *Neurourol Urodyn* 2014; 33(Suppl 3): S14–20.
103. Ferrandiz-Huertas C, Mathivanan S, Wolf CJ, Devesa I, Ferrer-Montiel A. Trafficking of ThermoTRP Channels. *Membranes (Basel)* 2014; 4(3): 525–64.
104. de Groat WC, Griffiths D, Yoshimura N. Neural control of the lower urinary tract. *Compr Physiol* 2015; 5(1): 327–96.
105. Apostolidis A, Popat R, Yiangou Y, Cockayne D, Ford AP, Davis JB, Dasgupta P, Fowler CJ, Anand P. Decreased sensory receptors P2X3 and TRPV1 in suburothelial nerve fibers following intradetrusor injections of botulinum toxin for human detrusor overactivity. *J Urol* 2005; 174(3): 977–82; discussion 982-3.
106. Hanna-Mitchell AT, Wolf-Johnston AS, Barrick SR, Kanai AJ, Chancellor MB, de Groat WC, Birder LA. Effect of botulinum toxin A on urothelial-release of ATP and expression of SNARE targets within the urothelium. *Neurourol Urodyn* 2015; 34(1): 79–84.
107. Smith CP, Gangitano DA, Munoz A, Salas NA, Boone TB, Aoki KR, Francis J, Somogyi GT. Botulinum toxin type A normalizes alterations in urothelial ATP and NO release induced by chronic spinal cord injury. *Neurochem Int* 2008; 52(6): 1068–75.
108. Sanderfoot AA, Raikhel NV. The specificity of vesicle trafficking: Coat proteins and SNAREs. *Plant Cell* 1999; 11(4): 629–42.
109. Shimizu T, Shibata M, Toriumi H, Iwashita T, Funakubo M, Sato H, Kuroi T, Ebine T, Koizumi K, Suzuki N. Reduction of TRPV1 expression in the trigeminal system by botulinum neurotoxin type-A. *Neurobiol Dis* 2012; 48(3): 367–78.
110. Dolly JO, Aoki KR. The structure and mode of action of different botulinum toxins. *Eur J Neurol* 2006; 13(Suppl 4): 1–9.
111. Brady CM, Apostolidis A, Yiangou Y, Baecker PA, Ford AP, Freeman A, Jacques TS, Fowler CJ, Anand P. P2X3-immunoreactive nerve

fibres in neurogenic detrusor overactivity and the effect of intravesical resiniferatoxin. *Eur Urol* 2004; 46(2): 247–53.
112. Brady CM, Apostolidis AN, Harper M, Yiangou Y, Beckett A, Jacques TS, Freeman A, Scaravilli F, Fowler CJ, Anand P. Parallel changes in bladder suburothelial vanilloid receptor TRPV1 and pan-neuronal marker PGP9.5 immunoreactivity in patients with neurogenic detrusor overactivity after intravesical resiniferatoxin treatment. *BJU Int* 2004; 93(6): 770–6.
113. Liu HT, Chancellor MB, Kuo HC. Urinary nerve growth factor levels are elevated in patients with detrusor overactivity and decreased in responders to detrusor botulinum toxin-A injection. *Eur Urol* 2009; 56(4): 700–6.
114. Chapple C, Sievert KD, MacDiarmid S, Khullar V, Radziszewski P, Nardo C, Thompson C, Zhou J, Haag-Molkenteller C. OnabotulinumtoxinA 100 U significantly improves all idiopathic overactive bladder symptoms and quality of life in patients with overactive bladder and urinary incontinence: A randomised, double-blind, placebo-controlled trial. *Eur Urol* 2013; 64(2): 249–56.
115. Nitti VW, Dmochowski R, Herschorn S, Sand P, Thompson C, Nardo C, Yan X, Haag-Molkenteller C, ES Group. OnabotulinumtoxinA for the treatment of patients with overactive bladder and urinary incontinence: Results of a phase 3, randomized, placebo controlled trial. *J Urol* 2013; 189(6): 2186–93.
116. Sievert KD, Chapple C, Herschorn S, Joshi M, Zhou J, Nardo C, Nitti VW. OnabotulinumtoxinA 100U provides significant improvements in overactive bladder symptoms in patients with urinary incontinence regardless of the number of anticholinergic therapies used or reason for inadequate management of overactive bladder. *Int J Clin Pract* 2014; 68(10): 1246–56.
117. Nitti V, DeRidder D, Sussman D et al. Durable reductions in UI with long-term onabotulinumtoxinA treatment in patients with overactive bladder syndrome. *Final results of 3.5-year study. Presented at the Annual Meeting of the American Urinary Association*. May 15–19, 2015, New Orleans, LA.
118. Cruz F, Herschorn S, Aliotta P, Brin M, Thompson C, Lam W, Daniell G, Heesakkers J, Haag-Molkenteller C. Efficacy and safety of onabotulinumtoxinA in patients with urinary incontinence due to neurogenic detrusor overactivity: A randomised, double-blind, placebo-controlled trial. *Eur Urol* 2011; 60(4): 742–50.
119. Ginsberg D, Gousse A, Keppenne V, Sievert KD, Thompson C, Lam W, Brin MF, Jenkins B, Haag-Molkenteller C. Phase 3 efficacy and tolerability study of onabotulinumtoxinA for urinary incontinence from neurogenic detrusor overactivity. *J Urol* 2012; 187(6): 2131–9.
120. Kennelly M, Dmochowski R, Ethans K, Karsenty G, Schulte-Baukloh H, Jenkins B, Thompson C, Li D, Haag-Molkenteller C. Long-term efficacy and safety of onabotulinumtoxinA in patients with urinary incontinence due to neurogenic detrusor overactivity: An interim analysis. *Urology* 2013; 81(3): 491–7.
121. Kennelly M, Dmochowski R, Schulte-Baukloh H et al. Efficacy and safety of onabotulinumtoxinA therapy are sustained over 4 years of treatment in patients with neurogenic detrusor overactivity: Final results of a long-term extension study. *Neurourol Urodyn*, 2017; 36(2): 368–75.
122. Whitcup SM, Turkel CC, DeGryse RE, Brin MF. Development of onabotulinumtoxinA for chronic migraine. *Ann N Y Acad Sci* 2014; 1329: 67–80.
123. Burstein R, Zhang X, Levy D, Aoki KR, Brin MF. Selective inhibition of meningeal nociceptors by botulinum neurotoxin type A: Therapeutic implications for migraine and other pains. *Cephalalgia* 2014; 34(11): 853–69.
124. Welch MJ, Purkiss JR, Foster KA. Sensitivity of embryonic rat dorsal root ganglia neurons to Clostridium botulinum neurotoxins. *Toxicon* 2000; 38(2): 245–58.
125. Durham PL, Cady R, Cady R. Regulation of calcitonin gene-related peptide secretion from trigeminal nerve cells by botulinum toxin type A: Implications for migraine therapy. *Headache* 2004; 44(1): 35–42; discussion -3.
126. Paterson K, Lolignier S, Wood JN, McMahon SB, Bennett DL. Botulinum toxin-A treatment reduces human mechanical pain sensitivity and mechanotransduction. *Ann Neurol* 2014; 75(4): 591–6.
127. Dodick DW, Turkel CC, DeGryse RE, Aurora SK, Silberstein SD, Lipton RB, Diener HC, Brin MF, PCMS Group. OnabotulinumtoxinA for treatment of chronic migraine: Pooled results from the double-blind, randomized, placebo-controlled phases of the PREEMPT clinical program. *Headache* 2010; 50(6): 921–36.
128. Aurora SK, Winner P, Freeman MC, Spierings EL, Heiring JO, DeGryse RE, VanDenburgh AM, Nolan ME, Turkel CC. OnabotulinumtoxinA for treatment of chronic migraine: Pooled analyses of the 56-week PREEMPT clinical program. *Headache* 2011; 51(9): 1358–73.
129. Deinhardt K, Schiavo G. Endocytosis and retrograde axonal traffic in motor neurons. *Biochem Soc Symp* 2005; 72: 139–50.
130. Antonucci F, Rossi C, Gianfranceschi L, Rossetto O, Caleo M. Long-distance retrograde effects of botulinum neurotoxin A. *J Neurosci* 2008; 28(14): 3689–96.
131. Restani L, Giribaldi F, Manich M, Bercsenyi K, Menendez G, Rossetto O, Caleo M, Schiavo G. Botulinum neurotoxins A and E undergo retrograde axonal transport in primary motor neurons. *PLoS Pathog* 2012; 8(12): e1003087.
132. Wang T, Martin S, Papadopulos A et al. Control of autophagosome axonal retrograde flux by presynaptic activity unveiled using botulinum neurotoxin type a. *J Neurosci* 2015; 35(15): 6179–94.
133. Aoki KR, Brin MF, Whitcup SM. Is botulinum toxin really moving into the CNS like tetanus toxin? *J Neurosci* 2008; available at: http://www.jneurosci.org/cgi/eletters/28/14/3689.
134. Lawrence GW, Ovsepian SV, Wang J, Aoki KR, Dolly JO. Extravesicular intraneuronal migration of internalized botulinum neurotoxins without detectable inhibition of distal neurotransmission. *Biochem J* 2012; 441(1): 443–52.
135. Cai BB, Francis J, Brin MF, Broide RS. Botulinum neurotoxin type A-clearved SNAP25 is confined to primary motor neurons and localized on the plasma membrane following intramuscular toxin injection. *Neuroscience* 2017; 352: 155–69.
136. Zbinden G, Flury-Roversi M. Significance of the LD50-test for the toxicological evaluation of chemical substances. *Arch Toxicol* 1981; 47(2): 77–99.
137. Hunt T, Clarke K. Potency evaluation of a formulated drug product containing 150-kd botulinum neurotoxin type A. *Clin Neuropharmacol* 2009; 32(1): 28–31.
138. Blome MC, Yowler BC, O'Keeffe R, Panjwani N, Pickett AM, Schengrund C-L. Use of surface plasmon resonance to characterise binding of botulinum type A toxin-haemagglutinin complex to gangliosides. *The Botulinum J* 2008; 1(1): 88–99.
139. Dressler D, Mander G, Fink K. Measuring the potency labelling of onabotulinumtoxinA (Botox®) and incobotulinumtoxinA (Xeomin®) in an LD50 assay. *J Neural Transm* 2012; 119(1): 13–5.
140. Sesardic D, Leung T, Gaines Das R. Role for standards in assays of botulinum toxins: International collaborative study of three preparations of botulinum type A toxin. *Biologicals* 2003; 31(4): 265–76.
141. Hunt T, Clarke K. Potency evaluation of a formulated drug product containing 150-kd botulinum neurotoxin type A. *Clin Neuropharmacol* 2009; 32: 28–31.

142. Fernandez-Salas E, Wang J, Molina Y, Nelson JB, Jacky BP, Aoki KR. Botulinum neurotoxin serotype A specific cell-based potency assay to replace the mouse bioassay. *PLoS One* 2012; 7(11): e49516.
143. Hunt T, Clarke K. Potency of the botulinum toxin product CNBTX-A significantly exceeds labeled units in standard potency test. *J Am Acad Dermatol* 2008; 58(3): 517–8.
144. Chertow DS, Tan ET, Maslanka SE et al. Botulism in 4 adults following cosmetic injections with an unlicensed, highly concentrated botulinum preparation. *JAMA* 2006; 296(20): 2476–9.
145. Beer K, Rothschild K. Importing injectables. *J Drugs Dermatol.* 2014; 13: 1156–8.
146. Beer K. Importing injectables. *The Dermatol.* 2013; 3: 24–5.
147. Goschel H, Wohlfarth K, Frevert J, Dengler R, Bigalke H. Botulinum A toxin therapy: Neutralizing and nonneutralizing antibodies–therapeutic consequences. *Exp Neurol* 1997; 147(1): 96–102.
148. Frevert J. Pharmaceutical, biological, and clinical properties of botulinum neurotoxin type A products. *Drugs R D* 2015; 15(1): 1–9.
149. Brin MF, Comella CL, Jankovic J, Lai F, Naumann M. Long-term treatment with botulinum toxin type A in cervical dystonia has low immunogenicity by mouse protection assay. *Mov Disord* 2008; 23(10): 1353–60.
150. Allergan, Inc. BOTOX® (onabotulinumtoxinA) Prescribing Information. Irvine CA, January 2013.
151. Ipsen Biopharm Ltd. Dysport® (abobotulinumtoxinA) Prescribing Information. May 2012.
152. Dolimbek BZ, Aoki KR, Steward LE, Jankovic J, Atassi MZ. Mapping of the regions on the heavy chain of botulinum neurotoxin A (BoNT/A) recognized by antibodies of cervical dystonia patients with immunoresistance to BoNT/A. *Mol Immunol* 2007; 44(5): 1029–41.
153. Dolimbek BZ, Steward LE, Aoki KR, Atassi MZ. Immune recognition of botulinum neurotoxin B: Antibody-binding regions on the heavy chain of the toxin. *Mol Immunol* 2008; 45(4): 910–24.
154. Oshima M, Aoki KR, Atassi MZ. Regions recognized on the light chain of botulinum neurotoxin type A by T lymphocytes of SJL and BALB/c mice primed with inactivated toxin. *Immunobiology* 2014; 219(12): 950–7.
155. Naumann M, Boo LM, Ackerman AH, Gallagher CJ. Immunogenicity of botulinum toxins. *J Neural Transm* 2013; 120(2): 275–90.
156. Frevert J, Dressler D. Complexing proteins in botulinum toxin type A drugs: A help or a hindrance? *Biologics* 2010; 4: 325–32.
157. United States Food and Drug Administration. Approval Package for Xeomin® (2010) (incobotulinumtoxinA) Injection. vol Application Number 125360. http://www.accessdata.fda.gov/drugsatfda_docs/nda/2010/125360s0000TOC.cfm. Accessed January 21, 2014.
158. Naumann M, Carruthers A, Carruthers J et al. Meta-analysis of neutralizing antibody conversion with onabotulinumtoxinA (BOTOX®) across multiple indications. *Mov Disord* 2010; 25(13): 2211–8.

3 Pharmacology and immunology of non-complexed botulinum toxin

Juergen Frevert

INTRODUCTION

Botulinum toxin (BoNT) for therapeutic use was pioneered by Alan Scott. His first experiments to treat strabismus were carried out with the botulinum complex of *Clostridium botulinum* type A,[1] which was prepared by Edward Schantz and Eric Johnson, and at that time was known as crystalline botulinum toxin.[2] The production process starts with the fermentation of *C. botulinum* under anaerobic conditions using a complex medium consisting of several ingredients, including peptides and sugars. This produces a complex of several proteins, one of which is the botulinum toxin, the active substance of all BoNT formulations. Besides serotype A, six further distinct serotypes are known: B, C1, D, E, F, and G.[3] Only serotypes A and B have been developed for human use. Further numerous subtypes exist,[4] for example, for serotype A subtypes A1–A8, and all together, more than 40 subtypes have been described to date. The currently marketed products for aesthetic medicine are all of serotype A1. The subtype of the type B product that is approved only for neurological indications has not been described in the literature.

In 1989, the product developed by Scott was approved for the treatment of strabismus, hemifacial spasm, and blepharospasm. Several other toxins are now licensed in different countries for various indications. A major breakthrough in aesthetic medicine came when Jean and Alastair Carruthers discovered that botulinum toxin could be used for the treatment of wrinkles.[4]

Currently, three products are approved for aesthetic use in Western markets, and all are approved by the FDA: onabotulinumtoxin A (OnaBTX-A; BOTOX®/Vistabel®, Vistabex Allergan Inc., Irvine, CA), abobotulinumtoxin A (AboBTX-A; Dysport®/Azzalure®, Ipsen, Paris, France), and incobotulinumtoxin A (IncoBTX-A; Xeomin®/Bocouture®, Merz Pharmaceuticals GmbH, Frankfurt, Germany).[5–10] There are also several BoNT products originating and approved in Asian countries: in Korea Neuronox® (Medytox Inc.), Nabota® (Daewoong, Inc), and Botulax® (Hugel), and from China BTXA™ or Lantox® (Lanzhou Institute). They are all similar to OnaBTX-A and claim to be based on the 900 kD BoNT complex, but some are formulated with different excipients. They will not be further discussed in this chapter because they contain complexing proteins. In contrast to OnaBTX-A and AboBTX-A and all other botulinum products, IncoBTX-A is the only approved botulinum product free from complexing proteins containing only the pure 150 kD botulinum toxin (here: BoNT), the protein which is responsible for the therapeutic effect. Another non-complexed BoNT known as Purtox® was under development, but has been discontinued for unknown reasons. The company Revance Inc. has stopped developing a purified botulinum toxin product (daxibotulinumtoxinA) as a topical agent but is developing an injectable product (RT002). The botulinum toxin is formulated with peptides that are supposed to bind to the botulinum toxin. It is not known whether this formulation influences the immunogenic potential and pharmacological characteristics of the botulinum toxin.

In the last couple of years, BoNT-A injections have become the most popular cosmetic procedures, especially among dermatologists and plastic surgeons.[11] IncoBTX-A differs in its content of bacterial proteins and in its formulation, which could have an effect on therapy. For optimal use, it is desirable that physicians are aware of the properties of products with complexing proteins and those with pure neurotoxin only. This chapter will describe the similarities and differences between the BoNT products with special regard to IncoBTX-A and examine whether the complexing proteins have any function in BoNT therapy.

MECHANISM OF ACTION OF BoNT

The molecular composition and mechanism of action of BoNTs are described in excellent reviews and are only briefly summarized here.[3,12] The active moiety in all BoNT products is the botulinum toxin, a 1296 amino acid protein with a relatively high molecular weight of 150 kD.[3,12–14] For comparison, insulin, a small protein, has a molecular weight of 5.8 kD.

BoNT is synthesized as a single chain protein, which is nicked into two subunits by a clostridial protease, resulting in two subunits: a heavy chain and a light chain, linked by a disulfide bridge. The C-terminal domain of the heavy chain binds the molecule highly specifically to receptor molecules on the presynaptic membrane of cholinergic neurons. The heavy chain has two binding domains, one for special glycolipids (GT1b) and one for a protein receptor called SV2.[15] The receptor-bound BoNT is taken up into the nerve cell by endocytosis. The second domain of the heavy chain then facilitates the translocation of the light chain into the cytosol, the interior of the neuron. The light chain is a highly specific protease which cleaves a protein, SNAP25, required for the secretion of acetylcholine. Cleaved SNAP25 can no longer function in the secretory process. As a result, the acetylcholine-containing secretory vesicle cannot fuse with the presynaptic membrane, acetylcholine is not secreted, and so the muscle cell is no longer activated and becomes paralyzed.[16] By this mechanism, BoNT blocks cholinergic muscular innervation of striated and smooth muscles as well as the innervation of exocrine glands. The mode of action is identical for all BoNT products (Figure 3.1).

MANUFACTURE OF BoNT PRODUCTS

This is divided into two steps: the manufacture of the drug substance or active pharmaceutical ingredient (API), a highly concentrated solution with the botulinum toxin, and the manufacture of the final drug or drug product, which requires a high dilution, addition of excipients, filling into vials, and a final drying process.

The manufacture of the active pharmaceutical ingredient of all products starts with the fermentation of the anaerobic spore forming *C. botulinum* type A.[2] The details of the fermentation process and of the purification procedure are proprietary and not known in detail. All products use a so-called Hall strain, originally isolated by the microbiologist Ivan Clifford Hall. However, as he kept several *C. botulinum* type A strains, it is not known which is the actual Hall strain. IncoBTX-A is produced with the strain ATCC 3502, which is a defined strain distributed and controlled by the American Type Culture Collection (ATCC). The production strain for OnaBTX-A is called "Hall hyper," which is claimed to produce a higher toxin concentration and not to form spores,[17] although this might be due to fermentation conditions. The identity of the Hall strain used for AboBTX-A has not been published and it is only named "a Hall strain."[18] In any event, the amino acid sequence of the neurotoxin in all products appears to be identical. Of course, one cannot exclude the possibility that the applied strain influences the quality of the product by producing different proteins and therefore a different purity profile, which might also influence

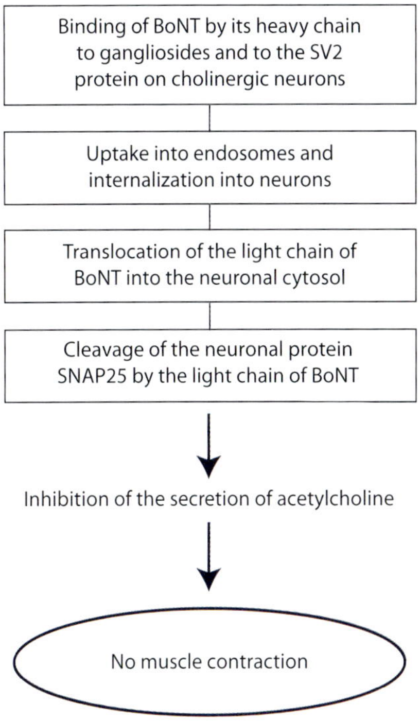

Figure 3.1 Mode of action of BoNT.

the folding of the BoNT molecule and have an effect on its immunological properties (epitope structure).

After fermentation, the biomass is precipitated and the neurotoxin extracted. OnaBTX-A is further purified by precipitation steps (ethanol precipitation) and finally by precipitation with ammonium sulfate, which provides the so-called "crystalline complex" with a molecular weight of about 900 kD.[19,20] Instead of precipitation ("crystallization") steps, the manufacture of AboBTX-A uses chromatography and dialysis,[18] resulting in a drug substance containing complexing proteins accompanied by partly degraded complexing proteins and some impurities, that is, flagellin and a clp protease.[18] The proportion of the different complexing proteins is not consistent with any complex described in the literature. It might be a mixture of complexes (300 and 500 kD), but the complex composition has never been published. For IncoBTX-A, the complexing proteins and other impurities are removed from the neurotoxin in a series of chromatographic steps to end up with the pure neurotoxin.[21] The manufacturing process providing the pure neurotoxin is illustrated in Figure 3.2.

To prepare the final drug product, excipients are added to the diluted drug substance. All products contain human serum albumin (HSA), but in different amounts (Table 3.1). HSA is required to stabilize the tiny amount of drug substance (picogram to nanogram quantities). The molecular effect of HSA is not really understood. It was initially thought that it would block the adsorption of the botulinum toxin to the walls of the vial or other surfaces, but this has never been demonstrated. The addition of sodium chloride during the OnaBTX-A drying process destabilizes the BoNT; it has been shown that sodium chloride causes a loss of activity.[22] If a proportion of the botulinum toxin is inactivated during the drying step, this might be the reason why OnaBTX-A contains a higher amount of botulinum toxin protein,[23] that is, about 50% more or 150 U must be processed to end up with 100 U in the final product. OnaBTX-A is vacuum dried, which means that the solution is not frozen, but only cooled and a low vacuum applied to prepare a thin film on the bottom of the vial. AboBTX-A and IncoBTX-A are produced by freeze drying (lyophilization) providing a loose "cake."

COMPLEXES AND COMPLEXING PROTEINS

OnaBTX-A and AboBTX-A contain the 150 kD BoNT as well as other proteins, known as complexing proteins or neurotoxin-associated proteins (NAPs). It is claimed that these proteins form a complex with the botulinum toxin, which can influence their pharmaceutical properties.[24] The complex agglutinates red blood cells—an activity

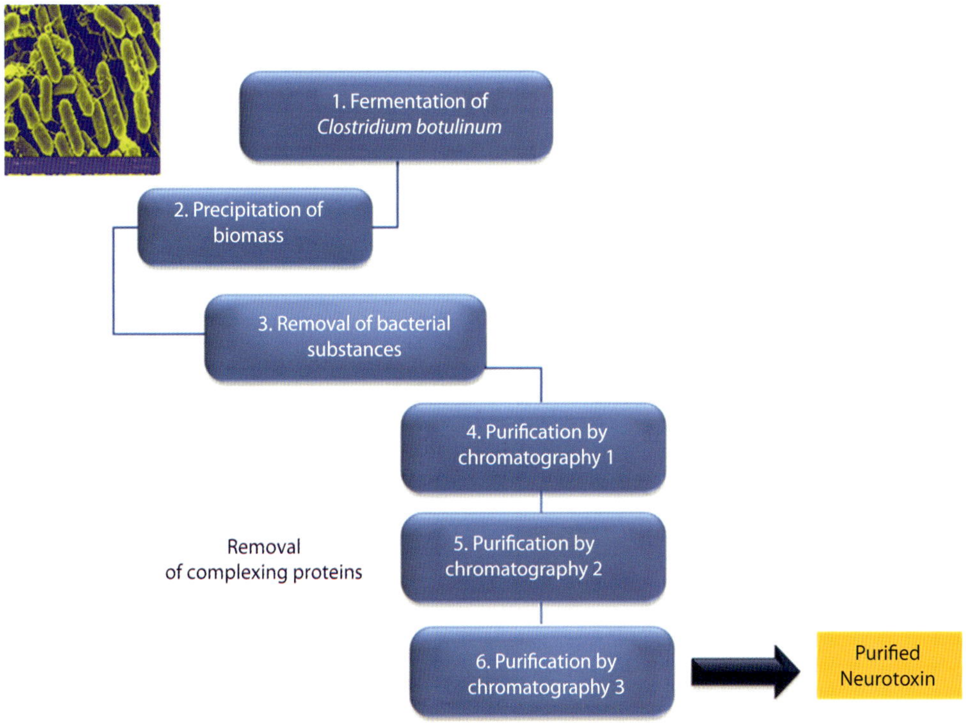

Figure 3.2 Flow diagram of the manufacturing of the purified BoNT.

Table 3.1 Comparison of BoNT-A Formulations

Botulinum toxin type A	AboBTX-A	OnaBTX-A	IncoBTX-A
Brand names	Dysport®, Azzalure®	BOTOX®, Vistabel®	Xeomin®, Bocouture®
Approved aesthetic indication	Moderate to severe glabellar lines	Moderate to severe glabellar lines and crow's feet	Moderate to severe glabellar lines and crow's feet
Presentation	Freeze-dried (lyophilized) powder for reconstitution	Vacuum-dried powder for reconstitution	Freeze-dried (lyophilized) powder for reconstitution
Isolation process	Precipitation and chromatography	Precipitation	Precipitation and chromatography
Composition	*Clostridium botulinum* type A neurotoxin HA and non-HA proteins	*Clostridium botulinum toxin* type A HA and non-HA proteins	*Clostridium botulinum* type A neurotoxin
Excipients	500 U vial[a]: 125 μg human serum albumin 2.5 mg lactose	100 U vial[a]: 0.5 mg human serum albumin 0.9 mg NaCl	100 U vial[a]: 1 mg human serum albumin 4.6 mg sucrose
Molecular weight (neurotoxin), kD	Not published (150)	900 (150)	150
Approximate total clostridial protein content‡	4.35 ng (500 U)	5.0 ng (100 U)	0.44 ng (100 U)
Neurotoxin protein load (neurotoxin per 100 U[a])	0.65 ng	0.73 ng	0.44 ng
Specific neurotoxin potency	154 U/ng	137 U/ng	227 U/ng
Shelf-life	2°C–8°C 2 years	2°C–8°C 2–3 years[b] (or freezer)	Room temperature 3–4 years[b]
Storage (post-reconstitution)	2°C–8°C 4 hours	2°C–8°C 24 hours	2°C–8°C 24 hours

[a] Units of measurement for the three commercially available BoNT-A preparations are proprietary to each manufacturer and are not interchangeable.
[b] Depending on the number of units per vial. HA, hemagglutinin.

certainly not necessary for BoNT therapy—and some of these different molecular weight proteins are therefore called hemagglutinins: HA50, HA34, HA20, and HA17 (slightly different names exist in the literature, e.g., HA34 is also named HA33) In addition, a protein known as non-toxic non-hemagglutinating protein (NTNH) is the direct binding protein for BoNT in the complex.[25] Together, these proteins form a complex under acid conditions (around pH = 5) with the 150 kD neurotoxin.[26] The integration of BoNT into a complex is required for its action as a food poison: the BoNT complex is protected against the hostile conditions of the gastrointestinal tract (low pH, protease attack).[26] The hemagglutinins may also play an important role in the absorption of BoNT from the gastrointestinal tract. They are sugar-binding proteins (lectins), and can bind to E-cadherin and allow BoNT to pass through the mucosa of the intestine and be transported into the blood or lymph.[27,28]

The BoNT progenitor complexes isolated from *C. botulinum* type A cultures adopt three sizes: 900, 500, and 300 kD.[19] It is claimed that the complex size for OnaBTX-A is 900 kD[20] (Table 3.1). The complexes present in AboBTX-A have not been published, but data have shown that complexing proteins are present as both full-length proteins and as a succession of fragments.[18] As most of the NTNH is truncated in AboBTX-A, one can infer that there is little or no 500 kD and no 900 kD complex, and that the 300 kD complex is probably the most abundant.

To determine the identity of the complexes in a vial, the reconstituted products were analyzed by an ultracentrifugation technique, which allows the separation of proteins and complexes of different sizes.[29] According to these data, the botulinum toxin dissociates immediately after reconstitution from the complex in OnaBTX-A, with ≥85% of BoNT present as the 150 kD free form prior to injection into target tissues[29] (Figure 3.3). Data for AboBTX-A show the botulinum toxin completely dissociated from the complexing proteins prior to injection.[29] It can be concluded that molecular weight or protein complex size do not affect biological activity and pharmacological properties, as the BoNT-A botulinum toxin rapidly dissociates from the complexing proteins after reconstitution of the preparation.[29]

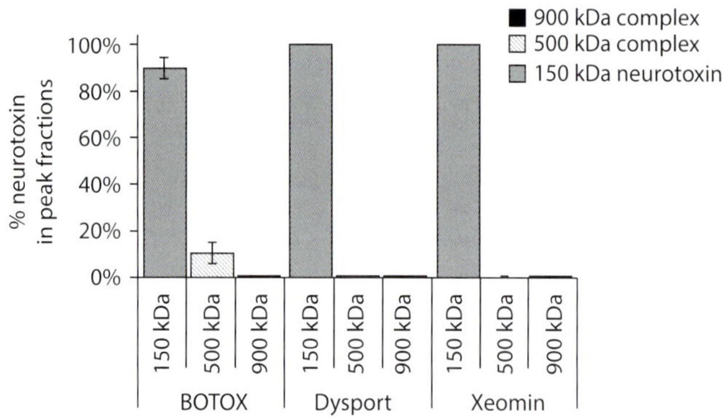

Figure 3.3 Presence of botulinum toxin in complexes after reconstitution of vials.[29] Vials were reconstituted with saline and the complex size determined by sedimentation velocity analysis followed by immunoassay analysis of the botulinum toxin and complexing proteins. (Reproduced from *Toxicon*, 57, Eisele KH et al., Studies on the dissociation of botulinum neurotoxin type A complexes, 555–65, Copyright 2011, with permission from Elsevier.)

BENEFICIAL ROLE OF COMPLEXING PROTEINS?

In the early days of BoNT therapy, it was claimed that it was unlikely that the pure botulinum toxin would ever be used in a clinical setting because pure botulinum toxins "are inactivated on dilution, formulation, and drying."[2] This has certainly been refuted since IncoBTX-A, the botulinum toxin free from complexing proteins, was licensed in Germany. Indeed, IncoBTX-A is the most stable of the BoNT products.

Although complexing proteins do not play a role in the mechanism of action, it was argued that they influence the diffusion or spread of the botulinum toxin out of the injected muscle into other adjacent muscles not intended for treatment.[24] Due to their high specificity for cholinergic neurons (motor neurons and certain neurons that activate glands, e.g., sweat gland, salivary gland), all treatment-related adverse events of BoNT therapy are related to migration of the botulinum toxin in the muscle tissue.

Discussions on botulinum toxin spread and diffusion are hampered by inconsistent use of terminology.[30] Spread occurs when the injected molecule travels from the original injection site, which is determined by the injection technique, volume of injection, needle size, and by the size of the traveling molecule. In contrast, the physical term diffusion indicates the passive movement of botulinum toxin along a concentration gradient within a fluid.[30] According to Fick's law, the diffusion of molecules is proportional to their molecular mass: a molecule with a higher molecular weight migrates slower than one with a lower molecular weight. This suggests that the complex with the high molecular weight of 900 kD would have a reduced tendency to leave the muscle compared with the markedly smaller non-complexed botulinum toxin, and one would expect a lower rate of off-target effects. However, this has never been demonstrated; the adverse event profile in all head-to-head studies with OnaBTX-A and IncoBTX-A is very similar.[31–33]

Recent studies, which have compared the spread of BoNT-A products by measuring the size of anhidrotic halos following injection of identical volumes and equipotent doses into the forehead of patients, reveal a similar spread, suggesting that there are no differences in migration properties.[34,35] A comparison of OnaBTX-A and AboBTX-A, using dose ratios of 1:2.5, 1:3, and 1:4, showed that the area of anhidrosis was larger with AboBTX-A in 93% of comparisons at all dose ratios and identical injection volumes.[36] A separate study, which used a dose ratio of 1:2.5, observed no significant difference between the mean size of halos produced by the two products.[37] There were no differences in product spread when the same dose was injected with the same technique.[34]

The reason why the complexing proteins do not affect the migration of botulinum toxin in the tissue is very simple: the botulinum toxin is already dissociated from the complexing proteins when it is injected into patients.[29] Even if the complex was still intact, it would immediately dissociate when injected into the muscle because it would not be stable at the tissue pH of 7.3.[26] Similar migration properties have also been demonstrated in a clinical study by intramuscular injection of equivalent doses in the same volume of OnaBTX-A and IncoBTX-A (5 U) or AboBTX-A (12.5 U) into two sites of the forehead of volunteers (split face).[35] After 6 weeks and again after 6 months, the area of anhidrosis was made visible with iodine starch stain (Figure 3.4) and analyzed. The area of anhidrosis was similar for OnaBTX-A and IncoBTX-A, indicating that the complexing proteins do not influence spread of the toxin.[35] The area of anhidrosis for AboBTX-A was larger, but this might have been due to the applied dose ratio. These results were confirmed in a preclinical study in mice, in which spread was visualized by analyzing the expression of a protein (N-CAM). This protein is only detectable in paralyzed muscle and showed no difference between the products.[38] It can be concluded that, in all products, the botulinum toxin migrates unhindered, and that the tendency of the botulinum toxin to leave the injected muscle is the same.

Based on the observation that being part of a complex protects the botulinum toxin against the harsh conditions in the environment, it was hypothesized that the complexing proteins were required to ensure the stability of the BoNT product during storage. This would mean that IncoBTX-A should have a shorter storage stability or more restricted storage conditions than the other products. This has proved not to be the case. Whereas IncoBTX-A has a shelf-life of 3 or 4 years at room temperature, AboBTX-A has a shelf-life of 2 years at 2°C–8°C, and OnaBTX-A can be stored for 2 or 3 years at 2°C–8°C (depending on the number of units) or in the freezer. After reconstitution, IncoBTX-A and OnaBTX-A are stable for 24 hours at 2°C–8°C, and AboBTX-A is stable for 4 hours at 2°C–8°C.[5–10] A recent study, which compared the efficacy of freshly reconstituted IncoBTX-A with IncoBTX-A that had been reconstituted and stored for 1 week at 25°C, has provided further confirmation of the stability of IncoBTX-A.[39] In a split-face design, 10 U of the two formulations were injected into the crow's feet of 21 subjects. Over 4 months of follow-up, there was

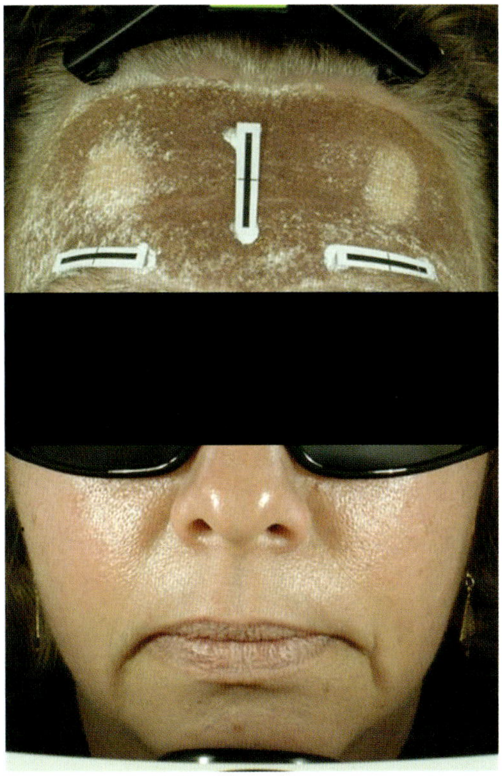

Figure 3.4 Determination of the spread of complexed versus non-complexed BoNT products in a split-face study.[35] 5 U of OnaBTX-A (left side) or 5 U of IncoBTX-A were injected intramuscularly into the forehead of volunteers. After 6 weeks, the anhidrotic halo was made visible with iodine starch stain. (With kind permission from Springer Science+Business Media: *Arch Dermatol Res*, Comparison of the spread of three botulinum toxin type A preparations, 304, 2012, 155–61, Kerscher M et al.)

no statistically significant difference in either efficacy or longevity between the fresh and stored products. The prolonged shelf-life and less stringent temperature restrictions displayed by IncoBTX-A (Table 3.1) and (Figure 3.5) suggest that complexing proteins are not required for BoNT-A stability.[39] It has also been demonstrated that storage of IncoBTX-A at 60°C for 4 weeks does not cause inactivation.[40]

POTENCY AND CLINICAL EFFICACY

The potency of BoNT products is measured in the LD50 assay and given in units. One unit is defined as the dose capable of killing 50% of mice in comparison to a standard preparation of BoNT, which is

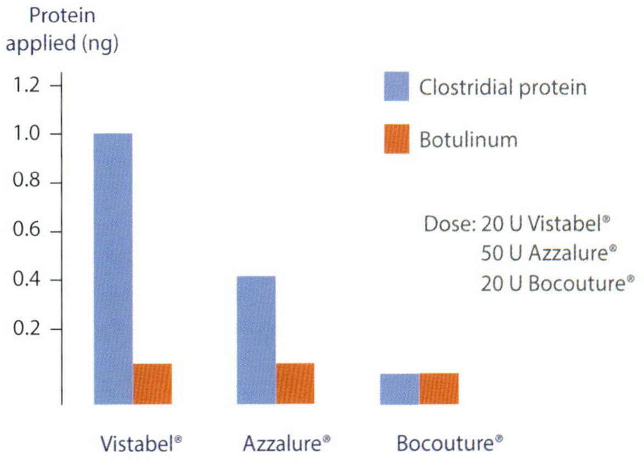

Figure 3.5 Amount of clostridial and botulinum toxin protein (ng) in the treatment of glabellar lines. Dose: 20 U Vistabel®, 20 U Bocouture®, 50 U Azzalure®.

also analyzed in every assay (parallel line assay). The dose for treating patients is related to the LD50 units and therefore an accurate LD50 assay is required. The assays used by the companies differ in various aspects, including dilution procedure, diluents, and stabilizing agents: HSA (IncoBTX-A), gelatin (AboBTX-A), or no stabilizing agent (OnaBTX-A).[41] As the calculation of units depends on the methods that each manufacturer uses in non-standardized assays,[42] a comparison of potency based solely on the units is problematic. This underlines the importance of clinical head-to-head studies to evaluate treatment effects. Interestingly, the potency assay for IncoBTX-A using HSA in the diluent and simulating conditions in the clinic has shown a 1:1 ratio between IncoBTX-A and OnaBTX-A.[43] The LD50 is now being replaced by cell-based assays, which must be cross-validated with the LD50 assay. The manufacturer of OnaBTX-A uses a sensitive neuronal cell line (SiMa cells)[44] approved in different countries, whereas the manufacturer of IncoBTX-A has recently obtained FDA approval for an assay based on differentiated induced pluripotent stem cells.[45] Both procedures quantitate the amount of cleaved SNAP25. The assays are extensively validated before they can replace the animal assay. It would be interesting to analyze the BoNT products with both assays.

The respective amounts of botulinum toxin per 100 U, measured using a high sensitivity ELISA technique, were 0.73 ng for OnaBTX-A, 0.65 ng for AboBTX-A, and 0.44 ng for IncoBTX-A (Table 3.1).[23,46] The specific botulinum toxin potency or biological activity (U) per mass of botulinum toxin protein was calculated based on the overall mean concentration of BoNT-A neurotoxin, giving IncoBTX-A the highest specific biological activity (U/ng botulinum toxin) at 227 U/ng compared with 137 U/ng for OnaBTX-A and 154 U/ng for AboBTX-A.[23] IncoBTX-A contains no other clostridial proteins and, therefore, the specific biologic potency relative to the total clostridial protein is 227 U/ng. As the reported clostridial protein content per 100 U of OnaBTX-A is 5 ng[47] and of AboBTX-A is 4.35 ng, the equivalent specific biologic potency relative to the total clostridial protein load for OnaBTX-A is 20 U/ng and for AboBTX-A is 115 U/ng. The units of AboBTX-A are different from those of OnaBTX-A and IncoBTX-A. However, comparing OnaBTX-A and IncoBTX-A, which have demonstrated similar clinical activity, the findings suggest that 0.44 ng of IncoBTX-A has the same biological activity as 0.73 ng of OnaBTX-A. It is hypothesized that part of the botulinum toxin in OnaBTX-A may be inactived or denatured due to the vacuum drying process used in the manufacture of the final drug in the presence of sodium chloride.[23,48] Figure 3.6 shows the amount of clostridial protein and botulinum toxin protein injected into a patient treated for glabellar lines with 20 U OnaBTX-A or IncoBTX-A, or 50 U of AboBTX-A. Patients treated with products containing complexing proteins are loaded with a markedly higher amount of bacterial protein; for OnaBTX-A the amount is about 10-fold higher.

The complexing proteins do not influence the mode of action of the botulinum toxin. Only the botulinum toxin binds unhindered and independently of any other components to gangliosides (GT1b) and the protein receptor (SV2) of cholinergic neurons and is then taken up by endosomes, followed by translocation of the light chain into the cytosol of the nerve cell. No step in the mode of action requires the presence of other proteins. Although all products contain the botulinum toxin as the active substance, it has been debated whether the biological activity of the products is comparable. Several clinical head-to-head studies in different aesthetic indications (glabellar frown lines, crow's feet) have demonstrated comparable clinical efficacy of IncoBTX-A compared with OnaBTX-A, suggesting a 1:1 conversion ratio between the products (Figure 3.7).[33,49–52] These studies also showed that there was no difference in side effect profile. Comparable efficacy was confirmed in a recent split-face, cross-over study with the same dosage of OnaBTX-A and IncoBTX-A in the treatment of crow's feet (Figure 3.8).[50] Furthermore, the duration of effect was not different in a study comparing OnaBTX-A, IncoBTX-A, and AboBTX-A in the treatment of glabellar frown lines.[53] Several evidence-based consensus reviews on BoNT-A application in aesthetic indications have recapped the evidence confirming a 1:1 conversion ratio between OnaBTX-A and IncoBTX-A.[54–57,58]

A conversion ratio between AboBTX-A and OnaBTX-A or IncoBTX-A is still debated and has not been finally established.[59] A recent consensus review suggests that a conversion ratio of 1:2.5 (IncoBTX-A:AboBTX-A) may be assumed in aesthetic indications.[58] A consensus review from Asia suggests a ratio of 1:2–1:4 (OnaBTX-A:AboBTX-A).[57] RimabotulinumtoxinB (RimaBTX-B), which is based on the botulinum toxin type B complex, is not approved for aesthetic indications and a conversion ratio IncoBTX-A:RimaBTX-B has not been published.

IMMUNOLOGICAL PROPERTIES

BoNT is a bacterial protein and is therefore foreign to the human immune system and an antigen per se. Like any other therapeutic protein product administered repeatedly, BoNT products can elicit the formation of antibodies directed against the botulinum toxin and/or the complexing proteins in the case of OnaBTX-A and AboBTX-A. The immune system might therefore produce antibodies against the foreign

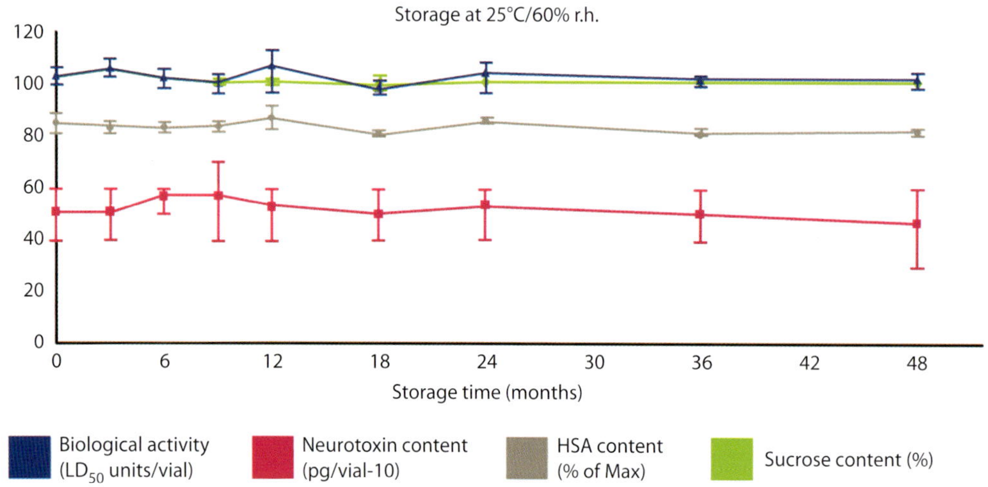

Figure 3.6 Stability of IncoBTX-A at 25°C.[40]

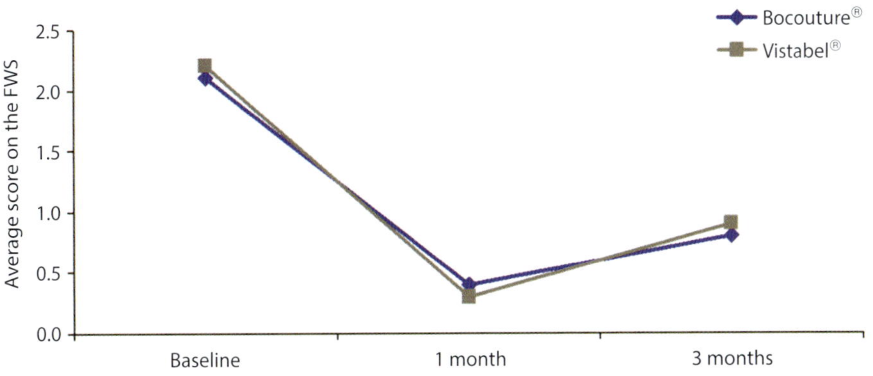

Figure 3.7 Head-to-head noninferiority study of IncoBTX-A (Bocouture®) versus OnaBTX-A (Vistabel®) in the treatment of glabellar frown lines.[33] The outcome of the injection was assessed by an independent rater after 4 and 12 weeks.

protein that will inhibit the therapy when the antibody titer is high enough, leading to a secondary non-response. It is clear that antibodies directed against the binding domain of the botulinum toxin heavy chain will inhibit the binding of the botulinum toxin to the neuron.[60,61] Antibodies directed against the enzymatic domain (light chain) can also neutralize the botulinum toxin's activity because of steric hindrance.[62]

Apart from patient-related factors (sensitivity of the patient's immune system), several product-related factors influence the immunogenicity of biological proteins (see Table 3.2). For BoNT products, these include the manufacturing process, the antigenic protein load, and the presence of complexing proteins as well as treatment-related factors, for example, the interval between injections, booster injections, and prior exposure. The first generation of OnaBTX-A applied in neurological indications contained 10 times more potentially antigenic protein (50 ng of clostridial protein) than the current formulation, which generated a high rate of antibody formation and secondary non-responders.[63] Physicians were advised to keep the dosing interval as long as acceptable for the patient to prevent the formation of antibodies.[63] The amount of botulinum toxin protein in OnaBTX-A has since been markedly reduced to 5 ng clostridial protein (see Table 3.1) and the rate of antibody formation has consequently also decreased.[64] The development of neutralizing antibodies is more common in therapeutic indications because of high doses of the antigen. It had been claimed that antibody production and secondary non-response was negligible in aesthetic indications because of the low doses applied. However, more and more reports about antibody formation in aesthetic indications are appearing in the literature.[65–69] There might also be a high number of unreported cases, as patients treated for aesthetic indications can change physicians or stop treatment when the therapy is not working. Physicians in the aesthetic field are also not as aware of secondary non-response as physicians in the therapeutic field.

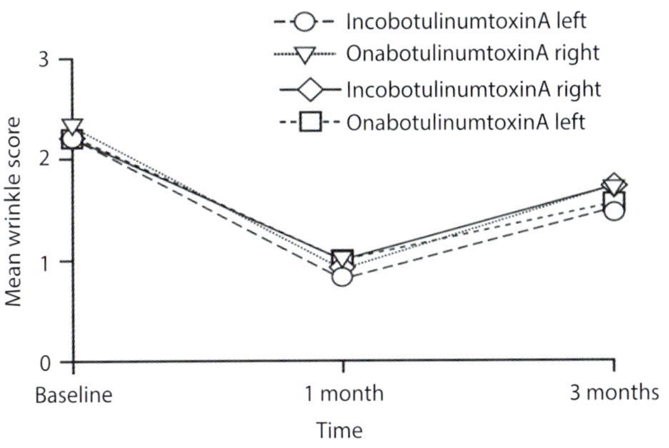

Figure 3.8 Head-to-head clinical trial of IncoBTX-A versus OnaBTX-A in the treatment of crow's feet.[50] A prospective, split face, subject- and rater-blinded, crossover evaluation in two consecutive treatment cycles with 12 U of IncoBTX-A or OnaBTX-A and a 6-month "wash out" between cycles. The graph illustrates pooled results from cycles 1 and 2, showing the mean score for crow's feet severity over time for both IncoBTX-A and OnaBTX-A on both sides of the face at maximum contraction. (Reproduced from Muti G, Harrington L. *Dermatol Surg* 2015; 41(Suppl 1): S39–46, with permission from Wolters Kluwer.)

Complexing proteins do not play a role in the mechanism of action of BoNT, and so antibodies directed against the complexing proteins cannot block the activity of BoNT. It has been reported that about 50% of patients (treated for a therapeutic indication) develop antibodies against the complexing proteins, but that this has no clinical relevance and is not linked to responsiveness.[70] From this standpoint, complexing proteins would be just inert proteins with no effect on BoNT therapy. However, new data suggest that this might not be the case. A growing body of evidence shows that complexing proteins might interact with the host immune system and therefore be clinically relevant.[71]

In contrast to OnaBTX-A and AboBTX-A, IncoBTX-A does not lead to the formation of antibodies in New Zealand white rabbits after repeated injection of high doses of the product and short treatment intervals.[72] While this study does not reflect the clinical application, it demonstrates that there are clear differences in the antigenic response related to the presence or absence of complexing proteins.

To initiate an immune response, the immune system must be activated. Not only the antigen must be present, but also an activating signal.[73] The first cells to recognize the antigen (i.e., BoNT) are dendritic cells. These present the antigen to T-lymphocytes, which are then activated by the dendritic cells. The activated T-lymphocytes

Table 3.2 Factors Influencing Immunogenic Response According to CHMP Guideline EMEA/CHMP/BMWP/14327/2006 (2008)

Factors that may influence the development of an immune response against a therapeutic protein
Patient and disease related factors
Genetic factors modulating the immune response
Genetic factors related to a gene defect
Age
Disease-related factors
Concomitant treatment
Duration, route of administration, treatment modalities
Previous exposure to similar or related proteins
Product-related factors of immunogenicity
Protein structure
Formulation
Aggregation and adduct formation
Impurities

subsequently activate B-lymphocytes to produce antibodies.[74] Dendritic cells have exposed pattern recognition receptors (Toll-like receptors), which react with different bacterial components, such as bacterial DNA, parts of the bacterial cell wall, and bacterial proteins such as flagellin.[74] Hemagglutinins are known to act as adjuvants, binding and activating dendritic cells.[75,76] It is known that hemagglutinin HA33 is the major immunoreactive protein in the BoNT complex.[69]

The first step of the binding to immune cells has been demonstrated by analyzing the interaction of BoNT, the BoNT complex, and BoNT free from complexing proteins with lymphoblasts, fibroblasts, and a human neuroblastoma cell line (as a control).[71] It was clearly shown that the complexing proteins and the BoNT complex reacted with the lymphoblasts, but not the pure BoNT.[71] Further, the release of inflammatory cytokines was not influenced by pure BoNT, but by BoNT complex and the complexing proteins.[71] It can be concluded that complexing proteins can affect the formation of antibodies against BoNT by stimulating cells of the immune system.[71]

The presence of antibodies in patients does not necessary lead to a secondary non-response, and it is not clear which titer is required to inhibit therapy. The variability in the reported rate of neutralizing antibodies and treatment failure can be attributed to study design, administered doses, indication, assay methodology, timing of serum sample testing, and treatment history.[77,78] Only antibodies that bind BoNT effectively so that its biological activity is sufficiently neutralized, will attenuate its effect on the neuromuscular junction. Thus, the formation of antibodies may have no effect on treatment, or may result in partial or complete clinical unresponsiveness to BoNT-A.[79,80] However, further injections might act as a booster and increase the titer leading to subsequent secondary non-response. This might become relevant given that patients are starting their aesthetic treatments at increasingly younger ages and for several single indications, resulting in an increased overall dose of botulinum toxin per treatment and a high frequency of use over a lifetime. For patients who have developed antibodies following aesthetic therapy, it could be disastrous if the patient later suffers from a stroke and cannot be treated for spasticity with botulinum toxin products.

Clinical studies and case reports in different indications show that a small proportion of patients develops neutralizing antibodies against BoNT after treatment with OnaBTX-A or AboBTX-A, with incidence rates ranging from 0.3% to 6%, which is dependent on the condition being treated and thus treatment dose.[77,81–88] In contrast, there have been no cases of antibody-induced therapy failure with IncoBTX-A in treatment-naïve patients. One case of antibody-induced therapy failure was reported in a patient with progressive hereditary juvenile onset generalized dystonia, whose immune system had already been sensitized by pretreatment with AboBTX-A for 15 years,[89] supporting the hypothesis of reduced immunogenicity with IncoBTX-A.[90] Furthermore, a prospective blinded study in 37 cervical dystonia patients previously treated with OnaBTX-A or AboBTX-A, who developed neutralizing antibodies and partial secondary non-responsiveness, reported that continuous treatment with IncoBTX-A with a high dose of 200 U every 3 months for 48 months, did not result in an increase in neutralizing antibody titer.[91] Despite a transient increase in 10 patients in the first 24 months, neutralizing antibodies in fact declined significantly below the initial titer in 84% of patients ($p < 0.001$), and 62% of patients became seronegative. The decline of the antibody titer was similar to the decline of the titer in a second group of patients who were not treated during that time period.[91] This demonstrates that the immune system did not recognize the neurotoxin molecule in IncoBTX-A as an antigen.

In addition to selecting a product with a low risk of immunogenicity, it is important to establish good practice to minimize the risk of neutralizing antibodies developing. Studies of BoNT-A formulations containing complexing proteins suggest that a higher dosing frequency, short treatment intervals, and greater number of injections may increase the likelihood of their development.[80,92–94]

CONCLUSIONS

BoNT therapies are biological products and their clinical pharmacology depends on many factors, including the bacterial strain used in production, methods of isolation and purification, and the presence or absence of complexing proteins. These factors vary for each commercially available BoNT product, exposing the patient to different proteins and to different quantities of molecules. The active moiety in all BoNT products is the botulinum toxin. The complexing proteins rapidly dissociate from the botulinum toxin on product reconstitution and do not play a role in any of the steps involved in blockade of neurotransmitter release. They are also not required for either the stability of the toxin complex or for limiting the spread of the botulinum toxin. IncoBTX-A is the only pure BoNT commercially available product, free from complexing proteins. It has the lowest amount of foreign protein of all available BoNT preparations, and contains only the purified botulinum toxin as the active substance. BoNT preparations with the lowest amount of proteins provide the best chance for long-term and repeated therapy by minimizing the potential of the patient to form neutralizing antibodies and the possibility of secondary treatment failure. Therapies with a biological product like BoNT are naturally subject to inherent variability. To ensure safe and effective dosing, each batch of BoNT-A must be tested for potency before it can be released onto the market and applied for human use. The potency assays for evaluating the biological activity of currently available BoNT therapies are different, and therefore the products can only be truly compared in clinical head-to-head trials. Results from these have shown that IncoBTX-A and OnaBTX-A are clinically equivalent in terms of efficacy and safety at a 1:1 conversion ratio, confirming findings observed in clinical practice.

REFERENCES

1. Scott AB. Botulinum toxin injection of eye muscles to correct strabismus. *Trans Am Ophthalmol Soc* 1981; 79: 734–70.
2. Schantz EJ, Johnson EA. Properties and use of botulinum toxin and other microbial neurotoxins in medicine. *Microbiol Rev* 1992; 56: 80–99.
3. Rossetto O, Pirazzini M, Montecucco C. Botulinum neurotoxins: Genetic, structural and mechanistic insights. *Nat Rev Microbiol* 2014; 12: 535–49.
4. Carruthers JD, Carruthers JA. Treatment of glabellar frown lines with C. botulinum-A exotoxin. *J Dermatol Surg Oncol* 1992; 18: 17–21.
5. Azzalure (Galderma). *Summary of Product Characteristics*. United Kingdom, 2010.
6. Bocouture (Merz). *Summary of Product Characteristics*, United Kingdom, 2012.
7. BOTOX (Allergan). *Summary of Product Characteristics*, United Kingdom, 2013.
8. Dysport (Ipsen), *Summary of Product Characteristics*, United Kingdom, 2012.
9. Vistabel (Allergan), *Summary of Product Characteristics*, United Kingdom, 2013.
10. Xeomin (Merz), *Summary of Product Characteristics*, United Kingdom, 2012.
11. International Society of Aesthetic Plastic Surgeons. ISAPS International Survey on Aesthetic/Cosmetic Procedures Performed in 2013. Available from http://www.isaps.org/news/isaps-global-statistics. Last accessed August 2014.

12. Montal M. Botulinum neurotoxin: A marvel of protein design. *Annu Rev Biochem* 2010; 79: 591–617.
13. Aoki KR, Guyer B. Botulinum toxin type A and other botulinum toxin serotypes: A comparative review of biochemical and pharmacological actions. *Eur J Neurol* 2001; 8(Suppl 5): 21–9.
14. Poulain B, Lonchamp E, Jover E et al. Mecanismes d'action des toxines et neurotoxines botuliques. *[Mechanisms of action of botulinum toxins and neurotoxins]. Ann Dermatol Venereol* 2009; 136(Suppl 4): S73–6.
15. Brunger AT, Rummel A. Receptor and substrate interactions of clostridial neurotoxins. *Toxicon* 2009; 54: 550–60.
16. Popoff MR, Poulain B. Bacterial toxins and the nervous system: Neurotoxins and multipotential toxins interacting with neuronal cells. *Toxins (Basel)* 2010; 2: 683–737.
17. Dineen SS, Bradshaw M, Johnson EA. Neurotoxin gene clusters in Clostridium botulinum type A strains: Sequence comparison and evolutionary implications. *Curr Microbiol* 2003; 46: 345–52.
18. Panjwani N, O'Keeffe R, Pickett A. Biochemical, functional and potency characteristics of type A botulinum toxin in clinical use. *Botulinum J* 2008; 1: 153–66.
19. Inoue K, Fujinaga Y, Watanabe T et al. Molecular composition of Clostridium botulinum type A progenitor toxins. *Infect Immun* 1996; 64: 1589–94.
20. Lietzow MA, Gielow ET, Le D, Zhang J et al. Subunit stoichiometry of the Clostridium botulinum type A neurotoxin complex determined using denaturing capillary electrophoresis. *Protein J* 2008; 27: 420–5.
21. Park J, Lee MS, Harrison AR. Profile of Xeomin(R) (incobotulinumtoxinA) for the treatment of blepharospasm. *Clin Ophthalmol* 2011; 5: 725–32.
22. Goodnough MC, Johnson EA. Stabilization of botulinum toxin type A during lyophilization. *Appl Environ Microbiol* 1992; 58: 3426–8.
23. Frevert J. Content of botulinum neurotoxin in Botox®/Vistabel®, Dysport®/Azzalure®, and Xeomin®/Bocouture®. *Drugs R D* 2010; 10: 67–73.
24. Aoki KR, Ranoux D, Wissel J. Using translational medicine to understand clinical differences between botulinum toxin formulations. *Eur J Neurol* 2006; 13(Suppl 4): 10–19.
25. Gu S, Rumpel S, Zhou J et al. Botulinum neurotoxin is shielded by NTNHA in an interlocked complex. *Science* 2012; 335: 977–81.
26. Chen F, Kuziemko GM, Stevens RC. Biophysical characterization of the stability of the 150-kilodalton botulinum toxin, the nontoxic component, and the 900-kilodalton botulinum toxin complex species. *Infect Immun* 1998; 66: 2420–5.
27. Lee K, Zhong X, Gu S et al. Molecular basis for disruption of E-cadherin adhesion by botulinum neurotoxin A complex. *Science* 2014; 344(6190): 1405–10.
28. Sugawara Y, Fujinaga Y. The botulinum toxin complex meets E-cadherin on the way to its destination. *Cell Adh Migr* 2011; 5: 34–6.
29. Eisele KH, Fink K, Vey M et al. Studies on the dissociation of botulinum neurotoxin type A complexes. *Toxicon* 2011; 57: 555–65.
30. Pickett A. Dysport: Pharmacological properties and factors that influence toxin action. *Toxicon* 2009; 54: 683–9.
31. Benecke R, Jost WH, Kanovsky P et al. A new botulinum toxin type A free of complexing proteins for treatment of cervical dystonia. *Neurology* 2005; 64: 1949–51.
32. Roggenkamper P, Jost WH, Bihari K et al. Efficacy and safety of a new botulinum toxin type A free of complexing proteins in the treatment of blepharospasm. *J Neural Transm* 2006; 113: 303–12.
33. Sattler G, Callander MJ, Grablowitz D et al. Noninferiority of incobotulinumtoxinA, free from complexing proteins, compared with another botulinum toxin type A in the treatment of glabellar frown lines. *Dermatol Surg* 2010; 36(Suppl 4):2146–54.
34. Brodsky MA, Swope DM, Grimes D. Diffusion of botulinum toxins. *Tremor Other Hyperkinet Mov (N Y)* 2012; 2.
35. Kerscher M, Roll S, Becker A et al. Comparison of the spread of three botulinum toxin type A preparations. *Arch Dermatol Res* 2012; 304: 155–61.
36. Trindade de Almeida AR, Marques E, de Almeida J et al. Pilot study comparing the diffusion of two formulations of botulinum toxin type A in patients with forehead hyperhidrosis. *Dermatol Surg* 2007; 33: S37–43.
37. Hexsel D, Dal'Forno T, Hexsel C et al. A randomized pilot study comparing the action halos of two commercial preparations of botulinum toxin type A. *Dermatol Surg* 2008; 34: 52–9.
38. Carli L, Montecucco C, Rossetto O. Assay of diffusion of different botulinum neurotoxin type a formulations injected in the mouse leg. *Muscle Nerve* 2009; 40: 374–80.
39. Soares DJ, Dejoseph LM, Zuliani GF et al. Impact of postreconstitution room temperature storage on the efficacy of incobotulinumtoxinA treatment of dynamic lateral canthus lines. *Dermatol Surg* 2015; 41: 712–7.
40. Grein S, Mander GJ, Fink K. Stability of botulinum neurotoxin type A, devoid of complexing proteins. *The Botulinum J* 2011; 2: 49–58.
41. Adler S, Bicker G, Bigalke H et al. The current scientific and legal status of alternative methods to the LD50 test for botulinum neurotoxin potency testing. *The Report and Recommendations of a ZEBET Expert Meeting.* Altern Lab Anim 2010; 38: 315–30.
42. Hambleton P, Pickett AM. Potency equivalence of botulinum toxin preparations. *J R Soc Med* 1994; 87: 719.
43. Dressler D, Mander G, Fink K. Measuring the potency labelling of onabotulinumtoxinA (BOTOX®) and incobotulinumtoxinA (Xeomin®) in an LD50 assay. *J Neural Transm* 2012; 119: 13–5.
44. Fernández-Salas E, Wang J, Molina Y et al. Botulinum neurotoxin serotype A specific cell-based potency assay to replace the mouse bioassay. *PLoS One* 2012; 7(11):e49516.
45. Pellett S, Du ZW, Pier CL et al. Sensitive and quantitative detection of botulinum neurotoxin in neurons derived from mouse embryonic stem cells. *Biochem Biophys Res Commun* 2011; 404: 388–92.
46. Whitemarsh RC, Strathman MJ, Chase LG et al. Novel application of human neurons derived from induced pluripotent stem cells for highly sensitive botulinum neurotoxin detection. *Toxicol Sci* 2012; 126: 426–35.
47. Jankovic J, Vuong KD, Ahsan J. Comparison of efficacy and immunogenicity of original versus current botulinum toxin in cervical dystonia. *Neurology* 2003; 60(7): 1186–8.
48. Bigalke H. Properties of pharmaceutical products of botulinum neurotoxins. In: Jankovic J, Albanese A, Atassi MZ et al. (eds). *Botulinum Toxin: Therapeutic Clinical Practice and Science.* Philadelphia (PA): Saunders Elsevier; 2009, 389–97.
49. Prager W, Wissmuller E, Kollhorst B et al. Comparison of two botulinum toxin type A preparations for treating crow's feet: A split-face, double-blind, proof-of-concept study. *Dermatol Surg* 2010; 36(Suppl 4): 2155–60.
50. Muti G, Harrington L. A prospective rater- and subject-blinded study comparing the efficacy of incobotulinumtoxinA and onabotulinumtoxinA to treat crow's feet: A clinical crossover evaluation. *Dermatol Surg* 2015; 41(Suppl 1): S39–46.
51. Prager W, Huber-Vorländer J, Taufig AZ et al. Botulinum toxin type A treatment to the upper face: Retrospective analysis of daily practice. *Clin Cosmet Investig Dermatol* 2012; 5: 53–8.
52. Yeilding RH, Fezza JP. A prospective, split-face, randomized, double-blind study comparing onabotulinumtoxinA to

incobotulinumtoxinA for upper face wrinkles. *Plast Reconstr Surg* 2015; 135: 1328–35.
53. Rappl T, Parvizi D, Friedl H et al. Onset and duration of effect of incobotulinumtoxinA, onabotulinumtoxinA, and abobotulinumtoxinA in the treatment of glabellar frown lines: A randomized, double-blind study. *Clin Cosmet Investig Dermatol* 2013; 6: 211–9.
54. Lorenc ZP, Kenkel JM, Fagien S et al. Consensus Panel's assessment and recommendations on the use of 3 botulinum toxin type A products in facial aesthetics. *Aesthet Surg J* 2013; 33: 35S–40S.
55. Carruthers J, Fournier N, Kerscher M et al. The convergence of medicine and neurotoxins: A focus on botulinum toxin type A and its application in aesthetic medicine—a global, evidence-based botulinum toxin consensus education initiative: Part II: Incorporating botulinum toxin into aesthetic clinical practice. *Dermatol Surg* 2013; 39: 510–25.
56. Poulain B, Trevidic P, Clave M et al. Clinical equivalence of conventional OnabotulinumtoxinA (900 kD) and IncobotulinumtoxinA (neurotoxin free from complexing proteins—150 kD): 2012 multidisciplinary French consensus in aesthetics. *J Drugs Dermatol* 2013; 12: 1434–46.
57. Ahn BK, Kim YS, Kim HJ et al. Consensus recommendations on the aesthetic usage of botulinum toxin type A in Asians. *Dermatol Surg* 2013; 39: 1843–60.
58. Yutskovskaya Y, Gubanova E, Khrustaleva I et al. IncobotulinumtoxinA in aesthetics: Russian multidisciplinary expert consensus recommendations. *Clin Cosmet Investig Dermatol* 2015; 8: 297–306.
59. Ravenni R, De Grandis D, Mazza A. Conversion ratio between Dysport and Botox in clinical practice: An overview of available evidence. *Neurol Sci* 2013; 34: 1043–8.
60. Dolimbek BZ, Aoki KR, Steward LE et al. Mapping of the regions on the heavy chain of botulinum neurotoxin A (BoNT-A) recognized by antibodies of cervical dystonia patients with immunoresistance to BoNT/A. *Mol Immunol* 2007; 44: 1029–41.
61. Atassi MZ, Dolimbek BZ. Mapping of the antibody-binding regions on the HN-domain (residues 449–859) of botulinum neurotoxin A with antitoxin antibodies from four host species. Full profile of the continuous antigenic regions of the H-chain of botulinum neurotoxin A. *Protein J* 2004; 23: 39–52.
62. Takahashi T, Joshi SG, Al-Saleem F et al. Localization of the sites and characterization of the mechanisms by which anti-light chain antibodies neutralize the actions of the botulinum holotoxin. *Vaccine* 2009; 27: 2616–24.
63. Jankovic J, Schwartz K. Response and immunoresistance to botulinum toxin injections. *Neurology* 1995; 1743–6.
64. Jankovic J, Vuong KD, Ahsan J. Comparison of efficacy and immunogenicity of original versus current botulinum toxin in cervical dystonia. *Neurology* 2003; 60: 1186–8.
65. Lee S-K. Antibody-induced failure of botulinum toxin type A therapy in a patient with masseteric hypertrophy. *Dermatol Surg* 2007; 33(1 Spec No): S105–S10.
66. Dressler D, Wohlfahrt K, Meyer-Rogge E et al. Antibody-induced failure of botulinum toxin a therapy in cosmetic indications. *Dermatol Surg* 2010; 36(Suppl 4): 2182–7.
67. Stengel G, Bee EK. Antibody-induced secondary treatment failure in a patient treated with botulinum toxin type A for glabellar frown lines. *Clin Interv Aging* 2011; 6: 281–4.
68. Torres S, Hamilton M, Sanches E et al. Neutralizing antibodies to botulinum neurotoxin type A in aesthetic medicine: Five case reports. *Clin Cosmet Investig Dermatol* 2013; 7: 11–7.
69. Stephan F, Habre M, Tomb R. Clinical resistance to three types of botulinum toxin type A in aesthetic medicine. *J Cosmet Dermatol* 2014; 13: 346–8.
70. Göschel H, Wohlfarth K, Frevert J et al. Botulinum A toxin therapy: Neutralizing and nonneutralizing antibodies—therapeutic consequences. *Exp Neurol* 1997; 147: 96–102.
71. Wang L, Sun Y, Yang W et al. Type A botulinum neurotoxin complex proteins differentially modulate host response of neuronal cells. *Toxicon* 2014; 82: 52–60.
72. Blümel J, Frevert J, Schwaier A. Comparative antigenicity of three preparations on botulinum neurotoxin A in the rabbit. *Neurotox Res* 2006; 9: 238.
73. Kukreja R, Chang TW, Cai S et al. Immunological characterization of the subunits of type A botulinum neurotoxin and different components of its associated proteins. *Toxicon* 2009; 53: 616–24.
74. Iwasaki A, Medzhitov R. Regulation of adaptive immunity by the innate immune system. *Science*. 2010; 327: 291–5.
75. Sharon N, Lis H. History of lectins: From hemagglutinins to biological recognition molecules. *Glycobiology* 2004; 14: 53R–62R.
76. Jung ID, Jeong SK, Lee CM et al. Enhanced efficacy of therapeutic cancer vaccines produced by co-treatment with Mycobacterium tuberculosis heparin-binding hemagglutinin, a novel TLR4 agonist. *Cancer Res* 2011; 71(8): 2858–7077.
77. Dressler D, Adib Saberi F. New formulation of Botox: Complete antibody-induced treatment failure in cervical dystonia. *J Neurol Neurosurg Psychiatry* 2007; 78: 108–9.
78. Benecke R. Clinical relevance of botulinum toxin immunogenicity. *BioDrugs* 2012; 26: e1–9.
79. Kranz G, Sycha T, Voller B et al. Neutralizing antibodies in dystonic patients who still respond well to botulinum toxin type A. *Neurology* 2008; 70: 133–6.
80. Lange O, Bigalke H, Dengler R et al. Neutralizing antibodies and secondary therapy failure after treatment with botulinum toxin type A: Much ado about nothing? *Clin Neuropharmacol* 2009; 32: 213–8.
81. Yablon SA, Brashear A, Gordon MF et al. Formation of neutralizing antibodies in patients receiving botulinum toxin type A for treatment of poststroke spasticity: A pooled-data analysis of three clinical trials. *Clin Ther* 2007; 29: 683–90.
82. Brin MF, Comella CL, Jankovic J et al.; CD-017 BoNTA Study Group. Long-term treatment with botulinum toxin type A in cervical dystonia has low immunogenicity by mouse protection assay. *Mov Disord*. 2008; 23: 1353–60.
83. Schulte-Baukloh H, Bigalke H, Miller K et al. Botulinum neurotoxin type A in urology: Antibodies as a cause of therapy failure. *Int J Urol* 2008; 15: 407–15.
84. Mohammadi B, Buhr N, Bigalke H et al. A long-term follow-up of botulinum toxin A in cervical dystonia. *Neurol Res* 2009; 31: 463–6.
85. Muller K, Mix E, Adib Saberi F et al. Prevalence of neutralising antibodies in patients treated with botulinum toxin type A for spasticity. *J Neural Transm* 2009; 116: 579–85.
86. Naumann M, Carruthers A, Carruthers J et al. Meta-analysis of neutralizing antibody conversion with onabotulinumtoxinA (BOTOX®) across multiple indications. *Mov Disord* 2010; 25: 2211–8.
87. Dressler D. Complete secondary botulinum toxin therapy failure in blepharospasm. *J Neurol* 2000; 247: 809–10.
88. Hefter H, Spiess C, Rosenthal D. Very early reduction in efficacy of botulinum toxin therapy for cervical dystonia in patients with subsequent secondary treatment failure: A retrospective analysis. *J Neural Transm* 2014; 121: 513–9.
89. Dressler D, Adib Saberi F, Bigalke H. IncobotulinumtoxinA (Xeomin®) can produce antibody-induced therapy failure in a patient pretreated with abobotulinumtoxinA (Dysport®). *J Neural Transm* 2014; 121: 769–71.

90. Dressler D. Five-year experience with incobotulinumtoxinA (Xeomin®): The first botulinum toxin drug free of complexing proteins. *Eur J Neurol* 2012; 19: 385–9.
91. Hefter H, Hartmann C, Kahlen U et al. Prospective analysis of neutralising antibody titres in secondary non-responders under continuous treatment with a botulinumtoxin type A preparation free of complexing proteins—a single cohort 4-year follow-up study. *BMJ Open* 2012; 2.
92. Dressler D. Clinical presentation and management of antibody-induced failure of botulinum toxin therapy. *Mov Disord* 2004; 19(Suppl 8): S92–S100.
93. Greene P, Fahn S, Diamond B. Development of resistance to botulinum toxin type A in patients with torticollis. *Mov Disord* 1994; 9: 213–7.
94. Herrmann J, Geth K, Mall V et al. Clinical impact of antibody formation to botulinum toxin A in children. *Ann Neurol* 2004; 55: 732–5.

4 Topical botulinum toxin*

Richard G. Glogau

INTRODUCTION

Ten years after the first publication describing the use of botulinum neurotoxin type A (BoNT-A) for the treatment of glabellar lines,[1] BoNT-A was approved in the United States for the "temporary improvement in the appearance of moderate to severe glabellar lines associated with corrugator and/or procerus muscle activity."[2] This was the first cosmetic indication for a botulinum toxin that had previously been approved for therapeutic use only (cervical dystonia, strabismus, and blepharospasm). BoNT-A is now used widely in facial aesthetics not only for glabellar lines but also for many other dynamic facial lines including lateral canthal lines (crow's feet), radial lip lines, horizontal forehead lines, and marionette lines (down-turned corners of the mouth).[3] The target muscles for these areas are the lateral orbicularis oculi, orbicularis oris, frontalis, and depressor anguli oris, respectively.[3] The safety and effectiveness of using BoNT-A in these muscles has now been well established over many years.

At the time of writing, three BoNT-As are available in the United States and Canada (onabotulinumtoxinA [OnaBTX-A], abobotulinumtoxinA [AboBTX-A], and incobotulinumtoxinA [IncoBTX-A]) while injectable daxibotulinumtoxinA [DaxiBTX-A] is in clinical development. All of these agents are administered by injection and therefore have the potential to cause needle anxiety and injection site reactions such as erythema, bruising, discomfort, tenderness, pain, and infection.[4] In an effort to avoid these potential issues, attempts have been made to develop formulations that are suitable for topical delivery.

CURRENT TRANSEPIDERMAL DELIVERY MECHANISMS

Most transepidermal drug delivery systems that have been developed to date are inefficient and can only transport small molecules such as nicotine, progesterone, and scopolamine. As a result, many macromolecules (including insulin, antibodies, and growth hormone) still need to be administered by injection.

In keeping with the skin's primary function—to exclude chemical assaults from the external environment—the stratum corneum and upper layers of the epidermis are lipid-rich barriers that block the entry of most large molecules and so the flux of most proteins across the skin barrier is essentially zero. The stratum corneum and upper layers of the epidermis are essentially a multilayered arrangement of the mature and differentiated horny cells of the epidermis that are interwoven with a lipid matrix that itself has a lamellar structure. Passage through the stratum corneum is less likely to be successful for highly ionic and/or aqueous molecules than lipophilic molecules, and it is also less efficient for larger molecules than smaller molecules. Furthermore, the process is heavily influenced by time and by the concentration of the relevant molecule.

Most attempts to enhance transepidermal delivery by manipulating drug structure have been rudimentary from a biochemical standpoint—because, for example, conjugating a drug to a carrier can compromise its activity and permeation enhancers may disrupt protein linkages and tertiary structures vital to the biological activity of a protein. Iontophoresis has also been explored as an alternative mechanism for drug delivery. Utilizing a direct current of relatively low amplitude, iontophoresis involves placing an active electrode in the drug formulation. The ionic charge imparted to the target molecule allows the drug to be driven into the skin as indifferent ions are pulled from the skin by the indifferent electrode to complete the circuit. However, few molecules are amenable to being delivered by iontophoresis, especially lipophilic molecules. Although it has been reported to be successful with botulinum toxin,[5,6] iontophoretic delivery lacks targeting and delivery specificity, is often painful, and is heavily influenced by time and by drug concentration.

A NOVEL TRANSEPIDERMAL DELIVERY SYSTEM FOR BOTULINUM TOXIN

A novel transepidermal drug delivery system has been developed that may allow BoNT-A to be available commercially as a topical formulation. The investigational product DaxiBTX-A topical gel (RT001, Revance Therapeutics, Inc., Newark, California) consists of a 150-kDa highly purified BoNT-A and a proprietary carrier peptide that binds to BoNT-A electrostatically and then enables it to be delivered transcutaneously. Topical delivery of BoNT-A in this way may be popular with patients because it avoids the need for injections.

The development of the proprietary peptide in DaxiBTX-A topical gel stemmed from the study of a human immunodeficiency virus (HIV) gene called "TAT" (the "transactivator of transcription" gene) that was originally characterized in 1988.[7,8] TAT has within it a protein transduction domain that is capable of penetrating cell membranes and is functionally responsible for the propagation of the viral genome. It causes accelerated production of the HIV double-stranded RNA by binding to cellular factors, controlling their phosphorylation, and resulting in increased transcription of all the HIV genes.

The peptide in DaxiBTX-A topical gel is novel in that it combines a cationic poly-Lysine core with the residues of the TAT gene domain on each end, thus enabling noncovalent binding to the toxin. The peptide backbone (a sequence of consecutive lysines) binds to BoNT-A electrostatically, with the positive charge of the peptide attracted to the relative negative charge of the 150-kDa BoNT-A (Figures 4.1a and b).

The toxin forms a complex with the peptides, with the protein transduction domains directed outward where they are free to attach to cell surfaces. The peptide-covered toxin is absorbed through cell membranes, crosses the cytoplasm to the cell membrane on the other side, and passes out and into the next cell. This is an active energy transport system and is not specific to botulinum toxin—it is a variant of induced macropinocytosis where the cell takes a "drink" of the surrounding media and conveys it out to the other side without harming the cell or the cell membrane.

Once the complex has traversed the cell, it moves through the next cell, and the next, until it exits the epidermis on the dermal side. At this point, the toxin is released from the carrier peptide and is free to exert its usual action on the SNAP-25 protein, producing the cholinergic blockade that is characteristic of BoNT-A. This action appears identical to the action of injected BoNT-A in every way except that the total dose delivered varies depending on the concentration of the toxin, the concentration of the peptide, and how long the complex is in contact with the skin.

* Adapted from Topical botulinum toxin, in *Botulinum Toxins: Cosmetic and Clinical Applications* (ed. Joel Cohen, MD), Wiley-Blackwell, Oxford UK, June 2017.

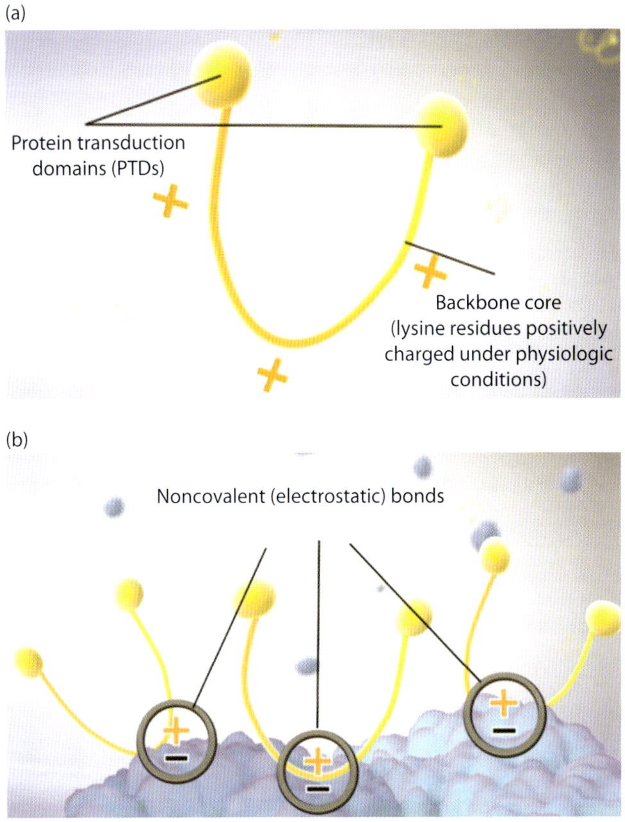

Figure 4.1 (a) Schematic representation of the proprietary peptide with the backbone of lysine residues and TAT domains that will noncovalently bond with the botulinum toxin. (b) The botulinum toxin is negatively charged at physiological pH. The backbone of the peptide then binds noncovalently to the toxin. The protein transduction domains are then projecting outward, available for binding to the cell wall. (With kind permission from Springer Science+Business Media: *Cell-Penetrating Peptides: Methods and Protocols. Methods in Molecular Biology*, Nonclinical and clinical experiences with CPP-based self-assembling peptide systems in topical drug development, 683, 2011, 553–72, Waugh JM et al., Humana Press.)

STUDIES EVALUATING TOPICAL DELIVERY OF BOTULINUM TOXIN

Animal studies first demonstrated the concept that BoNT-A could be transported through the skin and inhibit the contraction of a target muscle if it is applied in the presence of an appropriate peptide carrier[9]. This was evaluated using the digit abduction score assay,[10] which uses a startle reflex of the mouse. When a mouse is lifted up by its tail, its normal startle reflex is to extend its hind limbs and splay its toes apart. However, if the muscle contraction is first inhibited by BoNT-A, such movement is inhibited. Topical application of a peptide-botulinum complex to one leg produced almost complete inhibition of the reflex, compared with no inhibition in the other leg which received topical BoNT-A only without the carrier peptide.

The first reported evidence that topical application of a peptide-botulinum complex is effective in humans came from a randomized, blinded, vehicle-controlled study in patients with primary axillary hyperhidrosis.[11] Four weeks after a single topical application, the peptide-botulinum complex showed a significantly greater inhibition of sweating than vehicle (assessed gravimetrically and by Minor's starch-iodine test).

DaxiBTX-A topical gel was subsequently evaluated in a randomized, double-blind, parallel-group phase 2 study in subjects with moderate to severe primary axillary hyperhidrosis who produced at least 50 mg sweat/5 minutes.[12] The results of this study showed that a single application of DaxiBTX-A topical gel (25 or 50 ng) achieved a clinically meaningful reduction in sweat production—a mean of 214 and 166 mg/5 minutes with 25 and 50 ng, respectively, versus 66 mg/5 minutes with placebo.[13] Although the study was not powered to achieve statistical significance, the reduction in sweat was significantly greater in the higher dose group than the placebo group ($p = 0.003$). An additional important clinical finding was that, even though noninvasive treatments do not generally provide sufficient efficacy to treat severe hyperhidrosis, subjects with profound hyperhidrosis at baseline experienced an excellent reduction in sweating. Adverse events were generally mild, localized, and transient, with the most common treatment-related adverse events being erythema or pain at the application site and folliculitis. Photographic documentation of the effect of topical DaxiBTX-A is shown in Figure 4.2.

DaxiBTX-A topical gel has been studied most extensively in the treatment of lateral canthal lines. Topical delivery of BoNT-A would be highly desirable in this area given the thinness of the skin and the close relationship of the orbicularis oculi (the target muscle) to the skin's surface. Five dose-escalation studies have been performed evaluating the effects of DaxiBTX-A topical gel in the treatment of lateral canthal lines. As the dose of DaxiBTX-A increased, so did the proportion of lateral canthal areas attaining at least a 2-point improvement on the Investigator Global Assessment of Lateral Canthal Line severity scale (IGA-LCL)—8%, 18%, 26%, 34%, and 56% at concentrations of 3.3, 5.5, 11, 22, and 25 ng/mL, respectively.[14] This 5-point scale (of absent, minimal, mild, moderate, and severe) has been shown to be a reliable, appropriate, and clinically meaningful means of assessing lateral canthal line severity.[15] Photographic documentation of the efficacy of DaxiBTX-A topical gel is shown in Figure 4.3.

The escalating doses of DaxiBTX-A did not result in a dose-dependent increase in the severity or frequency of adverse events. Treatment-emergent adverse events were generally mild and transient and none of the studies revealed any safety signals of clinical relevance. Cranial nerve and ECG assessments showed no significant treatment- or dose-related findings and there were no treatment-related increases in antibody titers to the neurotoxin or the carrier peptide relative to predose serum samples.

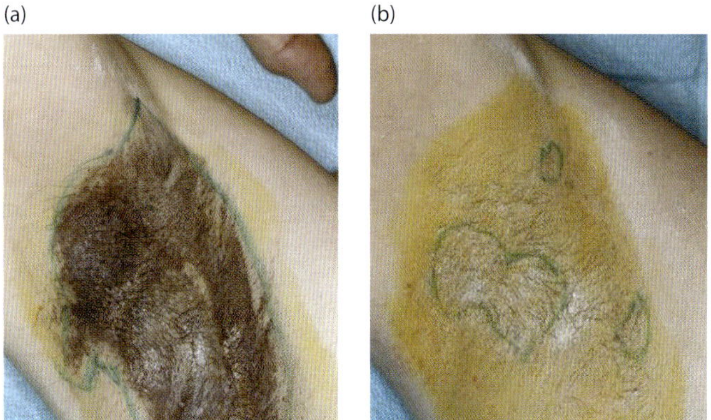

Figure 4.2 Result of Minor's starch-iodine test in a patient with axillary hyperhidrosis. (a) Baseline, (b) 4 weeks after topical application of 50 ng/mL of the peptide-botulinum complex to the axilla. (Reproduced with permission from Revance Therapeutics, Inc., Newark, California.)

(a)

(b)

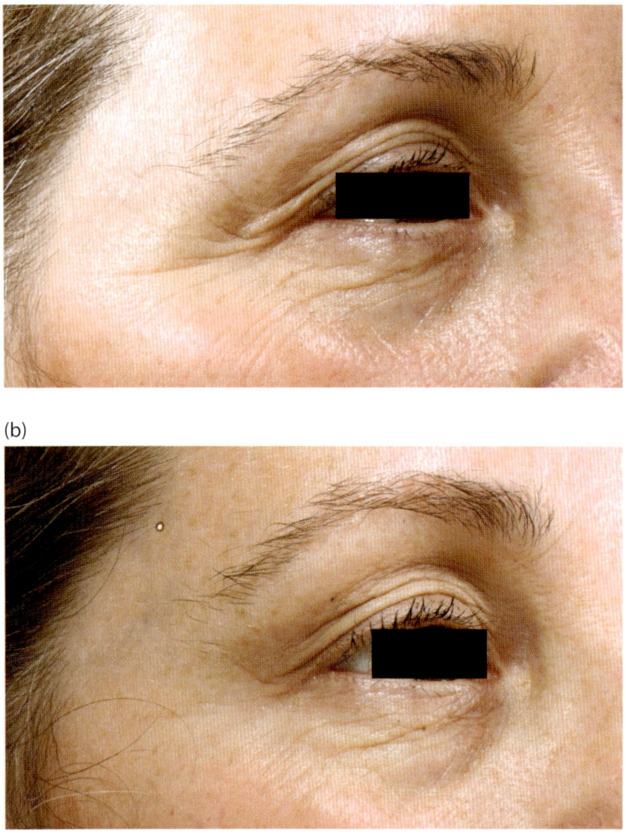

Figure 4.3 Representative appearance of lateral canthal lines treated with a single topical application of the peptide-botulinum complex that was left on the skin for 30 minutes. (a) Baseline, (b) 4 weeks post-treatment. (Reproduced with permission of Revance Therapeutics, Inc., Newark, California.)

A double-blind, placebo-controlled study involving 90 subjects with bilateral moderate or severe lateral canthal lines at rest confirmed the efficacy and tolerability of a single 25 ng dose of DaxiBTX-A (the dose subsequently evaluated in phase 3 studies).[16] A 30-minute topical application of DaxiBTX-A resulted in significantly greater efficacy than placebo for the primary efficacy endpoint (at least a 2-point improvement in both investigator and patient ratings of lateral canthal line severity in both lateral canthal areas at rest)—at week 4, 44% of subjects in the DaxiBTX-A group had achieved this endpoint compared with 0% in the placebo group ($p < 0.001$). DaxiBTX-A topical gel also achieved a significant efficacy advantage for each of five secondary endpoints (a 1- or 2-point improvement in IGA-LCL score in both lateral canthal areas, a 1- or 2-point improvement in patient rating of lateral canthal line severity, and a marked improvement on a patient global impression of change assessment). For example, the proportion of subjects with both lateral canthal areas showing at least a 1-point improvement in IGA-LCL score with DaxiBTX-A topical gel or placebo was 89% versus 28% ($p < 0.001$). For 2-point improvements, the proportions were 58% versus 14% ($p < 0.001$), respectively. A 1-point improvement in severity score was considered clinically relevant and a 2-point improvement was considered a marked improvement. DaxiBTX-A topical gel was found to be well tolerated, with no clinically meaningful or significant differences in safety outcomes observed between DaxiBTX-A topical gel and placebo.

Another double-blind, placebo-controlled study involved a repeat application of DaxiBTX-A topical gel (administered at baseline and again at 4 weeks).[17] At 8 weeks, the proportion of lateral canthal areas showing at least a 1-point improvement from baseline in IGA-LCL severity was 95% versus 15% after treatment with DaxiBTX-A topical gel and placebo, respectively ($p < 0.001$) (Figure 4.4). The corresponding proportions showing at least a 2-point improvement were 50% versus 0% with DaxiBTX-A topical gel and placebo, respectively ($p < 0.001$), (Figure 4.5). No treatment-related adverse events were reported. Photographic documentation illustrates the benefit of repeat dosing, with continued

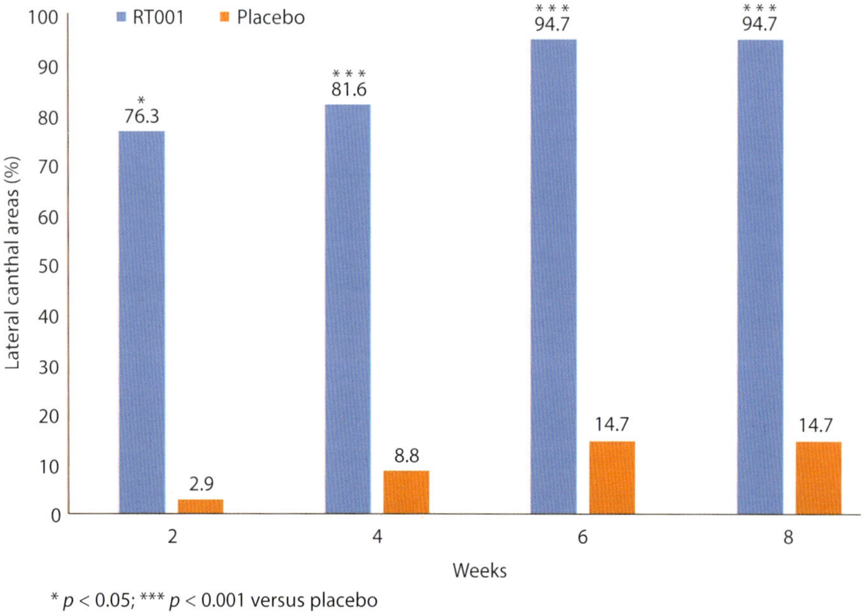

Figure 4.4 Compared with placebo, DaxiBTX-A topical gel resulted in a significantly greater proportion of lateral canthal areas showing at least a 1-point improvement in score on the Investigator's Global Assessment of Lateral Canthal Lines at Rest Severity Scale. Treatment was administered at baseline and repeated at week 4. (From Glogau R et al. *J Drugs Dermatol* 2012; 11: 38–45.)

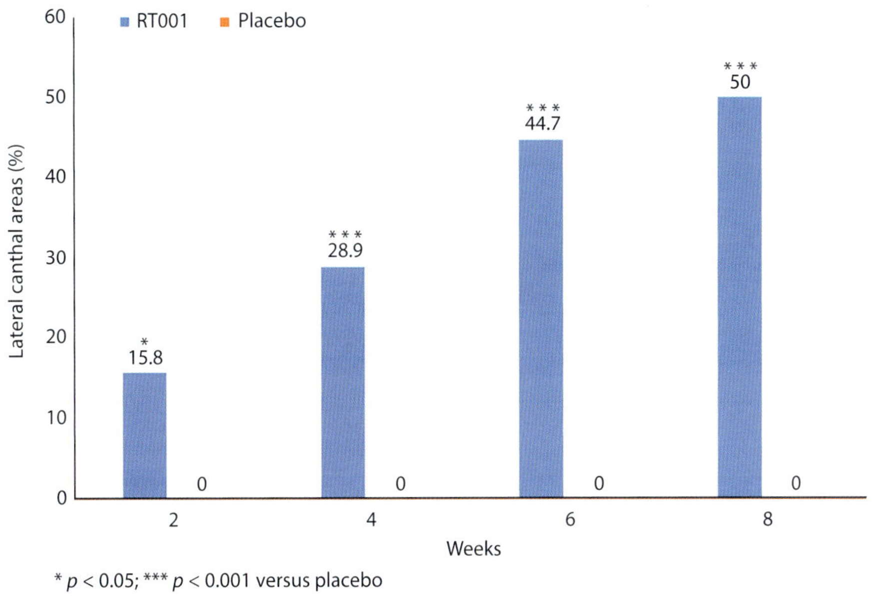

Figure 4.5 Compared with placebo, DaxiBTX-A topical gel resulted in a significantly greater proportion of lateral canthal areas showing at least a 2-point improvement in score on the Investigator's Global Assessment of Lateral Canthal Lines at Rest Severity Scale. Treatment was administered at baseline and repeated at week 4. (From Glogau R et al. *J Drugs Dermatol* 2012; 11: 38–45.)

improvement in lateral canthal lines after the second dose of DaxiBTX-A topical gel (Figure 4.6).

DaxiBTX-A topical gel has also been evaluated in a phase 3 study known as REALISE-1 (clinicaltrials.gov identifier NCT02580370).[18] In this randomized, multicenter, double-blind, placebo-controlled study, 450 subjects with moderate to severe lateral canthal lines received a single treatment with DaxiBTX-A or placebo. The co-primary efficacy endpoints in the trial were composite measurements of at least a 2-point and at least a 1-point improvement in lateral canthal lines between baseline and 28 days after treatment (graded by investigators using the IGA-LCL scale and subjects using the Patient Severity Assessment [PSA]). Results were reported in June 2016. Topical DaxiBTX-A generally appeared to be well tolerated but the co-primary efficacy endpoints were not achieved.[19] As a result, the clinical development of DaxiBTX-A topical gel is not being pursued further at this time for the treatment of lateral canthal lines or axillary hyperhidrosis.

DaxiBTX-A topical gel has also been evaluated for the prevention of chronic migraine headache. In a study conducted in Singapore, patients were considered responders if they had ≥50% improvement versus placebo in at least two of the following parameters (mean scores on the Headache Impact Test [HIT-6™], number of total migraine attacks, and intensity of migraine attacks) plus numerical superiority for the third parameter. At week 4, the proportion of responders was 43.8% with DaxiBTX-A versus 10.5% with placebo ($p < 0.05$).[20] Improvements were evident in the number and severity of headaches and in evaluations of headache-specific quality of life. Adverse events were generally mild. One report of a severe headache was considered serious and possibly related to treatment but resolved without sequelae.

FUTURE DIRECTIONS

Topical delivery of botulinum toxin to the skin could offer opportunities not only to treat areas that are difficult to manage with injectables but also to treat patients who want to avoid injections. Topical BoNT-A could also prove useful as an adjunctive or extender therapy in conjunction with injectable BoNT-A. Some of the most attractive targets for topical delivery may be the upper lip, forehead, and neck for aesthetic improvements, and the hands, scalp, and axillae in patients with hyperhidrosis. However, phase 3 results with DaxiBTX-A topical gel in the treatment of lateral canthal lines have been disappointing and clinical development is not currently being pursued for lateral canthal lines, axillary hyperhidrosis, or migraine.

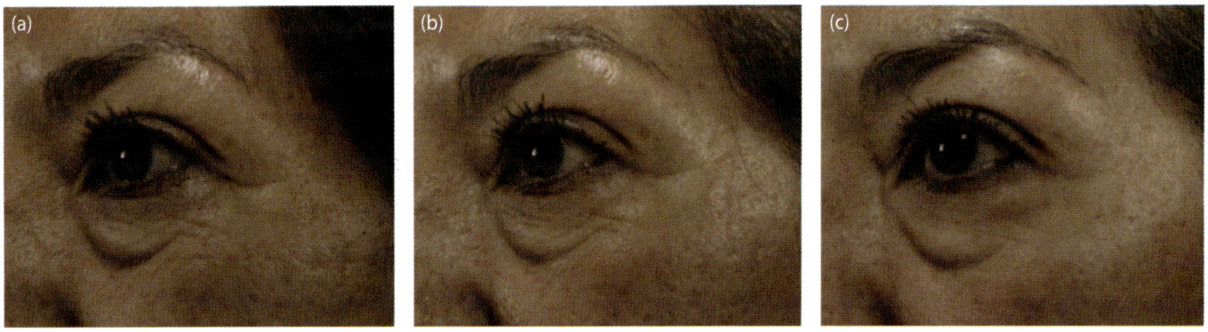

Figure 4.6 The clinical significance of this study is the demonstration of continued improvement with a second application of the topical peptide-toxin complex gel, observed over the 8-week study period. (a) Baseline, (b) 4 weeks after initial treatment, (c) 8 weeks after initial treatment (4 weeks after repeat treatment). (Reproduced with permission of Wolters Kluwer from: Brandt F et al. *Dermatol Surg* 2010; 36(Suppl 4): 2111–8.)

Importantly, the carrier peptide used in DaxiBTX-A has the potential to be joined to other molecules besides botulinum toxin and, as a result, could also deliver other drugs through the dermis. This could open opportunities for new treatment approaches in a variety of other areas of dermatology and beyond—including, for example, melasma, hyperpigmentation, acne, hirsutism, vitiligo, and peripheral neuralgias, e.g., post-herpetic neuralgia.

REFERENCES

1. Carruthers JD, Carruthers JA. Treatment of glabellar frown lines with C. Botulinum-A exotoxin. *J Dermatol Surg Oncol* 1992; 18: 17–21.
2. Goldenthal KL. Food and Drug Administration website. Department of Health & Human Services. Available at: http://www.fda.gov/downloads/Drugs/DevelopmentApprovalProcess/HowDrugsareDevelopedandApproved/ApprovalApplications/TherapeuticBiologicApplications/ucm088278.pdf. Accessed June 29, 2016.
3. Small R. Botulinum toxin injection for facial wrinkles. *Am Fam Physician* 2014; 90: 168–75.
4. Coté TR, Mohan AK, Polder JA, et al. Botulinum toxin type A injections: adverse events reported to the US Food and Drug Administration in therapeutic and cosmetic cases. *J Am Acad Dermatol* 2005; 53: 407–15.
5. Kavanagh GM, Oh C, Shams K. BOTOX delivery by iontophoresis. *Br J Dermatol* 2004; 151: 1093–5.
6. Solomon P. Delivery of Botox® by iontophoresis. *Br J Dermatol* 2005; 153: 1075.
7. Frankel AD, Pabo CO. Cellular uptake of the tat protein from human immunodeficiency virus. *Cell* 1988; 55: 1189–93.
8. Green M, Loewenstein PM. Autonomous functional domains of chemically synthesized human immunodeficiency virus that trans-activator protein. *Cell* 1988; 55: 1179–88.
9. Waugh JM, Lee J, Dake MD, Browne D. Nonclinical and clinical experiences with CPP-based self-assembling peptide systems in topical drug development. In: Langel Ü (ed). *Cell-Penetrating Peptides: Methods and Protocols. Methods in Molecular Biology*, vol 683. Humana Press, New York; 2011, 553–72. Available at: http://www.revance.com/pdfs/WaughJ_2011_Nonclinical-and-clinical-experiences-with-CPP-based-self-assembling-peptide-systems-in-topical-drug-development.pdf. Accessed June 3, 2016.
10. Aoki KR. A comparison of the safety margins of botulinum neurotoxin serotypes A, B, and F in mice. *Toxicon* 2001; 39: 1815–1820.
11. Glogau RG. Topically applied botulinum toxin type A for the treatment of primary axillary hyperhidrosis: Results of a randomized, blinded, vehicle-controlled study. *Dermatol Surg* 2007; 33: S76–S80.
12. Safety and efficacy of botulinum toxin type A topical gel for primary axillary hyperhidrosis. ClinicalTrials.gov website. https://clinicaltrials.gov/ct2/show/NCT02565732. Accessed June 13, 2016.
13. Revance announces positive phase 2 results for RT001 botulinum toxin type A topical gel to treat axillary hyperhidrosis [press release, Dec 23, 2015]. Revance Therapeutics website. Available at: http://investors.revance.com/releasedetail.cfm?releaseid=948101. Accessed June 23, 2016.
14. Waugh JM, Glogau RG. Topical neurotoxin. In: Carruthers A, Carruthers J (eds). *Botulinum Toxin, Procedures in Cosmetic Dermatology Series*. 3rd ed. Elsevier Saunders, Philadelphia; 2012, 67–71.
15. Kane MA, Blitzer A, Brandt FS et al. Development and validation of a new clinically-meaningful rating scale for measuring lateral canthal line severity. *Aesthet Surg J* 2012; 32: 275–85.
16. Glogau R, Blitzer A, Brandt F, Kane M, Monheit GD, Waugh JM. Results of a randomized, double-blind, placebo-controlled study to evaluate the efficacy and safety of a botulinum toxin type A topical gel for the treatment of moderate-to-severe lateral canthal lines. *J Drugs Dermatol* 2012; 11: 38–45.
17. Brandt F, O'Connell C, Cazzaniga A, Waugh JM. Efficacy and safety evaluation of a novel botulinum toxin topical gel for the treatment of moderate to severe lateral canthal lines. *Dermatol Surg* 2010; 36(Suppl 4): 2111–2118.
18. Safety and efficacy of botulinum toxin type A topical gel for lateral canthal lines (REALISE 1). ClinicalTrials.gov website. https://www.clinicaltrials.gov/ct2/show?term=revance&rank=3. Accessed June 27, 2016.
19. Revance reports results for RT001 topical phase 3 trial for lateral canthal lines [press release, Jun 13, 2016]. Revance Therapeutics website. Available at: http://investors.revance.com/releasedetail.cfm?releaseid=975537. Accessed June 27, 2016.
20. Data on file. Revance Therapeutics, Inc., Newark, California.

5 The different botulinum toxins and their clinical uses in the West

Gary Monheit and James Highsmith

OVERVIEW

Since 2001 there have been more than 11 million botulinum neurotoxin (BoNT) injections in the United States and probably double this amount worldwide. It thus represents the most common nonsurgical cosmetic procedure today. The FDA first approved it for glabellar lines, but it has been used off-label for many other aesthetic applications for aging skin of the face and neck.

Botulinum neurotoxin-A (BoNT-A) is the most commonly used serotype of BoNT, synthesized as a continuous 150 kDa protein. Initial proteolysis or nicking divides the polypeptide into 2 separate parts, a heavy chain (100 kDa) and a light chain (50 kDa). Each of these parts has a separate function in the deactivation of the synapse at the neuromuscular junction. This blockage at the SNARE complex stops the release of acetylcholine. The target for all type A serotype of BoNT is SNAP-25 regardless of commercial preparation.

In a natural setting, the BoNT-A exists as a complex with a protective shell of proteins.[1] These are known as toxin-associated proteins with 4 distinct hemagglutinin proteins and a nontoxic nonhemagglutinin protein. As botulinum toxin cultures differ, these complexes exist in 300, 500, and 900 kDa, and communal preparations vary with these different molecular weights.[2]

Neurotoxin associated proteins (NAPs) protect BoNT from degradation in the acidic gastrointestinal tract and promote toxin uptake by epithelial cells. The relevance of these proteins to aesthetic indications is still unknown.[3]

OnaBTX-A (BOTOX®) was first synthesized as Oculinum and first produced in 1979. It was produced by Allergan Pharmaceuticals as BOTOX® and first used for therapeutic, then cosmetic procedures.[4]

Several commercial preparations of BoNT serotype A (BoNT-A) and serotype B (BoNT-B) products have been manufactured for the treatment of a multitude of disorders. Initially, conditions involving excessive muscular contractions were targeted, such as dystonias, blepharospasms, and strabismus. At the same time in the early 1980s at the Centre for Applied Microbiology and Research (CAMR), United Kingdom, Dr. John Elston first used botulinum toxin clinically. The first marketing approval in the United Kingdom was for the treatment of blepharospasm. Dysport® was named for Dys (tonia) at (Port) on Down, the place where it was developed.[5] Aesthetic uses expanded remarkably when the Carruthers first investigated the usefulness of BoNT-A for glabellar frown lines.[6] Other mimetic muscles of expression on the face were then targeted for treatment of dynamic wrinkles and lines including forehead, marionette lines, and platysmal cords. Concomitant with these off-label indications in the United States, clinical researchers in Europe were performing similar on-label and off-label trials with Dysport®, or abobotulinumtoxinA (AboBTX-A).[7] More recently, nonmuscular uses began to be explored with conditions involving sebaceous glands, hair follicles, scars, chronic pain, and even depression. BoNT has evolved from the "most poisonous of all poisons" to one of the most widely applied medical drugs within the last 60 years.[8] Today, OnabotulinumtoxinA (OnaBTX-A) is approved for use in 78 countries with approximately 10.9 million vials sold in the United States alone since 2002.[9] Other toxins including Dysport®, Xeomin®, and others have evolved all over the world.

MECHANISM OF ACTION

After injection of BoNT, an endogenous protease snips the 150 kD BoNT polypeptide into two separate moieties, 100 and 50 kD, termed the heavy and light chains, respectively (Figure 5.1). These two chains are still bound together at this point by a single disulfide bridge which allows them to carry out distinct functions. The C-terminus of the heavy chain is responsible for binding the neurotoxin complex to specific receptors on the presynaptic nerve terminal. Internalization then occurs as the N-terminus of the heavy chain interacts with the receptor causing endocytosis. Next, the heavy chain forms a channel in the endosomal membrane of the vesicle as the disulfide bond is disintegrated by the acidic pH allowing the light chain to travel in the cytosol. This 50 kD light chain then cleaves **syn**aptosomal-**a**ssociated **p**rotein **25** (SNAP-25) preventing the docking and fusion of intracytoplasmic acetylcholine (Ach) vesicles. SNAP-25 is just one of many proteins that make up a superfamily of SNARE (**s**oluble **N**SF **a**ttachment protein **re**ceptors) proteins for exocytosis.[10] The mechanism for BoNT-B is nearly identical to BoNT-A except for the final SNARE target is synaptobrevin, also known as **v**esicle **a**ssociated **m**embrane **p**rotein (VAMP), which is cleaved thereby preventing neurotransmitter release. All type A BoNT act with the same mechanism at the SNARE receptor, whether they are a complex or free BoNT. Whether hemagglutinin (HA) protein assists the botulinum toxin-neurotoxin associated proteins (BoNT-NAP) complex to adhere to muscle and contribute to duration has been suggested by several investigators.[11]

Delivery has traditionally been done with an intramuscular injection using a 30-gauge needle on a tuberculin syringe. However, several topical formulations are being studied, including topical creams, liquids, and gels. These topicals are reviewed and discussed extensively in Chapters 4 and 6. Other delivery systems under investigation include topical application with microneedling or fractionated laser. Additionally, iontophoresis and phonophoresis have been studied to improve delivery without using needles.[12,13] Regardless of manufacturing differences, SNAP-25 is the molecular target for all of these new BoNT-A preparations.

PHARMACOLOGY

There are eight distinct serotypes of BoNT (A–H) but only BoNT-A and BoNT-B have been approved for human use (see Table 5.1). BoNT-A is the most commonly used form of BoNT for both clinical and aesthetic purposes but there are several variations in BoNT products. Regardless of the manufacturing process, the biologically active

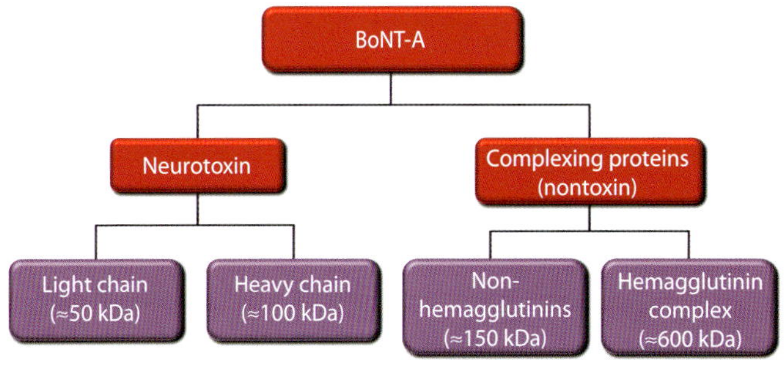

Figure 5.1 BoNT-A complexing proteins: the toxin (150 kDA) associates with nontoxin proteins to form large molecular weight complex (300, 500, or 900 kDa). (See further Dressler D et al., *Disabil Rehab* 2007; 29:1761–8; Hambleton P, *J Neurol* 1992; 239: 16–20; Inoue K, Fujinaga Y, Watanabe T. *Infect Immun* 1996; 64(5): 1589–94.)

Table 5.1 Summary of Available Botulinum Toxins for Cosmetic Usage

	BOTOX	Dysport	Xeomin	Myobloc	DWP—450	Meditoxin	Purtox	CosmeTox	RT001	RT002	CBTX-A	CNBTxA
Other names	Onabotulinum-toxinA, BOTOX Cosmetic, Vistabel, Vistabex	Abobotulinum-toxinA, Reloxin, Azzalure	Incobotulinum-toxinA, Bocouture	Rimabotu-linumtoxinB, Neurobloc	Evosyal, Nabota	Neuronox, Neu-BoNT/A			DaxibotulinumtoxinA topical gel	DaxibotulinumtoxinA	Prosigne, Lantox	
Company	Allergan Incorporated	Galderma Laboratories	Merz Pharmaceuticals	Solstice Neuroscience Incorporated	Evolus Incorporated of ALPHAEON Corporation	Medy-Tox Incorporated	Mentor Worldwide LLC	Transdermal Corporation	Revance Therapeutics Incorporated	Revance Therapeutics Incorporated	Lanzhou Institute of Biological Products	Nanfeng Medical Science and Technology Development Company
Units per vial	50; 100; or 200	300 or 500	50 or 100	2500; 5000; or 10,000	100	50; 100; or 200	n/a	n/a	n/a	unknown	50 or 100	55 or 100
Composition	Botulinum toxin type A human serum albumin, NaCl	Botulinum toxin type A human serum albumin, lactose, & may contain trace amount of cow's milk proteins	Botulinum toxin type A human serum albumin, sucrose	Botulinum toxin type B human serum albumin, NaCl, sodium succinate	Botulinum toxin type A	Botulinum toxin type A human serum albumin,	Botulinum toxin type A	Botulinum toxin type A INParT (proprietary ionic nanoparticle technology) in a topical cream	Botulinum toxin type A RTP004 (synthetic peptide) in a poloxamer gel	Botulinum toxin type A RTP004 (synthetic peptide)	Botulinum toxin type A bovine gelatin, dextran, sucrose	Botulinum toxin type A
SNARE complex cleavage site	SNAP 25	SNAP 25	SNAP 25	VAMP	SNAP 25	SNAP 25	SNAP 25	SNAP 25	SNAP 25	SNAP 25	SNAP 25	SNAP 25
Molecular Weight	900 kD	500—900 kD	150 kD	700 kD	900 kD	900—940 kD	150 kD		150 kD	150 kD	900 kD	unknown
U.S. FDA approval	Yes	Yes	Yes	Yes	No	No	No	No	No	No	No	No
Notable Research	Seeking indication for forehead lines, also studies to prevent keloids/ hypertrophic scars perioperatively, alopecia universalis and totalis	Decrease oil formation and pore size	Studies for lateral crow's feet, parkinson tremor, spasticity, sialorrhea, notalgia paresthetica, restless leg syndrome, and for pain after surgery	Hyperhidrosis, sialorrhea	Currently in phase 3 clinical trials	One phase 3 clinical trial completed, also studies for masseter hypertrophy	Phase 3 clinical trials completed but product currently discontinued	Facial rhytides, hyperhidrosis PMC2921740	Currently in phase 3 clinical trials	Currently recruiting for phase 2 clinical trials	Unknown	Potency may exceed labeled units
Approval in countries other than U.S.	Yes	Yes	Yes	Yes	Yes	Yes	No	No	No	No	Yes	No
Other uses	Raynauds phenomenon, bruxism, overactive bladder, depression, spasmodic dysphonia, chronic pelvic or scrotal pain, platysmal bands, sialorrhea	Decrease menopausal hot flashes, focal dystonia, hyperhidrosis, sialorrhea	Cervical dystonia, platysmal bands	Focal dystonia, hypertonia, sialorrhea	Glabellar lines	Blepharospasm, bruxism, equinus foot deformity/ spasticity, muscle spasticity, glabellar lines	Glabellar lines	Hyperpigmenta-tion	Crow's feet lines, hyperhidrosis	Glabellar lines	Blepharospasm, cervical dystonia, forehead lines, glabellar lines, hyperhidrosis, spasticity	Unknown

Source: Frevert J. *Drugs R D.* 2015; 15(1): 1–9. doi: 10.1007/s40268-014-0077-1.

150 kiloDalton (kD) portion remains the same for all of the BoNT-A products. However, some of the BoNT-A have a surrounding coat of associated proteins (NAPs), the hemagglutinin and nonhemagglutinin protective proteins. This significantly increases the molecular weight of these products up to 700 and 900 kD. Whether these weight differences are clinically relevant continues to be a point of debate between manufacturing companies (see Chapter 3).

Studies have demonstrated release of the biologically active 150 kD portion of the toxin from the NAPs when there is a change of the environment to a physiologic pH. This most likely occurs during reconstitution in the vial, well before being injected into the patient.[14,15] Surely if only the active 150 kD toxin protein is released at or before injection, then one would not expect a difference in diffusion and spread based on the weight of the toxin. While early studies showed differences in diffusion with halos on starch iodine test,[16] this has since been attributed to larger volumes and dosage variations as follow-up studies found safe and predictable results when these variants were corrected.[17,18] Thus, the molecular weight of the different complexes is probably not relevant in determining field of effect or spread.

Another concerning issue emerged regarding the stability of the BoNT-A as related to the complex size, NAPs, unique excipients, and stabilizing process. For example, OnaBTX-A is absorbed in saline and vacuum dried. AbobotulinumtoxinA (AboBTX-A) and IncobotulinumtoxinA (IncoBTX-A) use various sugars and are lyophilized (freeze dried). The NAPs of IncoBTX-A are dissociated on manufacturing unlike the others which occurs during reconstitution. Dr. Eisele tested the three U.S. commercially available BoNT-A products using standard stability tests and found no significant difference in potency or shelf life.[19]

It should be noted that all three of these commercial products are derived from the same Hall strain of *Clostridium botulinum*. The most important difference between these toxins is therefore the dosage or activity units as defined by the respective manufacturers. OnaBTX-A, for instance, uses BOTOX units (BU) while AboBTX-A uses Speywood units (SU). Incobotulinum toxin units are found to be similar to BOTOX units. New advances in science are leading a change from LD50 on murine models to a cell-based test. However, both currently use the mean lethal dose (LD_{50}) killing power on mice to define a unit. However, these LD_{50} assays are unique to each product using different substrates and diluents so they are not interchangeable. This contrasts with products such as injectable insulin which uses a standardized potency scale of international units (IUs) that are interchangeable among preparations regardless of manufacturer. Therefore, there is no direct conversion factor between units of the different BTX-A products and each manufacturer discourages equivalency conversion.

Nonetheless, practitioners have sought to define a conversion factor to guide less experienced injectors when transitioning from one BoNT-A to another. A summary of the dosage studies places OnaBTX-A roughly equivalent to IncoBTX-A.[20,21] However, ratios from AboBTX-A to OnaBTX-A have suggested between 2.5–3:1 for bioequivalence. When a lower dosage of AboBTX-A was used (1.25), then OnaBTX-A had greater longevity. However, when a ratio of 3:1 was used, AboBTX-A was found to have a longer duration of action.[22] Thus, we can see that dosage is really a determining factor regarding efficacy and duration. It is the authors' opinion that the primary differences in products seen, are most closely related to dosage unit differences and volume of reconstitution. It is not the molecular weight or intrinsic differences in the BoNT molecule or complex. In summary, dosage should be determined by physiologic response of individual units rather than comparing product units. Each of the manufactured neurotoxins has demonstrated full efficacy and safety in clinical studies both in the United States and Europe. Claims have been made by individual injectors as to advantages by definitive toxin in various areas of facial injections. But comparative clinical studies have not backed up the claims of superiority of any individual toxin. The experienced injector can use correct dosage and injection points to produce expected clinical results in all areas treated with each of the toxins (see Appendix 1 and Table 5.2).

Immunogenicity or neutralizing antibodies are potential factors in determining treatment failures in aesthetic use. It is known that BoNT-NAPs can induce the formation of neutralizing antibodies (NAbs). In reality, the present three toxins in the United States—AboBTX-A, OnaBTX-A, and IncoBTX-A—have little to no demonstrable antibody formation due to the low amount of protein load. The rates of immunogenicity or neutralizing antibodies for studies concerning glabellar injections are

- OnaBTX-A 0%
- AboBTX-A: 0%
- IncoBTX-A: 1.1%[23] (See Chapter 3)

In cervical dystonia and other uses for muscle disorders with a much higher dosage and more frequent injections the incidence of antibody induced nonresponders is 1.2%. There still are cases of nonresponders to BoNT which are probably due to factors other than

Table 5.2 Dosing Recommendations for Botulinum Toxins

	BOTOX	Dysport	Xeomin
Glabella	Women: 10–40 units Men: 20–50 units 5–7 injection points	Women: 50–70 units Men: 50–80 units 5 injection points	Women: 10–40 units Men: 20–50 units 5–7 injection points
Frontalis	5–20 units 4–10 injection points	20–60 units 4–6 injection points	5–20 units 4–10 injection points
Crow's feet	5–20 units per side 2–5 injection points	20–60 units per side 3 injection points	5–20 units per side 2–5 injection points
Lip lines	4–6 units 2–6 injection points	Upper: 5–10 units 2 or 4 injection points Lower: 5–10 units 2 injection points	4–6 units 2–6 injection points
DAO	5–7.5 units per side	4–10 units per side	5–7.5 units per side
Mentalis	4–10 units 1–2 injection points	5–25 units 1–2 injection points	4–10 units 1–2 injection points
Nefertiti lift	15–20 units per side	30–45 units per side	15–20 units per side
Platysma	30–60 units	30–120 units	30–60 units

antibody formation. These include inadequate dosing, poor technique for accurate needle injection, and treatment of nondynamic wrinkles for causes other than muscle activity. The question still arises as to whether long-term repeated use of BoNT for cosmetic use will lead to antibody formation and poor muscle response. At this time, there is no clinical evidence in controlled studies that this occurs.

FDA INDICATED NEUROTOXINS IN THE UNITED STATES

There are only four BoNT currently approved by the Food and Drug Administration (FDA) for use in the United States. BOTOX®, Dysport®, Myobloc®, and Xeomin® have all been approved for the treatment of cervical dystonia. BOTOX®, Dysport®, and Xeomin® are each indicated to treat moderate to severe glabellar lines in adults as well (Figure 5.2). However, blepharospasms are only indicated for treatment with either BOTOX® or Xeomin®. BOTOX® Cosmetic is the only U.S. FDA approved toxin for lateral canthal crow's feet. BOTOX® has also received other indications in the United States including chronic migraine headaches, neurogenic detrusor overactivity (urinary incontinence), upper limb spasticity, and severe primary axillary hyperhidrosis in adults. Clinical studies are underway for forehead and upper face FDA approval for BOTOX®.

The quest for the ideal cosmetic toxin has promoted research to alter the clinical properties. The properties of the ideal neurotoxin include:

1. Rapid time of onset
2. Stable pharmacological action throughout its time of activity
3. Toxin effect limited to muscle site of injection
4. Limited yet controlled diffusion or field of effect
5. Few drug-related side effects—pain, unwanted paresis, and so forth
6. Natural appearing response
7. Physiologic
8. Prolonged action—greater than 6 months

Of these ideal characteristics, duration appears to be the most important factor to both patient and clinician. The trial studies for all three toxins presently used in the United States for both efficacy and duration are glabellar studies. The OnaBTX-A and IncoBTX-A studies were performed for 5 months and the AboBTX-A studies for 6 months. All three have the same results when each efficacy measurement was evaluated up to 5 months. At this time, duration is determined by concentration, but with a cap at 5 months. The 6-month barrier still exists today, but new products are presently under study that may have a more prolonged activity.

BOTOX®, Vistabel®, or Vistabex® (OnabotulinumtoxinA)

The first toxin to ever be synthesized for therapeutic uses was the predecessor of today's BOTOX®. BOTOX® is the trade name for Allergan's proprietary formula of BoNT-A in the United States. Being the first in its class, OnaBTX-A revolutionized aesthetic medicine and led many consumers to refer to all botulinum toxins as "BOTOX". Over 75 other countries have approved BOTOX® for clinical use.[9] Studied conditions include bruxism, chronic anal fissures, chronic pelvic or scrotal pain, depression, overactive bladder, platysmal bands, Raynaud's phenomenon, and spasmodic dysphonia. New studies are currently being done on forehead lines which may lead to another U.S. FDA approved indication.

OnaBTX-A has also been studied in treating nonmuscular conditions such as sialorrhea and Frey's syndrome by inhibiting acetylcholine (Ach) release from postganglionic parasympathetic fibers to salivary glands.[24] Hypertrophic scars and keloids have been shown to improve by noncontractile means. This may seem counterintuitive initially as one may presume the improvement is a result of decreasing tension on the affected area by paralyzing nearby musculature but this does not seem to be the only mechanism. OnaBTX-A actually decreases transforming growth factor (TGF-β1), inhibits fibroblast proliferation, and induces apoptosis thereby improving hypertrophic scars. Established hypertrophic scars and keloids have improved and prevention with perioperative use has been studied with favorable results.[25–27] Improvement of chronic pain disorders may be achieved through muscle relaxation as well as interactions leading to a decrease in nociceptive neuropeptides but these pathways have not been fully elucidated.[28,29]

Dysport®, Reloxin®, or Azzalure® (AbobotulinumtoxinA) (See Appendix 1)

This formulation of BoNT-A was first studied to treat cervical dystonia in 1988 and was developed in Porton Down in the United Kingdom. The name is derived from combining the first part of the treated condition with the location of origin, **dys**tonia and **Port**on Down, yielding Dysport®. Dysport® received its first indication to treat cervical dystonia in 1991 and aesthetic indications have been granted in 57

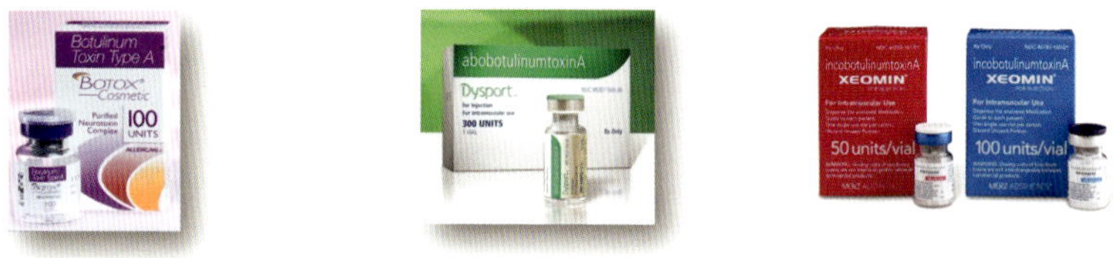

Figure 5.2 BoNT-As approved for aesthetic use in the U.S.

countries.[30] The U.S. FDA approved Dysport® for moderate to severe glabellar lines in April 2009. Dysport® has received many indications in different countries including blepharospasm, hemifacial spasm, spasmodic torticolis, and arm spasticity. Furthermore, AboBTX-A has been studied to treat other disorders including focal dystonia, hyperhidrosis, menopausal hot flashes, neurogenic detrusor overactivity (urinary incontinence), and sialorrhea. A 2013 study evaluated patients for forehead oily skin using a range from 30 to 45 SU of intradermal AboBTX-A on the forehead. Sebum production decreased at least 59% objectively and all patients improved subjectively at least 25% in skin oiliness by blocking lipid synthesis.[31,32]

Observation claims have been made for greater spread or diffusion of Dysport® after injection in the forehead area. The only objective clinical study has been the starch-iodine test for hyperhidrosis, but results have been nonconclusive by various clinicians. The fact that there is no direct conversion factor for standardized dosage between OnaBTX-A and AboBTX-A invalidates those results. The efficacy, field of effect, or diffusion as well as the duration seem directly affected by dosage, not differences in BTX molecules.

Xeomin®, Bocouture® (IncobotulinumtoxinA) (See Appendix 1)
Xeomin® is produced by Merz (Merz Pharma GMBH, Frankfurt am Main, Germany) and has been available in the United Kingdom since 2008 and the United States since 2010, for blepharospasms and cervical dystonia. It gained approval for cosmetic use in the United Kingdom (2010) and the United States (2011) for glabellar frown lines in adults, but is also indicated for crow's feet in Europe under the brand name Bocouture®. This patented version of BoNT-A is unique from the previously discussed toxins in that the molecular weight is lighter. The NAPs of IncoBTX-A are dissociated on manufacturing, unlike OnaBTX-A and AboBTX-A which occurs during reconstitution, but this difference does not appear clinically significant. Incobotulinum toxin thus has been stripped of any complexing proteins. With less protein load, claims have been made for less risk of allergenicity. In addition to the indications previously discussed, IncoBTX-A has been studied for platysmal neck bands, Parkinson tremors, spasticity, sialorrhea, notalgia paresthetica, and restless leg syndrome. IncoBTX-A was first reported in 2014 to be effective for patients that have refractory pain after radiation/surgery for cancer leading to current clinical trials.[33] Xeomin® has an even dose range with BOTOX® of 1:1 and clinical studies have documented equal efficacy and safety. Similar studies for spread or field of effect have been performed for IncoBTX-A as it relates to OnoA and AboBTX-A. These results also are inconclusive because of study design and conversion ratios. A comprehensive literature review concluded that neither molecular weight nor NAPs affect diffusion.[34]

Myobloc®, Neurobloc® (RimabotulinumtoxinB)
RimabotulinumtoxinB (RimaBTX-B) or Myobloc® or Neurobloc® is the only botulinum toxin product that is based on serotype B. It was approved by the FDA for the treatment of abnormal head positions and related pain of cervical dystonia in 2000. It has been found effective in other disorders and is also used in the aesthetic field for facial rhytides. It is produced as a uniform purified solution in ready-to-use vials injected as an intact complex. The units of activity differ from others with a concentration of 5000 U/mL, but the equivalency to BoNT-A-based units is a wide range of 1:125.[35]

Myobloc® is shown to be efficient in the treatment of hyperkinetic rhytides of the upper face including frown lines and forehead lines. It has a faster onset of effect, but a much shorter duration of effect than BoNT-A. Due to its broader effect it is thought to have more diffusion or spread. Because of side effects including pain of injection, headache and brow ptosis, and its shorter duration, it is less commonly used for cosmetic indications. It is not FDA approved for aesthetic purposes.

CURRENT NEUROTOXINS WITHOUT FDA APPROVAL (SEE CHAPTERS 4 AND 6)

Meditoxin®, Neuronox®, Neu-BoNT/A
Neuronox® is also derived from the Hall strain of *C. botulinum* and was approved in 2006 for the treatment of blepharospasms in South Korea. Since then, it has been studied and found to have a similar amino acid sequence to OnaBTX-A.[36] Additionally, Neuronox® has been shown to be equal to BOTOX with a 1:1 bioequivalence.[36,37] Neuronox® has completed phase 3 clinical trials for glabellar lines and has also been studied for masseter hypertrophy. Other studied conditions include blepharospasm, bruxism, equinus foot deformity, and muscle spasticity. Medytox Incorporated produces Neuronox®. It is approved under different brand names such as Botulift®, Siax®, Cunox®, and Meditoxin®. Though there is little molecular difference with OnaBTX-A, differences in manufacturing processes, such as purification and filtration, result in differences in molecular weight (925 kDa). It is also packaged as 100 mouse units per vial.[38]

Neuronox® has had extensive clinical trials for aesthetic usage in facial rhytides. In comparison to OnaBTX-A it has been found to have an efficacy-dosage of 1:1. Testing and clinical dose range studies have been performed for glabella, forehead, crow's feet, bunny lines and perioral rhytides. It is used commonly in Asia with similar patterns and dosage as OnaBTX-A.[39] A common usage in Asia is for masseter hypertrophy in which 10–40 units are used for each side. It has also been used to reduce the volume of muscles including temporalis, calf, and deltoid for cosmetic results. Medy-Tox Inc. has recently announced a liquid premixed injectable toxin as well, Innotox, but research studies are in progress.[40] This is being performed under a licensing agreement with Allergan, Inc. of Irvine, California.

Purtox®
Purtox was a promising new BoNT-A made by Mentor Worldwide LLC. Similar to Xeomin®, this product lacked NAPs and was a naked active neurotoxin. Purtox® was successful in clinical trials for glabellar lines and even completed phase 3 clinical trials in the United States. The clinical trials of this BoNT-A were very similar to findings with both OnaBTX-A and IncoBTX-A with onset, duration, and efficacy in frown lines. However, the manufacturer ultimately discontinued production in 2014 after acquisition by Johnson and Johnson.

Croma-Pharma
Croma-Pharma, founded in 1976 in Vienna, Austria innovates and distributes aesthetic products throughout the world. It has a BoNT-A now undergoing phase II clinical trials in the United States and Europe.

Evolus
Evolus is a BoNT-A produced in Santa Barbara, California by the company Evolus, Inc. and acquired by private equity firm, Strathspey Crown. It is partnered with Korean pharmaceutical company, Daewoong Pharmaceuticals, to manage clinical testing. Regulatory approval in the U.S. phase III testing of this BoNT-A product has just been completed with a glabellar line study.

RT001 (DaxibotulinumtoxinA [DaxiBTX-A])
The quest for a topically applied toxin has been promoted by many over the counter (OTC) cosmeceutical companies, but very little true research had been performed before Revance took the project seriously. Revance has developed a proprietary platform technology of a peptide that can carry molecules across the epidermal barrier (Figure 5.3). This will allow the transport of large molecular payloads across

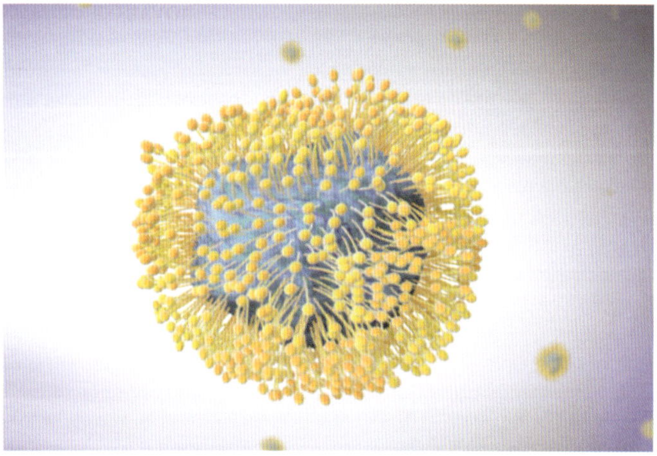

Figure 5.3 RT001 molecule including naked botulinum toxin plus peptide carrier.

the skin barrier. The proof of concept work has been performed with a variety of macromolecules including insulin, growth factors, and bioactive proteins. The 150 kD toxin molecule has also been successfully transported across the epidermal barrier through a combination of pathways including:

1. Lipid rafting; passive energy independent transcutaneous flux across non-living cells of the stratum corneum
2. Transcytosis; energy-dependent transport using micropinocytosis in and out of epidermal cells

This is accomplished by an excipient peptide carrier with covalent bands that carries the toxin molecule through the living epidermis. Once delivered to the dermis, the toxin will act the same as the injectable.[41] In clinical practice, the carrier and molecule are mixed and applied with a prototype applicator in the physician's office. The liquid which turns to a gel on the skin surface at room temperature should stay on the skin for 30 minutes and then washed off (Figure 5.4).

RT002 (DaxiBTX-A)

Revance has also tested the peptide carrier with its own proprietary 150 kD toxin as an injectable product. Initial studies as a glabellar frown line trial have been very favorable for both efficacy and safety. A phase 2 trial versus placebo demonstrated significant efficacy as well as duration over 6 months.[42] Various theories have been proposed to explain this result. The carrier protein may suspend the BoNT molecule for a longer duration surrounding the muscle sites creating a more prolonged action at the neuromuscular junctions. Further phase 3 studies are underway.

CBTX-A, Prosigne, Lantox

In 1993, the Chinese Ministry of Health approved CBTX-A for human use for a variety of neuromuscular conditions. CBTX-A received aesthetic approval for glabellar lines in 2012 by the Chinese Food and Drug Administration. However, this unique formulation of BoNT-A contains bovine gelatin, dextran, and sucrose and thus has an increased potential risk of allergenicity. In fact, at least two documented cases of adverse events have occurred and prior skin testing due to the bovine gelatin may be indicated before usage.[43,44] In one double-blind randomized crossover study, Prosigne demonstrated equal efficacy to OnaBTX-A.[45] However, another study suggested CBTX-A had greater diffusion using halos with Minor's test when compared to OnaBTX-A.[46] Although CBTX-A is also synthesized from the Hall strain of *C. botulinum*, more studies are needed in regard to safety, potency, diffusion, and bioequivalence.

CBTX-A has distribution in many countries including Korea, Brazil, Russia, and Ukraine (Esthetox-A). Clinical testing in Brazil found it to be favorable with BOTOX®.[47] It is not FDA approved for use in the United States.

CNBTxA

CNBTxA is produced by Nanfeng Medical Science and Technology Development Company and is not approved for use in any country. It is a superpotent BoNT-A that is known to be mislabeled. One study yielded 4.4 times higher concentration than the label claim when evaluated by a potency bioassay.[48] This mislabeling poses a significant health risk to patients. Patients treated with this product developed botulism as well as extended hospitalizations.[49,50] CNBTxA is not to be confused with CBTxA, although both are illegal in the United States along with any other unapproved BoNT products.

SUMMARY

There are only three BoNT-As approved by the FDA and presently available for cosmetic use in the United States. The clinician should be wary of nonapproved products which may be found on the Internet as cheaper or unusually compounded. These are illegal and more importantly dangerous as was found with the "TRI-toxin product," a rogue toxin promoted to doctors as a cheap mail-order product. Its usage in one Florida spa resulted in hospitalization of 4 patients due to extremely high dosage. Counterfeit products are also found on the Internet and these "knock offs" are either ineffective or dangerous (Figure 5.5).[51]

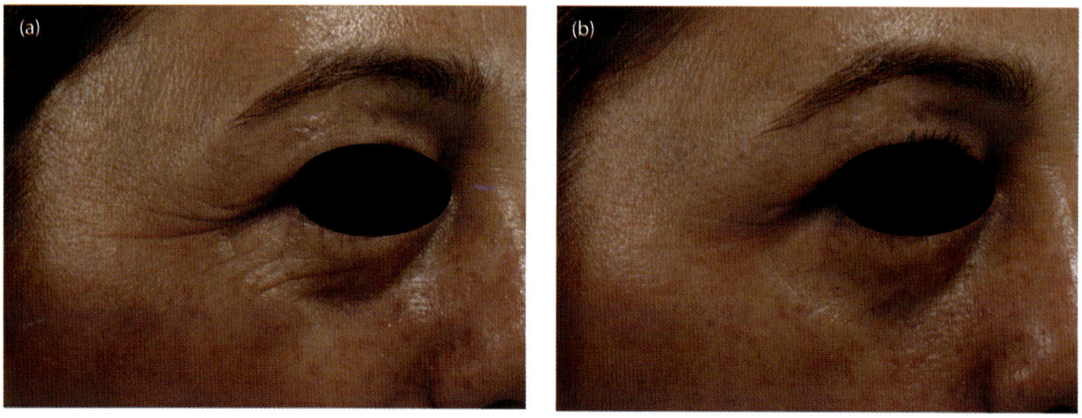

Figure 5.4 Topical application of the peptide-botulinum toxin complex for treatment of crows feet. Visible results: (a) Baseline; (b) 8 weeks post-treatment.

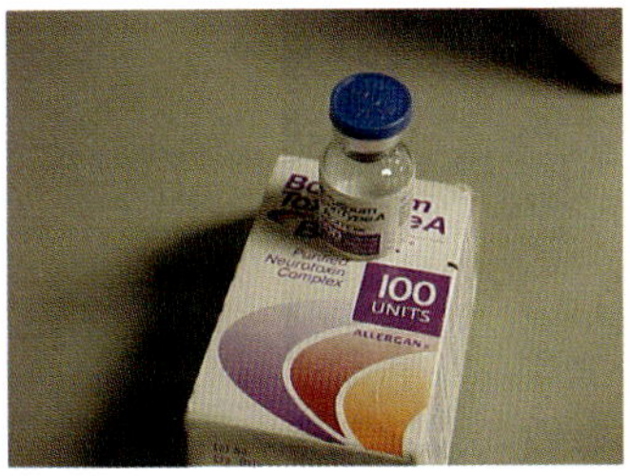

Discovered in Turkey and reportedly distributed through Russia (possibly manufactured in China). Product was evaluated at Allergan and found to yield low levels of BoNT-A

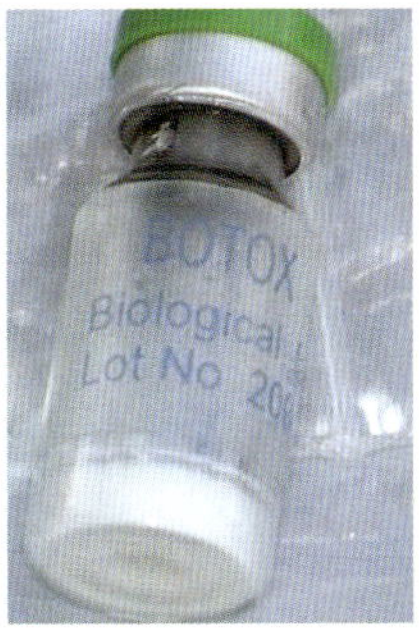

Found in the Philippines, apparently also from China

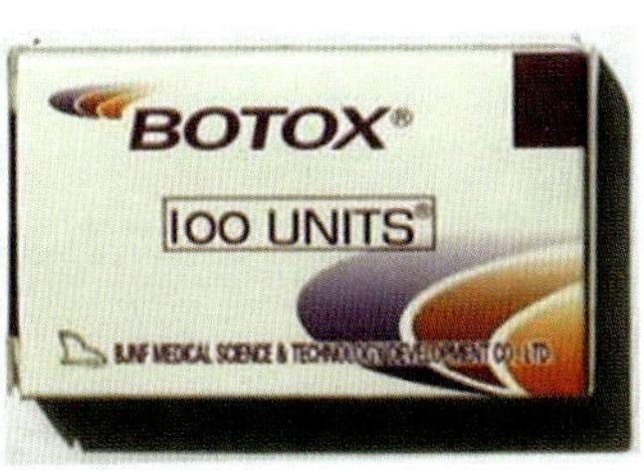

Advertised on the Internet as a "cheap" BOTOX from China, no actual product found yet

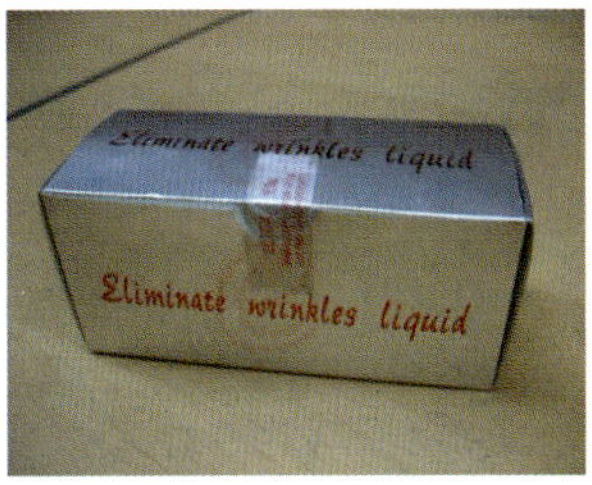

Discovered in Korea, appears to be of Chinese origin

Figure 5.5 Counterfeit products: a small but growing threat.

The research and development of new products and differences in future molecules is progressing around the world. The goals to increase duration, limit, or extend field of effect and increase efficacy with topical transcutaneous use will be a reality in the future as research continues. It is an exciting frontier with new horizons emerging regularly.

REFERENCES

1. Inoue K, Fujinaga Y, Watanabe T. Molecular composition of Clostridium botulinum type A progenitor toxins. *Infect Immun* 1996; 64(5): 1589–94.
2. Dasgupta BR. Botulinum neurotoxin: Studies on the structure and structure-biological activity relation. *Toxicon* 1979; 17: 41–101.
3. Cheng LW, Henderson TD II. Comparison of oral toxicological properties of botulinum neurotoxin serotypes A and B. *Toxicon* 2011; 58(1): 62–7.
4. Scott AB. Botulinum toxin injection into extraocular muscles as an alternative to strabismus surgery. *Ophthalmology* 1980; 87(10): 1044–9.
5. Pickett A. Dysport: Pharmacological properties and factors that influence toxin action. *Toxicon* 2009; 54(5): 683–9.
6. Carruthers JA, Lowe NJ, Menter MA, Gibson J, Nordquist M, Mordaunt J, Walker P, Eadie N. BOTOX Glabellar Lines I Study Group, a multicenter, double-blind, randomized, placebo-controlled study of the efficacy and safety of botulinum toxin type A in the treatment of glabellar lines. *J Am Acad Dermatol* 2002; 46(6): 840–9.
7. Ascher B, Zakine B, Kestemont P et al. A multicenter, randomized, double-blind, placebo-controlled study of efficacy and safety of 3 doses of botulinum toxin A in the treatment of glabellar lines. *J Am Acad Dermatol* 2004; 51(2): 223–33.
8. Schantz EJ, Johnson EA. Botulinum toxin: The story of its development for the treatment of human disease. *Perspect Biol Med* 1997; 40(3): 317–27.
9. Data on File. Allergan, Inc.; from Allergan Website: http://hcp.botoxcosmetic.com. Accessed July 19, 2015.
10. Binz T, Rummel A. Cell entry strategy of clostridial neurotoxins. *J Neurochem* 2009; 109(6): 1584–95.
11. Aoki KR, Ranoux D, Wissel J. Using translational medicine to understand clinical differences between botulinum toxin formulation. *European Journal of Neurology* 2006; 13: 10–9.
12. Kavanagh GM, Oh C, Shams K. Botox delivery by iontophoresis. *Br J Dermatol* 2004; 151(5): 1093–5
13. Andrade PC, Flores GP, Uscello Jde F, Miot HA, Morsoleto MJ. Use of iontophoresis or phonophoresis for delivering onabotulinumtoxinA in the treatment of palmar hyperhidrosis: A report on four cases. *An Bras Dermatol* 2011; 86(6): 1243–6.
14. Eisele KH, Taylor HV. Dissociation of the 900 kDa neurotoxin complex from c. botulinum under physiological conditions. *Toxicon* 2008; 51(supplement 1):10–10.
15. Eisele KH, Fink K, Vey M, Taylor HV. Studies on the dissociation of botulinum neurotoxin type A complexes. *Toxicon* 2011 Mar 15; 57(4): 555–65.
16. Trindade de Almeida AR, Marques E, de Almeida J, Cunha T, Boraso R. Pilot study comparing the diffusion of two formulations of botulinum toxin type A in patients with forehead hyperhidrosis. *Dermatol Surg* 2007; 33(1 Spec No.): S37–43.
17. Wohlfarth K, Schwandt I, Wegner F, Jürgens T, Gelbrich G, Wagner A, Bogdahn U, Schulte-Mattler W. Biological activity of two botulinum toxin type A complexes (Dysport and Botox) in volunteers: A double-blind, randomized, dose-ranging study. *J Neurol* 2008; 255(12): 1932–9.
18. Hexsel D, Dal'Forno T, Hexsel C, Do Prado DZ, Lima MM. A randomized pilot study comparing the action halos of two commercial preparations of botulinum toxin type A. *Dermatol Surg* 2008; 34(1): 52–9.
19. Eisele KH. Is there a role for complexing proteins in pharmaceutical neurotoxin formulations? *Presented at the International Masters Course on Aging Skin.* Jan 8–11, 2009. Paris, France.
20. Pickett A. Consistent biochemical data are essential for comparability of botulinum toxin type A products. *Drugs R D.* 2011; 11: 97–8.
21. Dressler D, Mander G, Fink K. Measuring the potency labelling of onabotulinumtoxinA (Botox(R)) and incobotulinumtoxinA (Xeomin (R)) in an LD50 assay. *J Neural Transm* 2012; 119: 13–5.
22. Karsai S, Adrian R, Hammes S, Thimm J, Raulin C. A randomized double-blind study of the effect of Botox and Dysport/Reloxin on forehead wrinkles and electromyographic activity. *Arch Dermatol* 2007; 143(11): 1447–9.
23. Brin MF, James C, Maltman J. Botulinum toxin type A products are not interchangeable: A review of the evidence. *Biologics: Targets & Therapy* 2014; 8: 227–41.
24. Benson J, Daugherty KK. Botulinum toxin A in the treatment of sialorrhea. *Ann Pharmacother* 2007; 41(1): 79–85.
25. Xiao Z, Qu G. Effects of botulinum toxin type A on collagen deposition in hypertrophic scars. *Molecules* 2012; 17(2): 2169–77. doi: 10.3390/molecules17022169
26. Gauglitz GG. Management of keloids and hypertrophic scars: Current and emerging options. *Clin Cosmet Investig Dermatol* 2013; 6: 103–14.
27. Zhibo X, Miaobo Z. Intralesional botulinum toxin type A injection as a new treatment measure for keloids. *Plast Reconstr Surg* 2009; 124(5): 275e–277e.
28. Gazerani P, Pedersen NS, Staahl C et al. Subcutaneous botulinum toxin type A reduces capsaicin-induced trigeminal pain vasomotor reactions in human skin. *Pain* 2009; 141: 60–9.
29. Walker TJ, Dayan SH. Comparison and overview of currently available neurotoxins. *J Clin Aesthet Dermatol* 2014; 7(2): 31–9.

30. Ipsen. *Dysport* Cosmesis Global Indications, May 2012. Data on file, Galderma Laboratories, L.P. from website https://www.dysportusa.com/what-is-dysport. Accessed August 23, 2017.
31. Rose AE, Goldberg DJ. Safety and efficacy of intradermal injection of botulinum toxin for the treatment of oily skin. *Dermatol Surg* 2013; 39(3 Pt 1): 443–8.
32. Ibrahim O, Keller EC, Arndt KA. Update on botulinum neurotoxin use in aesthetic dermatology. *Semin Cutan Med Surg* 2014; 33(4): 152–6.
33. Rostami R, Machado D, Richardson D, Jabbari B. Focal injection of Incobotulinum Toxin A improves refractory local cancer pain at the site of radiation/surgery. *Poster Session III, Neurologic Complications of Cancer*. April 29, 2014.
34. Brodsky MA, Swope DM, Grimes D. Diffusion of botulinum toxins. *Tremor and Other Hyperkinetic Movements* 2012; 2: tre-02-85-417-1.
35. Callaway JE. Botulinum toxin type B (Myobloc): Pharmacology and biochemistry. *Clin Dermatol* 2004; 22(1): 23–8.
36. Yang GH, Jung HH. A new botulinum toxin potentially bioequivalent to onabotulinumtoxinA: Are there any differences at all? *Dermatol Surg* 2013; 39(1 Pt 2): 165–70.
37. Won CH, Lee HM, Lee WS et al. Efficacy and safety of a novel botulinum toxin type A product for the treatment of moderate to severe glabellar lines: A randomized, double-blind, active-controlled multicenter study. *Dermatol Surg* 2013; 39(1 Pt 2): 171–8.
38. Yoon JS, Kim JC, Lee SY. Double-blind, randomized, comparative study of Meditoxin versus Botox in the treatment of essential blepharospasm. *Korean J Ophthalmol* 2009; 23(3): 137–41.
39. Rho NK, Kim HS, Kim YS et al. Botulinum toxin type A for facial wrinkles and benign masseter hypertrophy in Korean patients. *Korean J Dermatol* 2010; 48(10): 823–31.
40. Data on file, Medytox website; from Allergan website: http://www.medy-tox.co.kr/en_new/html/intro_1_04.php. Accessed July 26, 2015.
41. Kaplan IM, Wadia JS, Dowdy SF. Cationic TAT peptide transduction domain enters cells by macropinocytosis. *J Control Release* 2005; 102(1): 247–53.
42. Carruthers J, Solish N, Humphrey S, Rosen N, Muhn C, Bertucci V, Swift A et al. Injectable DaxibotulinumtoxinA for the treatment of glabellar lines: A Phase 2, randomized, dose-ranging, double-blind, multicenter comparison with OnabotulinumtoxinA and placebo. *Dermatol Surg*. 2017; Jun 12.
43. Wu CJ, Shen JH, Chen Y, Lian YJ. Comparison of two different formulations of botulinum toxin A for the treatment of blepharospasm and hemifacial spasm. *Turk Neurosurg* 2011; 21(4): 625–9.
44. Careta MF, Delgado L, Patriota R. Report of allergic reaction after application of botulinum toxin. *Aesthet Surg J* 2015; 35(5):NP102–5.
45. Rieder CR, Schestatsky P, Socal MP et al. A double-blind, randomized, crossover study of Prosigne® versus Botox® in patients with blepharospasm and hemifacial spasm. *Clin Neuropharmacol* 2007; 30(1): 39–42.
46. Jiang HY, Chen S, Zhou J, Leung KK, Yu P. Diffusion of two botulinum toxins type A on the forehead: Double-blinded, randomized, controlled study. *Dermatol Surg* 2014; 40(2): 184–92.
47. Talarico S. *Chinese Cosmetic Toxin*. International Masters Course on Aging Skin. Paris, January 28, 2012. Presentation.
48. Hunt T, Clarke K. Potency of the botulinum toxin product CNBTX-A significantly exceeds labeled units in standard potency test. *J Am Acad Dermatol* 2008; 58(3): 517–18.
49. Chertow DS, Tan ET, Maslanka SE et al. Botulism in 4 Adults following cosmetic injections with an unlicensed, highly concentrated botulinum preparation. *JAMA* 2006; 296: 2476–9.
50. Souayah N, Karim H, Kamin SS, McArdle J, Marcus S. Severe botulism after focal injection of botulinum toxin. *Neurology* 2006; 67: 1855–6.
51. Chertow DS, Tan ET, Maslanka SE, Schulte J, Bresnitz EA, Weisman RS, Bernstein J et al. Botulism in 4 adults following cosmetic injections with an unlicensed, highly concentrated botulinum preparation. *JAMA* 2006; 296(20): 2476–9.

6 The different botulinum toxins from around the world available for clinical use

Andy Pickett

INTRODUCTION

Botulinum toxin (BoNT) has been one of the most successful products ever developed in the world of pharmaceuticals. Since the first publication from Alan Scott in the 1970s[1] on the potential medical application of the molecule, use of BoNT products in both therapeutic and aesthetic treatments has grown year-on-year. Following the first licensure of the products in the late 1980s, nearly 30 years ago, their use has widened and expanded throughout the world. The applicability of BoNT to bringing real benefit to patients in a multitude of ways cannot be overstated. Although not life-saving, the BoNT products have clearly improved the quality of life of many people and have become a mainstay of many key and often untreatable areas of neurology, urology, and pain, as well as the aesthetic uses they have become equally famous for. New uses are regularly identified, especially in areas such as dermatology and these are almost universally shown to be of important clinical value for patient treatment.

The true size of the BoNT market is difficult to determine. Accurate data are available for therapeutic uses, but no equivalent data exist for the aesthetic marketplace. Estimates in the order of over $3 billion are currently available,[2] growing many times over the next decade.[3] However, the potential financial scale could be described as limitless, given the number of new uses emerging and the ever-growing routine use of the products across such a wide range of applications. Perhaps the only restriction on this growth is the time taken and data required for the official registration of each new indication with each country's regulatory authority.

There were initially two commercial BoNT products—Oculinum® and Dysport® (otherwise known as AbobotulinumtoxinA [AboBTX-A]). Oculinum® was pioneered by Alan Scott through his company Oculinum Inc., using the results he had obtained across a wide range of treatments he had given at the Smith-Kettlewell Institute, California.[4] Dysport®, pioneered through doctors and the Centre for Applied Microbiology and Research, was produced in the United Kingdom after several U.K. doctors had trained with Alan Scott and realized the significant potential of the product to treat difficult diseases, such as strabismus, which only had surgical interventions until then.[5] Oculinum was purchased by Allergan soon after licensing in the United States and became BOTOX® (otherwise known as OnabotulinumtoxinA [OnaBTX-A]). The background to how Oculinum came into being has been described recently.[6] BOTOX became firmly established in the United States and, shortly afterward, Europe and the rest of the world. Dysport did not reach the United States until 2009, for many reasons (not yet described), but this gave a virtual monopoly in the United States to Allergan for many years and enabled the brand to become world-dominant.

Both of these first-generation serotype A products contain the active toxin complexed with a range of other natural accessory proteins, often termed Neurotoxin-Associated Proteins (NAPs).[7] Despite much argument over many years between the companies who commercialize BoNT products, these NAPs have been found to clearly separate from the active BoNT on reconstitution in the vial, before injection[8] and have no known role for the pharmaceutical action or even stabilization of the active toxin components, notably when the products are used clinically. In addition, no detrimental effects or clinical significance have been identified to date from their presence. This is of course contrary to the role that NAPs have when toxin is ingested as a food poison.[9]

After the initial introduction of the two type A products, many years passed before another BoNT product became available. In fact, serotype F was the next new BoNT that went into clinical testing in several countries long before the advent of the type B product Neurobloc®/Myobloc®.[10] Several publications exist on the use of type F, but these development products had a short duration of action and the variant was never commercialized. Neurobloc®/Myobloc® has also not been an especially successful product mainly due to the high doses required and immuno resistance in many patients through repeated use. The scientific basis as to why serotype B BoNT is required in these high doses for clinical effects, has only recently been identified and this is due to inefficiencies in one of the receptors specifically in humans (and chimpanzees).[11] The product has been bought and sold several times by the owning companies during its history. Use of BoNT-B for aesthetic treatments has been reported,[12–14] but is not used in practice or licensed for this use and will not be considered further here.

In the early 2000s, a new serotype A product emerged from work in Germany by several scientists experienced in the field[15,16] and the product was finally assigned to the German company Merz. Their product, Xeomin® (otherwise known as IncobotulinumtoxinA [IncoBTX-A]), was first approved for commercial sale in Germany in 2006. Xeomin has since become available in 49 countries.[17] The product has distinguishing properties of being complex-protein free, with a high concentration of the stabilizer human serum albumin (HSA), and has been granted storage under qualified room temperature conditions (less than 25°C or 30°C, depending on the country of registration). As such, Xeomin could be considered a second-generation BoNT after the initial, complexed type A products.

CURRENT MAIN BoNT PRODUCTS

The three main serotype A products, BOTOX®, Dysport®, and Xeomin®, dominate the world market. Their characteristics have been reported many times in the literature as tables of so-called "key" product data. However, these data are often incorrect or irrelevant to the clinician using the products in practice.[18] Worse still, the apparent "differences" have been used commercially to distinguish one product from another and to attempt to demonstrate superiority of one product over another.[19] Such publications could be sponsored by the manufacturers of the products. Great care needs to be taken when reviewing such publications for useful information.

The characteristics of the main product families are presented in Table 6.1. The key aspect, without doubt, is that the potency units of each product are specific to that product family alone and cannot be readily interchanged between the products. There are no universally accepted "conversion factors" and, indeed, promotion of conversions by any company is strictly prohibited throughout the world by the regulatory authorities. For example, there have been many attempts in the past to say that one product has the same units as another, or that one product can be interchanged with another based on a certain "unit ratio". This has, however, not been borne out in routine, large-scale clinical use of the products as compared to what has been demonstrated in the (relatively) small clinical trials carried out for registration purposes. Much time and effort has really been wasted over the years in relation to these product unit conversions when simple, widescale clinical use is the key to this understanding.

Table 6.1 Major Botulinum Toxin Brands Worldwide Available for Aesthetic Use

Product™	Company	Country	Bacterial production strain	Process	u/vial (product specific)[a]	Excipients (in vial)[b]
Dysport/Dyslor/Azzalure	Ipsen/Galderma	France/Switzerland	Hall	Precipitation, dialysis, chromatography	125/300/500	0.125 mg HSA 2.5 mg lactose
BOTOX®/BOTOX® Cosmetic/Vistabel/Vistabex/Vista	Allergan Inc.	US/Ireland	Hall-hyper	Acid precipitations, dialysis	50/100/200	0.5 mg HSA 0.9 mg NaCl
Xeomin/Xeomin Cosmetic/Bocouture	Merz GmbH	Germany	Hall ATCC 3502	Unknown	50/100/200	1 mg HSA 4.7 mg sucrose

Source: By courtesy of Toxin Science Limited, 2017.
Note: All products are either freeze-dried (Dysport and Xeomin families) or vacuum-dried (BOTOX family).
[a]The potency units of each product are specific to that product and are not interchangeable with those for other BoNT products.
[b]HSA: human serum albumin.

Table 6.2 Botulinum Toxin Products from Asia, Current as of early 2017

Product™	Company	Country	Bacterial production strain	Process	u/vial (product specific)	Excipients (in vial)[a]
BTXA/Prosigne/Redux/Lantox/Lanzox/Liftox	Lanzhou Institute of Biological Products/Hugh Source International	China	Hall	Crystallization, dialysis	50/100 u	5 mg Gelatin 25 mg Dextran 25 mg Sucrose
Meditoxin/Neuronox/Siax/Botulift/Cunox	Medy-Tox Inc.	South Korea	Hall	Acid precipitations, dialysis	50/100/200 u	0.5 mg HSA 0.9 mg NaCl
Innotox/MT10109L (Liquid product)	Medy-Tox Inc.	South Korea	Hall	Unknown	25/50 u	No human serum albumin or animal products
Coretox/MT10107	Medy-Tox Inc.	South Korea	Hall	Unknown	100 u	Methionine Polysorbate 20 Sucrose
Botulax/Zentox/Regenox	Hugel Pharma	South Korea	CBFC26	Protamine sulphate DEAE sepharose chromatography	50/100/200 u	0.5 mg HSA 0.9 mg NaCl
Nabota/Evosyal (DWP 450)	Daewoong Pharmaceutical Co. Ltd.	South Korea	Hall	High-Pure Technology® (patented)	50/100/200 u	0.5 mg HSA 0.9 mg NaCl

Source: By courtesy of Toxin Science Limited, 2017.
[a]Concentrations of excipients may depend on the number of units in vial.

Contrary to certain statements and published information,[20] BoNT-A products are interchangeable in clinical use (even though the potency units are not) and many patients have been successfully changed between different products. The key to successful changeover is linked almost exclusively to the dose (number of units) given in treatment.

ASIAN BoNT PRODUCTS

Other BoNT-A products have steadily emerged as licensed products from certain countries throughout the world and have gradually gained market positions with the notable exception of Europe and North America, where they remain currently unavailable. Six of these products have come from Asia, five from South Korea alone (Table 6.2).

The oldest of the Asian BoNTs is BTXA™ from Lanzhou Institute of Biological Products in China (licensed since 1997). This product is unique in the world in using both dextran and gelatine as stabilizers instead of the traditional Human Serum Albumin (HSA) found in the majority of the other products. The presence of these stabilizers carries a degree of risk for the product and that is not the case with all the other BoNTs, namely the possibility of anaphylactic shock to the gelatin.[21] Significant side effects have been reported for this Chinese product.[22] Other issues related to, for example, the provenance of the bovine gelatin used, have not been adequately addressed in the limited supporting information available. Details on these aspects have to be sought from the main distributor's website.

Most of the five Korean BoNT products (Table 6.2) have been developed, as stated by those companies, as "copies" of BOTOX. Their formulations are similar or the same as BOTOX but the manufacturing processes are different and different strains of the production organisms are used.[23] Clinical trials of these products have slowly been published and often show that the potency units of the products are different to each other. Often, head-to-head aesthetic clinical trials, at the same dosage as BOTOX, have shown significant differences in results.[23] Unfortunately, these limited trials can be used by the manufacturers to claim somewhat improved results when compared to the reference product they have tested.[23] This only serves to emphasize the statement included on prescribing information and product literature for all licensed products worldwide, that the potency units of each product are specific to that product and are not interchangeable.

EMERGING BoNT PRODUCTS

Regional BoNT Products

In addition to the Asian toxins now available, there are other regional products that have arrived to find limited use in various countries. Typical examples are shown in Table 6.3.

Table 6.3 New Local Botulinum Toxin Products Currently Available, Late 2017

Product™	Company	Country	U/vial (product specific)	Excipients (in vial)
Masport	Masoondarou Company	Iran	500 U	0.5 mg HSA 2.5 mg Lactose
Relatox/ Relatoks	Microgen Company	Russia	50/100 U	6 mg Gelatin 5 mg Maltose
BOTOGENIE®	Bio Med Pvt. Ltd.	India	50/100 U	5 mg Lactose[a]
BTXA	Intas Pharmaceuticals Ltd.	India	100 U	Unknown

Source: By courtesy of Toxin Science Limited, 2017.
[a]Sterile saline diluent supplied with product.

There are limited clinical data for some of these products, but these data are difficult to obtain.[24–28] Further, very limited information is available from company websites. Sometimes, a video of a specific product use is posted on YouTube[29] or a clinical trial's database is useful for information[30] detailing trials used for registration purposes. There is no clear information available as to exactly why these regional products have been developed, but the main reason is believed to be the provision of a cheaper, local alternative to the main branded products through local manufacture.

Topical Products

One area of work directed toward aesthetic treatments is the development of so-called "topical" toxin products. The objective of all these products is to deliver sufficient BoNT by application to the skin in place of hypodermic injection.

Many companies were working in this area for many years (Table 6.4), the most notable being the Californian company Revance, who had been active in the field since 2002. Published data on their RT001 product has shown a limited efficacy for treatment of specific facial areas, notably lateral canthal lines (crow's feet).[31] The available clinical data are quite difficult to interpret especially regarding the dose applied to produce effects, but generally this is likely to be manyfold that of the dose effective by injection. The transport mechanism for BoNT across the dermal layers also appears to be highly inefficient, given the very high doses of active BoNT that are needed to achieve any effect[31,32]—equivalent to some 2500 AboBTX-A units per administration compared to approximately 60 units of an injected product. This is also true for other animal models where a topical product has been used (intranasal administration) and where doses have been very high (approximately 400 units/kg body weight for rats and 165,000 units/kg for guinea pigs).[33] Such high doses pose difficult issues about product safety and handling, perhaps adding to the reasons why no topical product has yet been approved for clinical use. Indeed, Revance had developed a proprietary device to prepare and administer their topical product to deal with these handling issues.

However, Revance announced in June 2016 that their RT001 topical product had unambiguously failed to meet the co-primary and other trial endpoints.[34] Consequently, the company decided to end their topical program for crow's feet and also their work on axillary hyperhidrosis. Instead, the company refocused on its injectable BoNT program, now only to be distinguished from other products on the different formulation being used.

The issue of the high dose needed for topical administration may also be one reason why, with a difficult regulatory path, Revance had earlier adopted a business model incorporating an injectable version of its product (RT002) with its carrier. Claims that this injectable version has an extended duration of action when compared to the other mainstream products, are not actually borne out when the clinical data are closely examined.[35] A recent publication has shown that, when the dose is *doubled* for treatment of glabellar lines (GL) (in comparison to an already licensed BoNT product), a marginal increase in duration of effect can be obtained.[35] This so-called "improvement" is likely to also be the case if doses are doubled with the already approved products. Indeed, more recent presentations (and now publication) of data from Phase 2 GL trials of RT002 by Revance investigators really do not show an advantage over an existing licensed product used as a comparator, even at much higher RT002 doses (and despite the various interpretations of data shown).[36,37] Revance has been the subject of much speculation and share price movement in response to its publicizing of its data over the years, but the certainty that a topical aesthetic BoNT will reach the market and, most importantly, be a useful and efficacious product over years, seems very unlikely. Other companies publicizing their work on topical toxins have yet to provide any substantial clinical trial data for peer review.

Towards Purified and Liquid Products

A clear development has started within the worldwide BoNT market for the next-generation of injectable products. These are generally based on higher purity BoNT, no HSA stabilizer and liquid format, or combinations of these.

The first of these products to reach the marketplace is Innotox® (also called MT10109L) from MedyTox in South Korea (Table 6.2), which has been licensed in South Korea. The product contains no HSA, is in a liquid format but is still a BoNT in the complexed form. Limited comparative clinical data have been published.[38] In January 2014, Allergan Inc. completed a license agreement with MedyTox for rights to develop and commercialize, if approved, certain products

Table 6.4 Development of Topical Botulinum Toxin Products Worldwide, 2017

Company	Country	Product name	Technology	Clinical data published	Comment
Revance	United States	RT001-RTT150	TransMTS®	Yes	Work stopped on topical products (June 2016)
Transdermal Corp.	Canada	CosmeTox	InParT (mixed micelles/ ionic nanoparticles)	Yes	
Anterios	United States	ANT-1207 lotion	Unknown	No	Company purchased by Allergan (January 2016)
Malvern Cosmeceutics Ltd	United Kingdom	MCL005-2 gel	Unknown	No	

Source: By courtesy of Toxin Science Limited, 2017.

from MedyTox including a liquid-format BoNT. The exact status of this product within Allergan's development portfolio is currently unclear, but no U.S. clinical trials of an Allergan liquid BoNT product have yet been initiated at the time of writing. This apparent lack of progress has just been recently (February 2017) highlighted by the CEO of Medytox.[39]

MedyTox has also developed a new product, Coretox® (also called MT10107), Table 6.2, which contains BoNT free from NAPs (complexing proteins) and in a formulation with no HSA; the product is freeze-dried with polysorbate 20, methionine, and sucrose as stabilizers[40]: doubtless a liquid version will be tested in the near future. Coretox was first licensed in South Korea in mid-2016.

Of the main players in the BoNT world, Ipsen has nearly completed the clinical testing of a liquid version of Dysport, labeled DNG (Dysport Next Generation). The product has completed Phase 2 and 3 clinical trials in cervical dystonia and Phase 2 trials for the treatment of GL. Phase 3 aesthetic trials are currently underway.[41,42] Unfortunately, the Phase 3 cervical dystonia trials did not meet their primary endpoint, indicating that DNG was in fact marginally inferior to the reference product tested, Dysport.[43] However, the product was efficacious and safe in the comparisons against placebo. No data are yet available from the Phase 3 aesthetic trials, but the Phase 2 data have been presented at an international meeting.[44]

The dermatology company Galderma, the partner to Ipsen for the marketing and distribution of Dysport and Azzalure in aesthetics, has also announced the clinical trials of a liquid, high purity BoNT product.[45–47] No clinical data are yet available for this product.

Based on these quite extensive new activities in the BoNT arena, the likelihood that liquid products could be considered the next generation of products to reach the marketplace must be high.

Alternative Administration Techniques

Alternative methods of BoNT injection are also receiving attention. In particular, the actual syringe injection method has been modified to utilize devices that can provide accurate dosing and more convenience to the injector.

The Swiss company Primequal[48] and the Dutch company TSK[49] have developed and marketed injection devices specifically for BoNT injections. TSK has additionally developed a range of very fine injection needles, down to 33 gauge and with a low dead-space hub, designed for BoNT aesthetic administration.[50] There is little doubt that very fine injection needles bring more comfort and less pain to the patient.[51,52] With respect to the injection devices, these are perhaps more targeted to the clinician just starting out with BoNT treatments. They can be helpful in ensuring the correct dosage is administered repeatedly and, if the clinician is using different products, can be adapted easily for the different injection volumes recommended by each BoNT manufacturer.

One alternative method has been to incorporate BoNT administration into jet nebulization to minimize patient pain, notably when given for different types of hyperhidrosis.[53,54] The results obtained demonstrate less pain for the patient than experienced by needle injection, but the issues surrounding aerosol generation of BoNT in solution require addressing.

FUTURE PROSPECTS FOR CLINICAL BoNT PRODUCTS

Some five new BoNT products are currently known to be in development in South Korea.[55] How many of these differ from existing products is currently unknown, although at least one of these (Hutox: Huons Global) is already publicizing their product as a purified BoNT complex again similar to BOTOX: the product has yet go through clinical trials and does not feature on the company website. Indeed, Huons have recently publicised that they are already selling their product in various overseas markets, despite not yet having secured approval from their home South Korean market for any indication.[56] One development product, Protox, from DSK, is making claims about a lower diffusion, but this has apparently only been demonstrated in animal models to date.[57]

In August 2017, the Californian company Bonti announced their Phase 2A clinical trial results of a new product based on serotype E used for GL treatment.[58] Bonti emerged early in 2016 as a company working in the field of BoNT, although having formed in 2015. The advantages of using serotype E, a fast acting but very short duration BoNT, for the treatment of an aesthetic condition such as GL, remains to be clarified since a long duration of effect is often a very important result that patients seek following treatment. Their data on onset have yet to be compared with those obtained for the already licensed serotype A products, to determine if onset of effect was faster or not.

Finally, the area of modified BoNT molecules with new or enhanced properties has been in vogue for many years. The company Syntaxin, now owned by Ipsen, originally spun out of the UK Centre for Applied Microbiology and Research, has been the most notable in the field with publications in the area going back 20 years. The main molecules under consideration are termed Targeted Secretion Inhibitors (TSI) and use modified BoNT molecules to retarget their activity to different cell types where normally BoNT is not active.[59] Two molecules from Syntaxin were in early clinical studies through their partnership with Allergan (one is named Senrebotase [AGN-214868]), but the doses of these modified molecules needed to obtain effects are considerably higher than the native BoNT.[60,61] As such, subjects such as the development of immunogenic responses, in response to a higher therapeutic protein load, will feature more heavily than for the native molecules, which use only nanograms of BoNT protein to gain significant effects. At the time of writing, Allergan is believed to have discontinued development of the product for both of the initially targeted indications, namely overactive bladder and post-herpetic neuralgia.[62]

A range of other, modified BoNT molecules are currently in development around the world for various targeted applications. Further discussion of these is beyond the scope of the present chapter.

From its early beginnings of few products, the global market for BoNT has grown significantly and now features a range of products, both global and local. There is also considerable research and development on new products for specific, targeted uses. The future of BoNT is therefore as bright today as it was in the very first years of availability, now over 30 years ago.

Note: The comments, statements and opinions expressed by Dr. Pickett are those of the author and Toxin Science Limited only.

REFERENCES

1. Scott AB, Rosenbaum A, Collins CC. Pharmacologic weakening of extraocular muscles. *Invest Ophthalmol* 1973; 12(12): 924–7.
2. http://www.grandviewresearch.com/industry-analysis/botulinum-toxin-market. Accessed March 3, 2017.
3. http://www.grandviewresearch.com/press-release/global-botulinum-toxin-market. Accessed March 3, 2017.
4. Scott AB. Botulinum toxin treatment of strabismus. *Am Orthop J* 1985; 35: 28–29.
5. Elston JS, Russell RW. Effect of treatment with botulinum toxin on neurogenic blepharospasm. *Br Med J (Clin Res Ed)* 1985; 290(6485), 1857-9.
6. Pickett A. Historical aspects of botulinum toxin used clinically: Part I: is that the right serotype? *Botulinum J* 2013; 2(3/4): 176–8.

7. Fu FN, Sharma SK, Singh BR. A protease-resistant novel hemagglutinin purified from type A Clostridium botulinum. *J Protein Chem* 1998; 17(1): 53–60.
8. Eisele KH et al. Studies on the dissociation of botulinum neurotoxin type A complexes. *Toxicon* 2011; 57(4): 555–65.
9. Fujinaga Y, Sugawara Y, Matsumura T. Uptake of botulinum neurotoxin in the intestine. *Curr Top Microbiol Immunol* 2013; 364: 45–59.
10. Pickett A. Historical aspects of botulinum toxin used clinically: Part II: overcoming resistance. *Botulinum J* 2015; 3(1): 34–40.
11. Strotmeier J. et al. Human synaptotagmin-II is not a high affinity receptor for botulinum neurotoxin B and G: increased therapeutic dosage and immunogenicity. *FEBS Lett* 2012; 586(4): 310–3.
12. Alster TS, Lupton JR. Botulinum toxin type B for dynamic glabellar rhytides refractory to botulinum toxin type A. *Dermatol Surg* 2003; 29(5): 516–8.
13. Sadick NS. Prospective open-label study of botulinum toxin type B (Myobloc) at doses of 2,400 and 3,000 U for the treatment of glabellar wrinkles. *Dermatol Surg* 2003; 29(5): 501-7; discussion 507.
14. Carruthers A et al. Dose-finding, safety, and tolerability study of botulinum toxin type B for the treatment of hyperfunctional glabellar lines. *Dermatol Surg* 2007; 33(1 Spec No.): S60-8.
15. Erdal E et al. Processing of tetanus and botulinum A neurotoxins in isolated chromaffin cells. *Naunyn Schmiedebergs Arch Pharmacol* 1995; 351(1): 67–78.
16. Friday D, Bigalke H, Frevert J. In vitro stability of botulinum toxin complex preparations at physiological pH and temperature. *International Conference on Basic and Therapeutic Aspects of Botulinum and Tetanus Toxins*. 2002.
17. http://www.xeomin.com/consumers/about-xeomin/experience-xeomin/. Accessed March 3, 2017.
18. Pickett A. Reviews of botulinum toxin products in aesthetic use must be accurate, clear and avoid speculation. *Clin Pharmacol* 2013; 5: 149–52.
19. Pickett A. Immunogenicity issues related to botulinum toxins in clinical use cannot be answered by speculation about product characteristics. *BioDrugs* 2013; 27(1): 83–4.
20. Brin MF, James C, Maltman J. Botulinum toxin type A products are not interchangeable: a review of the evidence. *Biologics* 2014; 8: 227–41.
21. Kamin W et al. Anaphylaxis after vaccination due to hypersensitivity to gelatin. *Klin Padiatr* 2006; 218(2): 92–4.
22. Careta MF, Delgado L, Patriota R. Report of allergic reaction after application of botulinum toxin. *Aesthet Surg J* 2015; 35(5): NP102-5.
23. Kim BJ et al. Double-blind, randomized non-inferiority trial of a novel botulinum toxin A processed from the strain CBFC26, compared with onabotulinumtoxin A in the treatment of glabellar lines. *J Eur Acad Dermatol Venereol* 2014; 28(12): 1761–7.
24. Elkin VD et al. Results of clinical trials of the safety and efficacy of the first Russian botulotoxinum type a Relatox® in the correction of mimic wrinkles [in Russian]. *Exp Clin Dermatocosmol* 2011; 6(2): 6–12.
25. Plotnikova EV, Elkin VD. Experimental and clinical test on safety and medical effectivness of native botulinic toxin of A-type Relatox® for correction of wrinkles [in Russian]. *Family Health - the 21st Century* 2011; 4.
26. Plotnikova, EV, Elkin, VD, Demchuk, ND, Mironov, AN. et al. Potentialities of esthetic correction of the face by botulotoxin A in complex with hemagglutinin [in Russian]. *Russian Journal of Skin and Venereal Diseases* 2013; 1: 54–7.
27. Plotnikova EV, Elkin VD. Results of Relatox treatment for cosmetic defects of the face [in Russian]. *Experimental & Clinical Dermatocosmology [Eksp Klin Dermatokosmetol]* 2013; 6: 3–6.
28. Churin AA et al. Study of Subchronic Toxicity of Relatox on Sexually Immature Animals. *Bull Exp Biol Med* 2015; 160(1): 53–6.
29. Botogenie from BioMed India. https://www.youtube.com/watch?v=Osd4TGEIGma. Accessed August 23, 2017.
30. Iranian clinical trials database http://www.irct.ir/searchresult.php?keyword=&id=14871&number=1&prt=5564&total=10&m=1. Accessed February 12, 2016.
31. Glogau R. et al. Results of a randomized, double-blind, placebo-controlled study to evaluate the efficacy and safety of a botulinum toxin type A topical gel for the treatment of moderate-to-severe lateral canthal lines. *J Drugs Dermatol* 2012; 11(1): 38–45.
32. Brandt F et al. Efficacy and safety evaluation of a novel botulinum toxin topical gel for the treatment of moderate to severe lateral canthal lines. *Dermatol Surg* 2010; 36(Suppl 4): 2111-8.
33. Zhu Z. et al. A novel botulinum neurotoxin topical gel: Treatment of allergic rhinitis in rats and comparative safety profile. *Am J Rhinol Allergy* 2012; 26(6): 450–4.
34. http://investors.revance.com/releasedetail.cfm?ReleaseID=975537. Accessed March 3, 2017.
35. Garcia-Murray E. et al. Safety and efficacy of RT002, an injectable botulinum toxin type A, for treating glabellar lines: Results of a Phase 1/2, open-label, sequential dose-escalation study. *Dermatol Surg* 2015; 41(Suppl 1): S47-55.
36. *Data presented at TOXINS 2017*, Madrid, Spain, January 2017 and IMCAS Paris, January 2017.
37. Carruthers J, Solish N, Humphrey S, Rosen N, Muhn C, Bertucci V et al. Injectable daxibotulinumtoxinA for the treatment of Glabellar lines: A phase 2, randomized, dose-ranging, double-blind, multicenter comparison with onabotulinumtoxinA and placebo. *Dermatol Surg.* 2017. doi: 10.1097/DSS.0000000000001206.
38. Kim JE et al. The efficacy and safety of liquid-type botulinum toxin type A for the management of moderate to severe glabellar frown lines. *Plast Reconstr Surg* 2015; 135(3): 732–41.
39. http://www.theinvestor.co.kr/view.php?ud=20170224000539. Accessed March 3, 2017.
40. Oh HM et al. Efficacy and safety of a new botulinum toxin type A free of complexing proteins. *Toxins (Basel)* 2015; 8(1). doi:10.3390/toxins8010001.
41. http://clinicaltrials.gov/ct2/show/NCT02353871?term=nct02353871&rank=1. Accessed February 14, 2016.
42. https://clinicaltrials.gov/ct2/show/NCT02493946?term=nct02493946&rank=1. Accessed February 14, 2016.
43. http://www.ipsen.com/wp-content/uploads/2014/02/05-02-2014-PR-Dysport-Next-Generation-EN.pdf 5th February 2014. Accessed February 14, 2016.
44. Ascher B et al. Efficacy and safety of a ready-to-use liquid formulation of abobotulinumtoxinA in moderate to severe glabellar lines: results of a phase II randomised, placebo controlled clinical trial. *Poster presented at Toxins 2015*, Lisbon, Portugal, January 14–17, 2015.
45. *Presentation by Humberto C. Antunes to IMCAS Annual Meeting*, IMCAS Paris, January 2014.
46. http://www.galderma.com/Media/Press-releases/articleType/ArticleView/articleld/40/Galderma-initiates-clinical-development-of-novel-muscle-relaxant 6th June 2013. Accessed February 14, 2016.
47. http://www.galderma.com/Media/Press-releases/articleType/ArticleView/articleld/70/Galderma-Initiates-US-Study-of-Novel-Muslce-Relaxant-for-Aesthetic-Dermatology-and-Cosmetic-Surgery 6th October 2014. Accessed February 14, 2016.
48. http://www.primequal.com/der_talent_bp.php. Accessed February 14, 2016.

49. https://tsklab.nl/bont-syringes/. Accessed February 14, 2016.
50. https://tsklab.nl/bont-needles/. Accessed February 14, 2016.
51. Sezgin B. et al. The effect of microneedle thickness on pain during minimally invasive facial procedures: A clinical study. *Aesthet Surg J* 2014; 34(5): 757–765.
52. Alam M. et al. Effect of needle size on pain perception in patients treated with botulinum toxin type A injections: A randomized clinical trial. *JAMA Dermatol* 2015; 151(11): 1194–9.
53. Nantel-Battista M, Vadeboncoeur S, Benohanian A. Selection of safe parameters for jet injection of botulinum toxin in palmar hyperhidrosis. *Aesthet Surg J* 2013; 33(2): 295–7.
54. Iannitti T. et al. A preliminary study of painless and effective transdermal botulinum toxin A delivery by jet nebulization for treatment of primary hyperhidrosis. *Drug Des Devel Ther* 2014; 8: 931–5.
55. Pickett A. Globalization of neurotoxins for facial aesthetics attracts new players. *Aesthetic Guide* 2017; 66–74.
56. http://www.theinvestor.co.kr/view.php?ud=20170814000756. Accessed August 14, 2017.
57. http://www.iprotox.com/mbs/protox/subview.jsp?id=protox_020200000000. Accessed March 3, 2017.
58. http://www.bonti.com/wp-content/uploads/2017/08/Bonti_EB-001-Phase-2A-GL-Topline-Results_Press-Release_FINAL_8.8.17.pdf. Accessed August 25, 2017.
59. Masuyer G et al. Engineered botulinum neurotoxins as new therapeutics. *Annu Rev Pharmacol Toxicol* 2014; 54: 27–51.
60. https://clinicaltrials.gov/ct2/show/NCT01157377?term=NCT01157377&rank=1. Accessed February 14, 2016.
61. https://clinicaltrials.gov/ct2/show/study/NC01129531?term-NCT01129531&rank=1. Accessed February 14, 2016.
62. http://www.ema.europa.eu/docs/en_GB/document_library/Other/2016/04/WC500204741.pdf. Accessed August 24, 2017.

7 Botulinum toxin used in conjunction with other injectables and devices for cosmetic purposes

Alastair Carruthers and Jean Carruthers

INTRODUCTION

Over the last 30 years, botulinum toxin type A (BoNT-A) has become the most popular minimally invasive cosmetic procedure in the United States.[1] When used alone, BoNT-A effectively reduces the appearance of dynamic rhytides and superficial lines, and is able to alter the contours of a face—widening the eyes, for example, or sculpting a jaw—but fails to address the underlying loss of volume or changes in skin texture or pigmentation that occur over time. As a result, toxins are increasingly used in conjunction with other interventions. Statistics show that nearly half of all cosmetic patients in the United States requesting minimally invasive interventions received multiple cosmetic procedures at the same time in 2014.[2] Combination therapy with BoNT-A, soft-tissue fillers, and light- or energy-based therapies often procures a kind of synergy, leading to enhanced aesthetic outcomes of greater duration.

THE ROLE OF FILLERS IN THE AGING FACE

The pan-facial treatment strategy signals a shift to a more three-dimensional approach to rejuvenation and is related, in part, to a deeper understanding of the aging process, a complex interplay of extrinsic and intrinsic factors, coupled with repetitive mimetic musculature, that exert significant changes in the appearance of the face over time. Extrinsic factors include photodamage, smoking, diet, and general health. Intrinsic factors are more profound: retaining ligaments loosen, and skin loses its youthful elasticity and begins to sag, bony landmarks resorb and retrude, altering the contours of the face, distinct fat compartments atrophy, and fat redistributes itself in the lower face, accumulating in the jowls and along the jaw.[3–5]

This greater understanding of the complexity of facial aging and recognition of the role of volume loss has led to a paradigm shift in facial rejuvenation, from the two-dimensional focus on hyperdynamic facial lines to a three-dimensional approach, incorporating volume restoration. Clinicians increasingly turn to the use of combined interventions targeting multiple aspects of the aging process—fillers to replace volume and add support deep in the soft tissues, along with BoNT-A for movement control and longer-lasting aesthetic outcomes.

Filler Formulations

Filling agents on the market are generally divided by their biodegradable characteristics. Proper choice of agent depends on experience and a careful understanding of the risks and benefits associated with each. Although ideal for patients seeking permanent changes, non-biodegradable fillers—polymethylmethacrylate (PMMA; Bellafill®, Suneva Medical Inc., San Diego, CA), and liquid injectable silicone (Silikon™ 1000, Alcon Pharmaceuticals, Fort Worth, TX, and ADATO™ SIL-ol 5000, Bausch and Lomb Surgical, San Dimas, CA)—are not readily broken down or reabsorbed and are associated with a higher risk of complications that can be more difficult to resolve.[6]

Biodegradable filling agents stimulate neocollagenesis but are eventually metabolized by the body, for a long-lasting but impermanent result. Although there are many formulations on the market, derivatives of hyaluronic acid (HA)—the most abundant glycosaminoglycans in human tissue—are by far the most popular for their ease of use, low incidence of adverse events, and reversibility (Table 7.1). In the skin, the body's natural HA functions as a key structural component within the extracellular matrix, binding collagen and elastin fibers, stabilizing intercellular structures and contributing to cell proliferation and migration.[7] In commercial preparations, HA consists of repeating polymer chains of polysaccharide cross-linked by various agents for greater durability. Commercial preparations of injectable HA increase volume by way of their space-filling properties—combining with the body's natural HA and binding to water—and by inducing neocollagenesis via changes in the structure and function of the extracellular matrix.[8–10]

Biodegradable particulate fillers include poly-L-lactic acid (PLLA; Sculptra®/Sculptra® Aesthetic; Galderma S.A., Lausanne, Switzerland), comprising synthetic, biodegradable polymer beads measuring 40–63 μm derived from the alpha-hydroxy-acid family[11] and calcium hydroxylapatite (CaHA; Radiesse®; Merz Aesthetics, Raleigh, NC), composed of spherical particles (25–45 μm in size) identical in composition to bone suspended in an aqueous sodium carboxymethylcellulose carrier gel.[12] After implantation, the particles induce histiocytic and fibroplastic response, stimulating the formation of new collagen at the site of implantation for a progressive increase in dermal volume that can last upwards of 12 months.

BOTULINUM TOXIN AND FILLERS

BoNT-A and fillers work by the dual mechanisms of reflation and relaxation—restoring volume and decreasing activity of the muscles of expression responsible for the creation of glabellar rhytides, lateral canthal rhytides, horizontal forehead lines, melomental folds and mouth frown, as well as lines and wrinkles around the mouth and in the neck.[13] Moreover, there is evidence of a synergistic effect: BoNT-A appears to increase the longevity of the filling agent and often leads to more satisfactory aesthetic outcomes, perhaps due to its reported smoothing effects on rhytides in repose.[14,15] Studies have shown that in addition to its effect on dynamic rhytides, BoNT-A appears to produce a kind of "glow," significantly decreasing skin roughness for a smoother and lighter appearance after treatment. This improvement on superficial skin texture is likely due to local relaxation of the transverse muscle cells, tissue remodeling in response to reduced muscle activity, or both.[15] This smoothing effect may be enhanced by the use of soft-tissue fillers, and vice-versa: BoNT-A extends the life of the filling agent by preventing repetitive muscular activity that hastens the absorption of the implant. Consensus recommendations provide detailed guidance on combination approaches in facial rejuvenation.[16]

Combination Therapy in the Upper face

In the upper face, dermal fillers are used to augment results achieved by BoNT-A alone. Most age-related changes in the forehead and periocular region occur because of photodamage and the effects of repetitive, mimetic musculature, rather than loss of volume. However, temporal hollowing may occur—sometimes associated with a drop in the tail of the brow that may be treated with a small amount of filler—and deeper, static rhytides in the forehead, glabella, and around the eyes sometimes require augmentation for optimal effect. Filler added to toxin gives a softer and more natural result, especially with filler reflation of the entire forehead and temples. Volumizing the glabella and medial forehead can lift the brow, soften forehead lines,

Table 7.1 Hyaluronic Acid Formulations in the United States

Trade name	Manufacturer	HA concentration (mg/mL)
Restylane® Restylane-L® Restylane® Silk	Galderma S.A., Lausanne, Switzerland	20
Perlane® Perlane-L®	Galderma S.A., Lausanne, Switzerland	20
Juvéderm® Ultra Juvéderm® Ultra XC	Allergan Inc., Irvine, CA	24
Juvéderm® Ultra Plus		24
Juvéderm® Ultra Plus XC		20
Juvéderm Voluma® XC		17
Juvéderm Volift®		15
Juvéderm Volbella®		
Hydrelle®	Anika Therapeutics, Bedford, MA	28
Prevelle™ Silk	Mentor Corporation, Santa Barbara, CA	5.5
BELOTERO BALANCE™	Merz Pharmaceuticals LLC, Greensboro, NC	22.5

elevate the root of the nose, and lessen horizontal procerus rhytides. Generally, injections of BoNT-A precede that of fillers by a week or two to assess the need for the treatment of residual static lines and deep folds.

Many studies have shown superior efficacy and patient satisfaction in association with a combination of fillers and botulinum toxin in the upper face, especially in individuals with deep resting rhytides. We first compared the efficacy of BoNT-A alone or in combination with HA in individuals with moderate-to-severe glabellar rhytides in two studies (Figure 7.1).[17,18] Combination therapy provided greater aesthetic benefit and extended the duration of the filling agent. Patel and colleagues found improved clinical effects of longer duration and greater patient satisfaction with BoNT-A and collagen for the treatment of glabellar rhytides compared to either therapy alone.[19] Dubina and colleagues showed that combination treatment produced longer-lasting results in dynamic forehead lines, and a greater reduction in static and dynamic glabellar rhytides up to 6 months after treatment.[20] Beer and colleagues evaluated BoNT-A and HA in individuals with mild-to-moderate temporal volume loss as well as glabellar and/or periorbital rhytides.[21] Combination therapy effectively rejuvenated the upper face, including the temples and periorbital region; 64% of subjects previously treated with BoNT-A rated the combined approach superior to treatment with botulinum toxin alone.

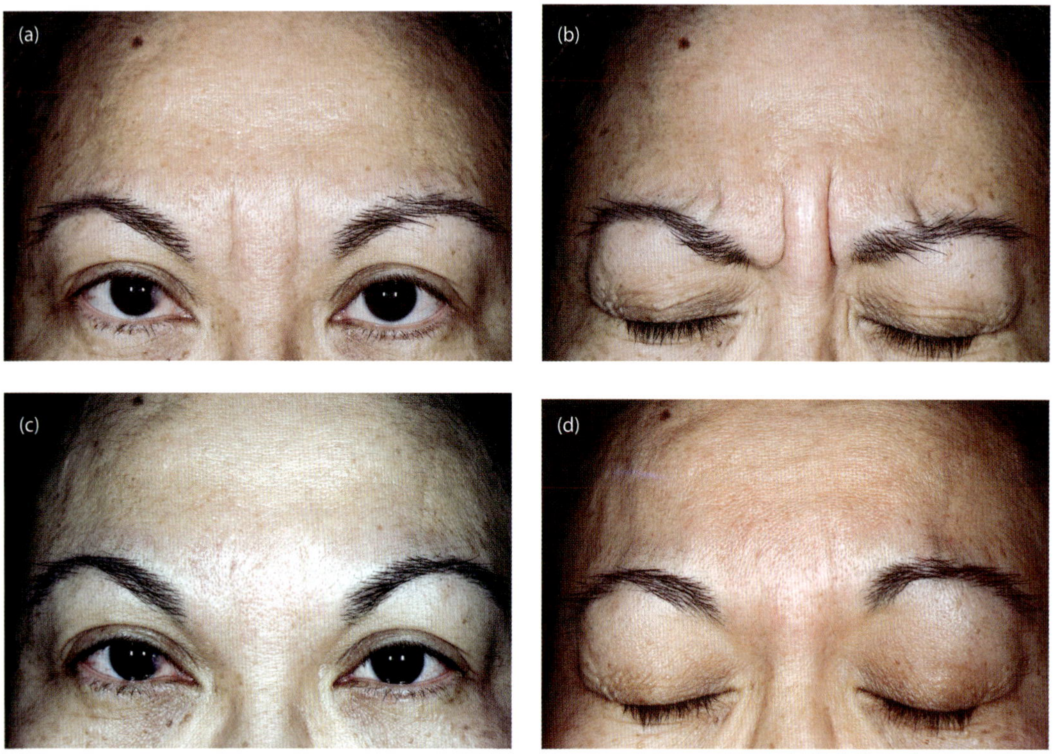

Figure 7.1 The combined effect of BoNT-A and filler on deep resting rhytides: (a) Deep resting glabellar furrows present prior to any treatment; (b) deep dynamic glabellar folds present prior to any treatment; (c) absence of resting folds after BoNT-A and HA filler; (d) full attempted frown after both BTX-A and HA filler. (Reproduced from Carruthers A, Carruthers J, *Dermatol Surg* 2003; 29: 802–9. With permission.)

Fillers and Botulinum Toxin in the Mid- and Lower Face

The use of soft-tissue fillers to restore volume in the midface is well documented and one of the tenets of the revised treatment paradigm.[22] Loss of volume and inferior descent of fat from within the superficial and deep fat compartments in the upper face contribute greatly to manifestations of aging in the lower face, including the nasolabial folds, marionette lines, and jowls. Restoring support and volume in the midface is often all that is required to produce a natural lift and to improve the appearance of more pronounced rhytides in the lower face.

The highly mobile perioral region is particularly susceptible to the signs of aging due to a number of factors: changes to the supporting structures around the mouth (loss of subcutaneous fat and elasticity, skin laxity, loosening of ligaments, gravitational pull, and resorption, rotation, and protrusion of the bony landmarks), compounded by photodamage and hyperdynamic muscle movement leading to dyspigmentation, irregular texture, and the appearance of radial lip lines.[23] It is also an area that is often difficult to treat: repetitive movement tends to undermine the effects of a filling agent on its own. Rejuvenation of the lower face involves the control of muscle movement as well as restoration of volume but, in some cases, neither BoNT-A nor HA filler alone will provide optimal results.[16]

Few trials have assessed the use of combination BoNT-A and soft-tissue fillers in the lower face. In a prospective, randomized trial of 90 we studied HA alone or in combination with BoNT-A for lip augmentation and the treatment of oral commissures and perioral rhytides as indicated by perioral and lip fullness, oral commissure assessments, and scores on the Cosmetic Improvement and Global Aesthetic Improvement Scales.[24] For all end points and most time points, combination therapy led to greater improvement from baseline than either single modality alone. Moreover, both therapies together proved better on three patient-reported outcomes (overall satisfaction, perioral/lipstick lines, and total satisfaction), although HA alone and in combination improved perceived age.[25]

COMBINATION THERAPY WITH LIGHT- AND ENERGY-BASED DEVICES

A proliferation of light- and energy-based systems has been developed to meet the demand for anti-aging treatments and has become an indispensable component for facial rejuvenation to treat the envelope of the skin, as well as tightening and lifting, improving texture, and correcting skin tone and discoloration. There is no evidence that the use of these devices adversely affects the efficacy or safety of BoNT-A, and the timing and sequence of treatments appear to be at the discretion of the clinician.[26]

Intense Pulsed Light (IPL)

A nonablative, broadband light source that emits a continuous spectrum ranging from 500 to 1200 nm, intense pulsed light selectively targets microvasculature and melanin components within the dermis by particular wavelengths and pulse durations while sparing the epidermis from thermal injury. The emitted heat improves hyperpigmentation through the destruction of melanin and hemoglobin and stimulates the formation of new collagen for positive changes in skin texture.[27] IPL is used for the treatment of photodamaged skin, reducing both lentigenes and vascular lesions, such as telangiectasias, port-wine stains, and poikiloderma, and improving skin texture, pore size, and fine wrinkles.[28,29] Results are often subtle and require multiple treatment sessions, and fine lines appear to respond better than deeper lines and furrows.[30]

Combination therapy with BoNT-A, however, increases the overall aesthetic benefit, with an improvement in texture and telangiectasis, along with a decrease in the appearance of rhytides. We compared IPL alone or in combination with BoNT for the treatment of moderate-to-severe bilateral canthal rhytides in 30 women.[31] Patients who received both modalities experienced a 15% improvement in overall aesthetic benefit—wrinkling, texture, and blemishes, at the 6-month evaluation. Similarly, Khoury and colleagues evaluated small wrinkles and fine lines, erythema, hyperpigmentation, pore size, skin texture, and overall appearance for 8 weeks in a randomized, split-face study in which patients were treated with botulinum toxin or saline plus IPL.[32] Adjunctive BoNT-A achieved a greater degree of improvement in small wrinkles and fine lines and erythema.

Radiofrequency (RF)

Monopolar and bipolar focused radiofrequency are noninvasive methods of skin tightening without significant recovery time or complications. RF devices use an electrical current rather than a light source to deliver uniform heat to the deep dermis and underlying tissue at a controlled depth, with concomitant surface skin cooling for immediate collagen contraction and a delayed wound healing response, with new collagen formation for 2–6 months post-treatment and subsequent skin tightening for up to a year.[33] Originally approved for periorbital skin rejuvenation, RF softens nasolabial folds, tightens the jowls, and provides lift to the brow and midface[34–39]

Although no controlled studies have assessed the combined approach with BoNT-A, post-treatment with botulinum toxin inhibits the underlying muscles from molding the newly formed collagen into additional wrinkles for a sustained aesthetic response and enhancing elevation when used for nonsurgical brow lift procedures.

Microfocused Ultrasound

Microfocused ultrasound with visualization (MFU-V; Ultherapy®; Ulthera Inc., Mesa, AZ/Merz Pharmaceuticals GmbH) delivers transcutaneous ultrasound energy to selectively heat dermal and subdermal tissues to greater than 60°C in a linear array of tightly focused thermal coagulation points (TCPs), stimulating long-term collagen remodeling and producing subsequent tissue tightening without any damage to the epidermal surface.[40,41] MFU-V has been shown to safely and effectively treat skin laxity in the face, neck, and décolleté, as well as other areas of the body, such as the knees, posterior arms, elbows, medial thighs, abdomen, and buttocks.[42–44] Treatment can be customized by adjusting energy (4–10 MHz) and focal depth (1.5–4.5 mm) of the emitted ultrasound.

CONCLUSION

A deeper understanding of the changes that occur in the face over time, has revolutionized the treatment approach to facial rejuvenation. Combination therapy reflects current clinical practice to address the many manifestations of aging. BoNT-A, fillers, and light- and energy-based devices combine for a synergistic effect to smooth rhytides, replace lost volume, correct surface imperfections, and tighten and lift the skin.

REFERENCES

1. American Society of Plastic Surgeons. *2014 Plastic Surgery Statistics Report*. 2015. http://www.plasticsurgery.org
2. American Society of Plastic Surgeons. 2015.
3. Lambros V. Models of facial aging and implications for treatment. *Clin Plast Surg* 2008; 35: 319–27.
4. Pessa JE, Slice DE, Hanz KR, Broadbent TH Jr, Rohrich RJ. Aging and the shape of the mandible. *Plast Reconstr Surg* 2008; 121: 196–200.
5. Rohrich RJ, Pessa JE. The fat compartments of the face: Anatomy and clinical implications for cosmetic surgery. *Plast Reconstr Surg* 2007; 119: 2219–27.
6. DeLorenzi C. Complications of injectable fillers, part I. *Aesthet Surg J* 2013; 33: 561–75.

7. Monheit GD, Narins RS, Mariwalla K. NASHA family. In: Carruthers J, Carruthers A (eds). *Procedures in Cosmetic Dermatology: Soft Tissue Augmentation*. New York: Elsevier; 2013, 10–12.
8. Wang F, Garza LA, Kang S, Varani J, Orringer JS, Fisher GJ, Voorhees JJ. In vivo stimulation of a de novo collagen production caused by cross-linked hyaluronic acid dermal filler injections in photodamaged human skin. *Arch Dermatol* 2007; 143: 155–63.
9. Turlier V, Delalleau A, Casas C et al. Association between collagen production and mechanical stretching in dermal extracellular matrix: In vivo effect of cross-linked hyaluronic acid filler: A randomised, placebo-controlled study. *J Dermatol Sci* 2013; 69: 187–94.
10. Quan T et al. Enhancing structural support of the dermal microenvironment activates fibroblasts, endothelial cells, and keratinocytes in aged human skin in vivo. *J Invest Dermatol* 2013; 133: 658.
11. Sterling JB, Hanke CW. Poly-L-Lactic acid as a facial filler. *Skin Therapy Letter* 2005; 10: 9–11.
12. Graivier MH, Bass LS, Busso M, Jasin ME, Rhoda, Narins S, Tzikas TL. Calcium hydroxylapatite (Radiesse) for correction of the mid- and lower face: Consensus recommendations. *Plast Reconstr Surg* 2007; 120: 55–66S.
13. Coleman KR, Carruthers J. Combination therapy with BOTOX and fillers: The new rejuvenation paradigm. *Dermatol Ther* 2006; 19: 177–88.
14. Dessy LA, Mazzocchi M, Rubino C et al. An objective assessment of botulinum toxin A effect on superficial skin texture. *Ann Plast Surg* 2007; 58: 469–73.
15. Carruthers A, Carruthers J, Lei X, Pogoda JM, Eadie N, Brin MF. OnabotulinumtoxinA treatment of mild glabellar lines in repose. *Dermatol Surg* 2010; 36(Suppl 4): 2168–71.
16. Carruthers JDA, Glogau RG, Blitzer A. Advances in facial rejuvenation: Botulinum toxin type A, hyaluronic acid dermal fillers, and combination therapies—consensus recommendations. *Plast Reconstr Surg* 2008; 121: 5S.
17. Carruthers J, Carruthers A, Maberley D. Deep resting glabellar rhytides respond to BTX-A and Hylan B. *Dermatol Surg* 2003; 29: 539–44.
18. Carruthers J, Carruthers A. A prospective, randomized, parallel group study analyzing the effect of BTX-A (Botox) and Nonanimal Sourced Hyaluronic Acid (NASHA, Restylane) in combination compared with NASHA (Restylane) alone in severe glabellar rhytides in adult female subjects: treatment of severe glabellar rhytides with a hyaluronic acid derivative compared with the derivative and BTX-A. *Dermatol Surg* 2003; 29: 802–9.
19. Patel MP, Talmor M, Nolan WB. Botox and collagen for glabellar furrows: Advantages of combination therapy. *Ann Plast Surg* 2004; 52: 442–7.
20. Dubina M et al. Treatment of forehead/glabellar rhytide complex with combination botulinum toxin A and hyaluronic acid versus botulinum toxin A injection alone: A split-face, rater-blinded, randomized control trial. *J Cosmet Dermatol* 2013; 12: 261–6.
21. Beer KR, Julius H, Dunn M, Wilson F. Remodeling of periorbital, temporal, glabellar, and crow's feet areas with hyaluronic acid and botulinumtoxin. *J Cosmet Dermatol* 2014; 13: 143–50.
22. Carruthers JDA, Glogau RG, Blitzer A. et al. Advances in facial rejuvenation: Botulinum toxin type a, hyaluronic acid dermal fillers, and combination therapies—consensus recommendations. *Plast Reconstr Surg* 2008; 121: 8S.
23. Sarnoff DS, Gotkin RH. Six steps to the "Perfect" lip. *J Drugs Dermatol* 2012; 11: 1081–8.
24. Carruthers A, Carruthers J, Monheit GD, Davis PG, Tardie G. Multicenter, randomized, parallel-group study of the safety and effectiveness of onabotulinumtoxina and hyaluronic acid dermal fillers (24-mg/mL smooth, cohesive gel) alone and in combination for lower facial rejuvenation. *Dermatol Surg* 2010; 36: 2121.
25. Carruthers A, Carruthers J, Monheit GD, Davis PG. et al. Multicenter, randomized, parallel-group study of the safety and effectiveness of onabotulinumtoxina and hyaluronic acid dermal fillers (24-mg/mL smooth, cohesive gel) alone and in combination for lower facial rejuvenation: Satisfaction and patient-reported outcomes. *Dermatol Surg* 2010; 36: 2135.
26. Cuerda-Galindo E, Palomar-Gallego MA, Linares-Garciavaldecasas R. Are combined same-day treatments the future for photorejuvenation? review of the literature on combined treatments with lasers, intense pulsed light, radiofrequency, botulinum toxin, and fillers for rejuvenation. *J Cosmet Laser Ther* 2015; 17: 49–54.
27. Goldberg DJ. New collagen formation after dermal remodeling with an intense pulsed light source. *J Cutan Laser Ther* 2000; 2: 59–61.
28. Sadick NS, Weiss R. Intense pulsed-light photorejuvenation. *Seminars in Cutaneous Med Surg* 2002; 21: 280–7.
29. Weiss RA, Weiss MA, Beasley KL. Rejuvenation of photoaged skin: 5 year results with intense pulsed light of the face, neck, and chest. *Dermatol Surg* 2002; 28: 1115–19.
30. Goldberg DJ. Current trends in intense pulsed light. *J Clin Aesthet Dermatol* 2012; 5: 45–53.
31. Carruthers J, Carruthers A. The effect of full-face broadband light treatments alone and in combination with bilateral crow's feet botulinum toxin type A chemodenervation. *Dermatol Surg* 2004; 30: 355–66.
32. Khoury JG, Saluja R, Goldman MP. The effect of botulinum toxin type a on full-face intense pulsed light treatment: A randomized, double-blind, split-face study. *Dermatol Surg* 2008; 34: 1062.
33. Hsu TS, Kaminer MS. The use of nonablative radiofrequency technology to tighten the lower face and neck. *Semin Cutan Med Surg* 2003; 22: 115–23.
34. Abraham MT, Ross EV. Current concepts in nonablative radiofrequency rejuvenation of the lower face and neck. *Facial Plast Surg* 2005; 21: 65–73.
35. Fitzpatrick R, Geronemus R, Goldberg D, Kaminer M, Kilmer S, Ruiz-Esparza J. Multicenter study of noninvasive radiofrequency for periorbital tissue tightening. *Lasers Surg Med* 2003; 33: 232–42.
36. Alster TS, Tanzi E. Improvement of neck and cheek laxity with a nonablative radiofrequency device: A lifting experience. *Dermatol Surg* 2004; 30: 503–7.
37. Koch RJ. Radiofrequency nonablative tissue tightening. *Facial Plast Surg Clin North Am* 2004; 12: 339–46.
38. Weiss RA et al. Monopolar radiofrequency facial tightening: A retrospective analysis of efficacy and safety in over 600 treatments. *J Drugs Dermatol* 2006; 5: 707–12.
39. Dover JS, Zelickson B. Results of a survey of 5,700 patient monopolar radiofrequency facial skin tightening treatments: Assessment of a low-energy multiple-pass technique leading to a clinical end point algorithm. *Dermatol Surg* 2007; 33: 900.
40. MacGregor JL, Tanzi EL. Microfocused ultrasound for skin tightening. *Semin Cutan Med Surg* 2013; 32:19.
41. Fabi SG. Noninvasive skin tightening: Focus on new ultrasound techniques. *Clin Cosmet Investig Dermatol* 2015; 8:47–52.
42. MacGregor JL, Tanzi EL. Microfocused ultrasound for skin tightening. *Semin Cutan Med Surg* 2013; 32: 20.
43. Alam M, White LE, Martin N, Witherspoon J, Yoo, S West DP. Ultrasound tightening of facial and neck skin: A rater-blinded prospective cohort study. *J Am Acad Dermatol* 2010; 62: 262–9.
44. Alster TS, Tanzi EL. Noninvasive lifting of arm, thigh, and knee skin with transcutaneous intense focused ultrasound. *Dermatol Surg* 2012; 38: 754–9.

8 Beyond the obvious: Beauty optimization with botulinum toxin

Arthur Swift, B. Kent Remington, and Steve Fagien

Neuromodulators based on the A strain of botulinum toxin (BoNT-A) were first introduced into the aesthetic arena in the early 1990s.[1] Their cosmetic use is now firmly entrenched and has classically been limited to the softening of undesirable dynamic facial lines, pathognomonic of the aging face. The true mandate of the cosmetic physician, however, when dealing with the feminine form, is to strive beyond rejuvenation into the realm of beauty maximization. Contrary to the common requests of patients to eliminate unsightly lines, affecting facial beauty goes far beyond wrinkles and furrows. Creating the best rather than a different version of the patient requires a comprehensive approach to restore lost volume, smooth contours, and enhance facial features naturally[2] (see Chapter 7).

Although truly the domain of autologous fat and pharmaceutically available "dermal" fillers, botulinum-based neuromodulators can also play a significant role in optimizing beauty by generating ideal proportions. The interplay of agonist and antagonist muscles, as modified with the application of BoNT-A, not only moderates dynamic expression, but the position of facial elements in the resting state through static muscle tension. When used in concert with filling agents, the effect is quite often synergistic, optimizing both the patient's experience and outcome. It is therefore incumbent upon injection specialists to have a deep understanding of beauty and the goals necessary to achieve a pleasing result. This chapter will focus on the artistic use of botulinum toxin to enhance facial beauty beyond the obvious indication of diminishing unsightly wrinkles.

UNDERSTANDING BEAUTY

True facial beauty arouses the senses to an emotional level of pleasure and evokes in the perceiver a high degree of attraction. Perception of beauty is innate, as borne out by numerous studies confirming that newborn infants prefer attractive faces.[3–5] Basic to our survival and evolution, we are attracted to beautiful traits implying unflawed health and robust reproductive abilities. Furthermore, in modern day culture there exists a "beauty premium" and a "plainness penalty"—attractive individuals are more likely to be hired, promoted, and to earn higher salaries than unattractive individuals.[6–8]

Extensive research has further shown that regardless of our racial background, we seem to have similar *subjective* ideas about what constitutes an attractive face.[9–11] Beauty pundits maintain that attractiveness is universal across race and culture but are unclear on what *objective* things we are assessing that allow us to determine one face as being more beautiful than another.[12,13] A clue may reside in the irrefutable fact that processing attractiveness takes milliseconds—we *look* with our eyes but we *see* with our brains. Is it possible that our brains act like supercomputers, mathematically assessing beauty? Leonardo Da Vinci, one of the world's most celebrated thinkers, insisted that there was a mathematical basis to all things beautiful, centered on specific ratios known as the Divine Proportion or Golden Ratio. Across the centuries, many other of the world's greatest intellectual minds, including Galileo, Michelangelo, and Einstein were in awe of the fact that natural beauty appeared dependent on this divine ratio.

The golden ratio is a mathematical ratio of 1.618:1, and the number 1.618 is called *Phi* (Φ) after the architect Phidias (fifth century BC), commonly regarded as one of the greatest of all classical Greek sculptors. In simple algebraic terms, the golden section is the only point dividing a line into two parts where the smaller segment in ratio to the larger segment is the same as the larger to the entire line (Figure 8.1). The significance of this divine ratio is that, true to Da Vinci's belief, *Phi* proportions are found over the entire beautiful face[2] (Figure 8.2). Our attraction to beauty may in part be hard-wired into our "computer" brains and based on how closely we subconsciously recognize *Phi* proportions. This may explain why across the world, regardless of their origin, most people seem to have similar subjective ideas of what constitutes an attractive face. Racial variations of skin color and diverse features then provide for an endless spectrum of *Phi* beauty that is unique for each individual. To paraphrase Hungerford, "beauty may actually reside in the *Phi* (eye) of the beholder".

Injection therapy restores youth by softening aging lines, reestablishing fullness of features, and smoothing contours with gradual transitions. However, creative use of botulinum toxin and fillers will also offer the opportunity to enhance attractiveness by pursuing ideal proportions. Individual ideal facial proportions can be obtained with the aid of a golden mean caliper—a tool for dynamically measuring the *Phi* ratio. Create *Phi* beauty, and youth accompanies it—but pursuing youth does not necessarily create beauty (Figure 8.3).

NEUROMODULATORS AND THE BEAUTIFUL UPPER FACE

The Beautiful Temple and Botulinum Toxin

Aesthetic injectors focusing purely on the presence of unsightly lines and creases often overlook the contribution of forehead and temple contour to overall beauty. An overly concave temple can detract from facial attractiveness, and signify a stigma of advancing age. Similarly, excess convexity in a female temple can portend a masculine look and distort the beautiful facial oval (or heart shape) preferred by most cultures.[14,15]

A female temple should be flat or only slightly concave/convex, offering a more balanced and harmonious look to the upper face. Facial width from the medial canthus to the ipsilateral cheek prominence should normally not exceed *Phi* (1.618) times the intercanthal distance for pleasing proportion (Figure 8.4).

Deposition of botulinum toxin into the temporalis muscle within its fossa can reduce upper facial bulkiness and provide the initial subtle concavity to the gentle S-shaped Ogee curve of the feminine form.

The temporalis muscle consists of superficial and deep parts that originate from the temporal bone and fascia in the temporal fossa of the parietal bone.[16] Deposition of botulinum toxin to reduce temporal volume must be placed into the deep portion which is the major contributor to temporal bulk, as isolated chemodenervation of the superficial temporalis muscle will lead to a hernia-type deformity of its untreated deeper counterpart (similar to masseteric hypertrophy). Two deep injection aliquots of BoNT-A (each 10 u of onabotulinum/incobotulinum; 25 u of abobotulinum toxin) spaced 2 cm apart into the maximum convexity of the muscle usually suffice, followed by several minutes of pressure to minimize the risk of bruising from the superficial vasculature in the region.

The aesthetic result is long lasting, typically requiring only biannual therapy. Furthermore, although maximal clench is diminished,[17] no detrimental effect on chewing has been observed, as the masseter and pterygoid muscles remain the principle contributors to mastication.

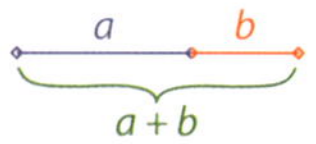

Figure 8.1 The Golden Ratio: The ratio of *b* (1.0) to *a* (1.618) is as a (1.618) is to *a* + *b* (2.618).

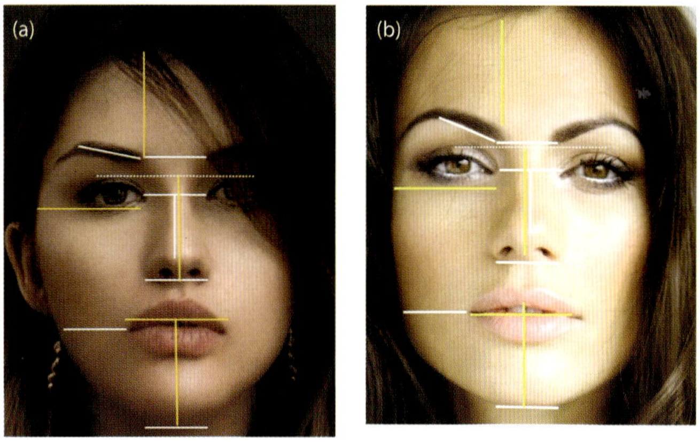

Figure 8.2 (a, b) Golden proportions are found all over the beautiful face, regardless of race.

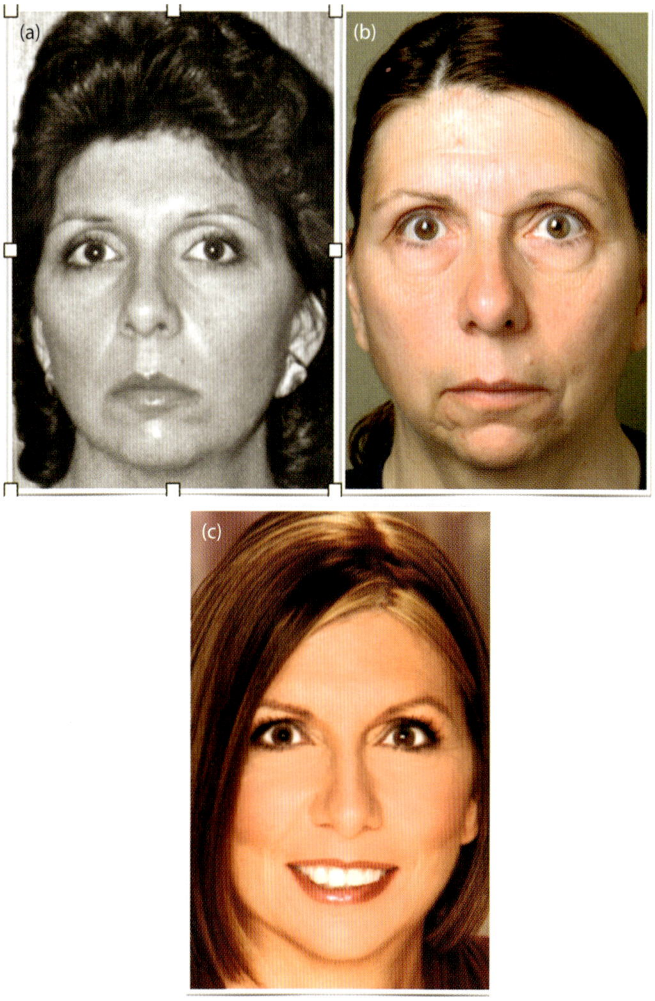

Figure 8.3 Creating beauty creates youth. (a) Patient aged 20. (b) Patient aged 45. (c) Lifestyle photo of patient aged 45, four weeks after botulinum toxin and filler treatment.

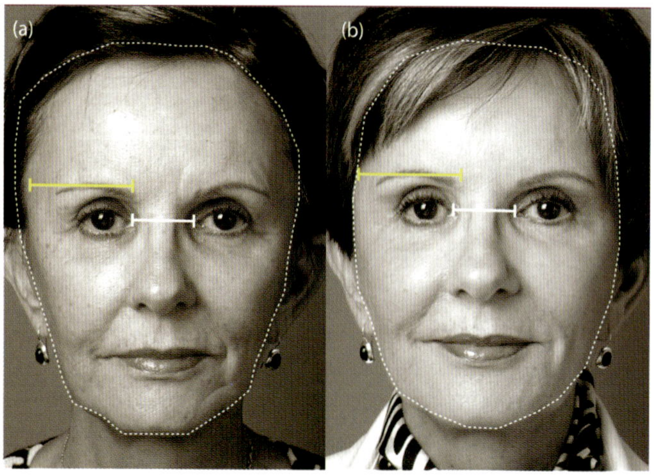

Figure 8.4 Patient before (a) and after (b) BeautiPHIcation™ demonstrating a pleasing reduction in bitemporal width to ideal proportions (white = 1.0; yellow = 1.618).

Surgical Anatomy Pearls: The temporalis muscle as a muscle of mastication must be strongly anchored to the underlying temporal bone to generate significant upward pull on the coronoid process of the mandible. As such, the superior portion of the muscle is firmly adherent to the underlying bone and devoid of interposing fascia. The periosteum and deep fascia of the forehead (galea aponeurotica) as they traverse the upper face under the frontalis muscle cannot continue under the temporalis muscle and as such lie over the muscle as the deep and superficial temporal fascia respectively. This anatomical oddity, of a deep fascia lying on the surface of the muscle which bears its name, provides a resistant plane that is appreciably felt when penetrating the region with a needle. Overlying this fascia in the posterior leaves of the superficial temporal fascia are the superficial temporal vessels (arteries and veins) and specifically the frontal ramus of the superficial temporal artery. Located in the depth of the muscle are the anterior and posterior deep temporal arteries (branches of the internal maxillary artery, second division), the middle temporal artery (connecting the deep and superficial arterial system), and the prominent middle temporal vein approximately 2 cm above the zygomatic arch. Deposition of botulinum toxin deep to the fascial layer is mandatory to access the bulky deep muscle as outlined above, and will require a 30-gauge needle of minimum ½ inch length. Prudent technique would require aspiration before injection of toxin into the temporal muscle to minimize the possibility of intravascular washout limiting the clinical result. Post-injection pressure for several minutes, regardless of the appearance of blood through the puncture site, will diminish the possibility of delayed unsightly bruising.

The Beautiful Glabella and Botulinum Toxin

Subtle differences in glabellar appearance have a profound effect on beauty and youthfulness. Aging skin changes and actinic exposure lead to the appearance of lines, creases, and dyschromias compounded with tissue atrophy and volume loss. Bone remodeling leads to an increase in glabellar height and width, which can often be evidenced by a paradoxical elevation of the medial brow in the elderly (Figure 8.5). This is to be distinguished from an elevated eyebrow resulting from increased frontalis activity as compensation for an upper eyelid partial levator dehiscence.

A beautiful glabella is not just about the absence of static or dynamic frown lines. Most BoNT injectors usually follow what everyone has done in the past, and limit their treatment to chasing

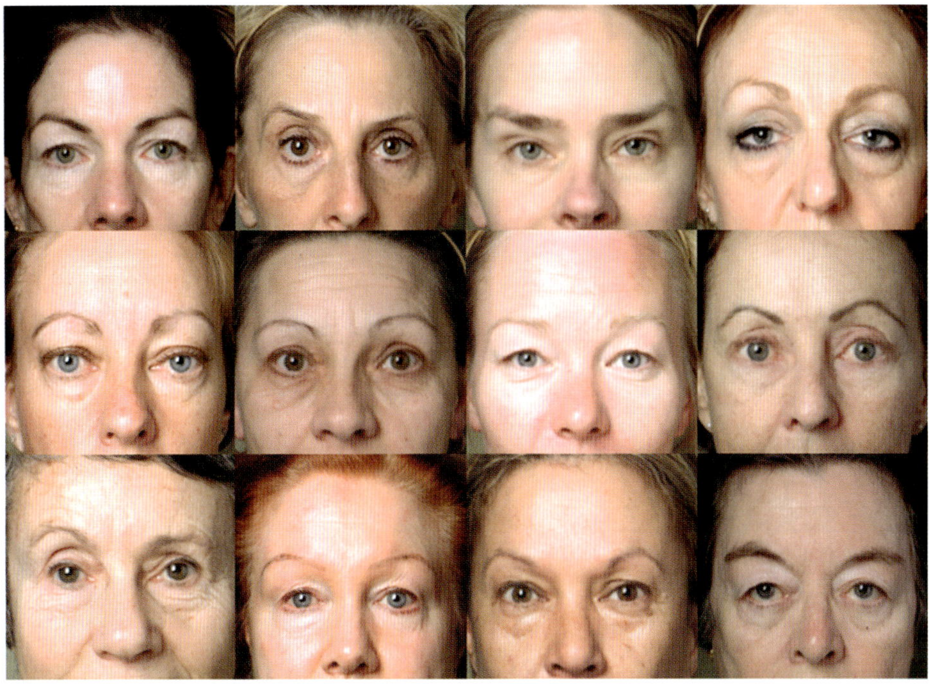

Figure 8.5 Elevated eyebrows commonly seen in the mature patient. All examples are devoid of botulinum toxin or brow-positioning surgery.

lines, occasionally causing medial brow splay or ptosis. However, the use of BoNT in this region affords the opportunity to enhance glabellar beauty by optimizing medial brow height and location to *Phi* proportions.

The glabellar complex consists of the interweaving of two superficial gliding muscles, the frontalis (elevator) and the procerus (depressor); and two deep brow depressor muscles, the paired corrugator and depressor supercilii. Through their soft tissue attachments into the skin of the region, these antagonistic muscles both animate the medial brow, and position it through resting tension depending on the individual's emotional state. The glabellar confluence of elevator and depressors is somewhat stratified as the frontalis blends superficially with the deeper depressors.

Delineation of each specific muscle within the central glabellar complex is clinically impossible; however, for practical purposes, function is stratified in that the elevator fibers of the frontalis remain sandwiched between the more superficial procerus fibers and the deeper corrugator/depressor fibers. Varying the height and depth of toxin deposition according to the muscle action being targeted can alter the resting position of the medial brow. *Phi* harmony in the upper face dictates that the medial brows begin in a vertical line above the medial canthii at a height of 0.618 (*phi*) of the intercanthal distance (Figure 8.6).

A more superficial (intermediate depth) slightly higher than normally planned injection of BoNT over the body of the corrugator (points **y** in Figure 8.7) will have a more profound effect on the frontalis muscle, dropping the height of an overly elevated medial eyebrow.

This technique is indicated when medial eyebrow position is too high *and* superior medial orbital hollowing is present to accommodate the potentially redundant skin that may occur as a result of treatment. Conversely, a slightly lower than planned deep injection of BoNT, targeting the corrugator belly and depressor supercilii muscles while avoiding the overlapping frontalis fibers, will potentially elevate a low-lying medial brow (Figure 8.8).

Unlike other regions of the face where *moderation* is desirable to maintain natural animation, it is often the goal of glabellar injection therapy to *obliterate* depressor function that is responsible for unsightly frown lines. Complete paralysis of the corrugator and depressor supercilii in the glabellar region, however, will eliminate eyebrow excursion inferomedially—the loss of resting tone in these muscles can cause a lateral drifting of the medial brow away from its ideal vertical position above the medial canthus. Simply stated, complete loss of the tethering effect of medial corrugator pull, in combination with the unopposed oblique pull of the frontalis muscle, can lead to unnatural eyebrow splay post-treatment (Figure 8.9). Patients at risk for this medial canthal splay after corrugator chemodenervation typically have mobile glabellar tissue that widens easily with digital manipulation during pretreatment assessment. Once these patients are identified, the addition of a small amount of toxin into the upper frontalis in the midpupillary line at initial glabellar treatment can

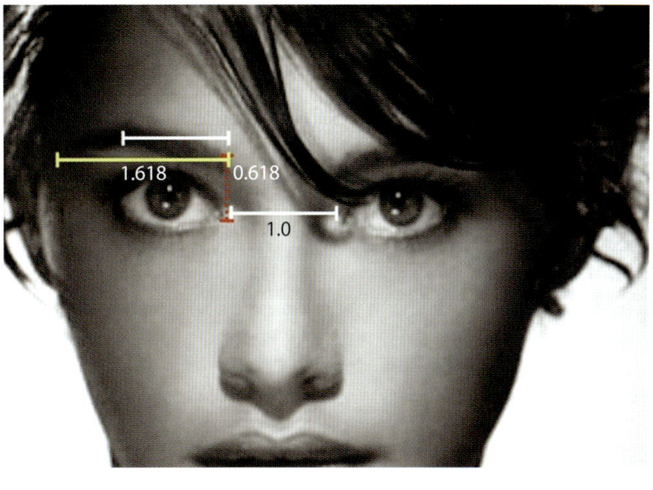

Figure 8.6 Golden Ratio proportions of the female brow. The medial eyebrow begins vertically above the medial canthus at a height equal to 0.618 (*Phi*) of the intercanthal distance. It then extends laterally at an angle of 10–20 degrees to a peak located *Phi* (equal to the intercanthal distance) of the entire length of the eyebrow (1.618 [*Phi*] of the intercanthal distance).

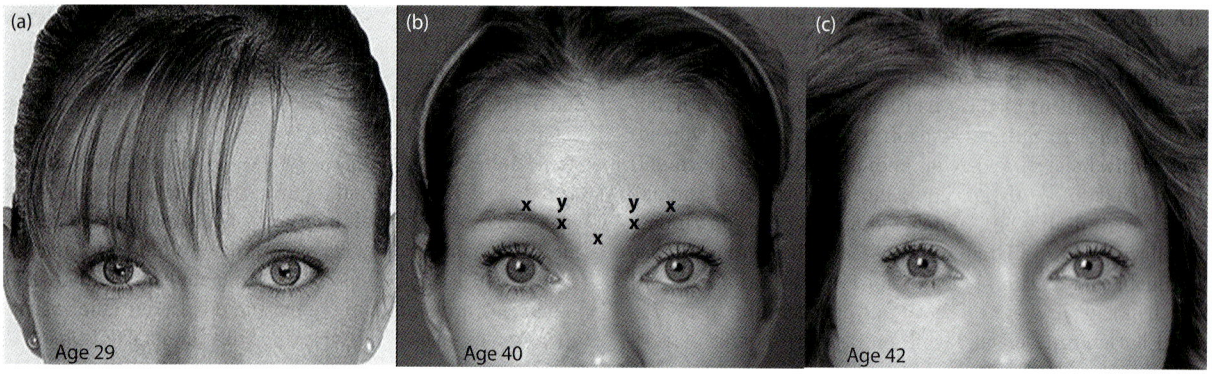

Figure 8.7 (a) Pleasing eyebrow position at age 29. (b) Elevated brow position at age 40. (c) Modification (slightly higher and more superficial injection points y) of BoNT-A results in resetting of the eyebrow to its more youthful position.

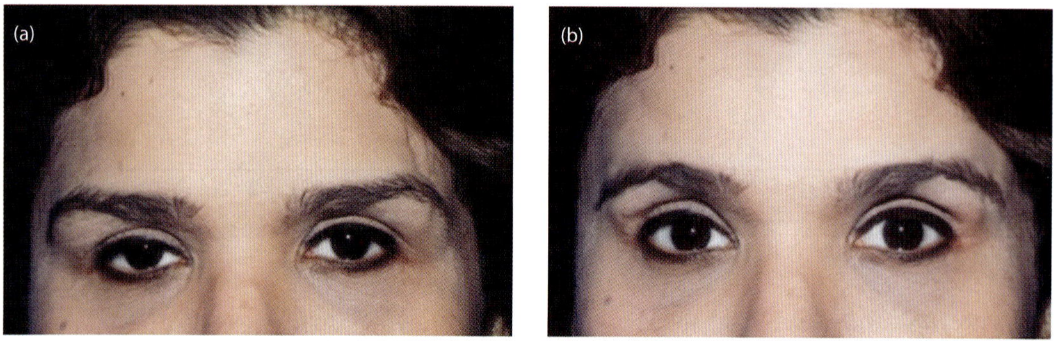

Figure 8.8 (a) Low-lying medial brow position. (b) Elevated medial brow after botulinum toxin treatment of the glabellar complex, targeting the corrugator and depressor supercilii (see text).

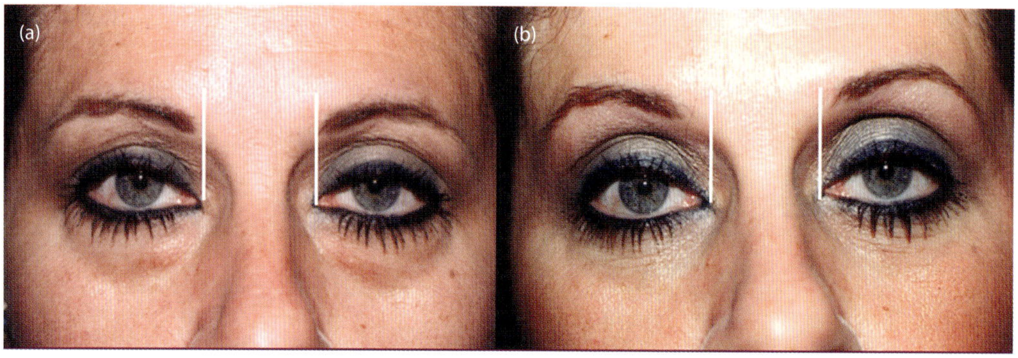

Figure 8.9 Patient pre-botulinum toxin treatment of glabella (a) exhibiting post-treatment medial eyebrow splay (b).

often dampen the deforming vectors responsible for unsightly glabellar spread (Figure 8.10).

In summary, thorough observation and palpation of the glabellar complex of muscles and overlying skin's resistance to spread is necessary in order to individualize the pattern of neurotoxin injections to optimize beauty in the region.

Surgical Anatomy Pearls: The arteries of the glabellar complex region (terminations of the intraorbital ophthalmic artery) are fairly consistent in their location as they exit the skull. The supraorbital artery (SOA) exits through a foramen or notch in the supraorbital rim within 1 mm from a line drawn vertically from the medial iris. The supratrochlear artery (STA) is commonly found 8–12 mm medial to the SOA under the most medial crease of the corrugator supercilii.[18,19] Needle injections of toxin in the region are best performed avoiding these exact topographical landmarks to minimize bruising.

The corrugator supercilii, depressor supercilii, and procerus act as medial depressors of the eyebrow. The corrugator supercilii runs from a deep osseous origin to a lateral superficial insertion into the dermis of the middle third of the eyebrow. The dimensions of the corrugator supercilii muscle are more extensive than previously described and can be easily delineated using fixed bony landmarks.[20] The muscle consists of two heads: the transverse and oblique.

The depressor supercilii muscle is distinct from the corrugator supercilii and medial head of the orbital portion of the orbicularis oculi muscle. It arises from the frontal process of the maxilla approximately at the level of the medial canthal tendon. The angular vessel is found anterior to the muscle. Insertion into the dermis is 13–14 mm superior to the medial canthal tendon. The triangular procerus is more superficial and can be considered as a musculoaponeurotic extension of the frontalis muscle onto the radix of the nose.

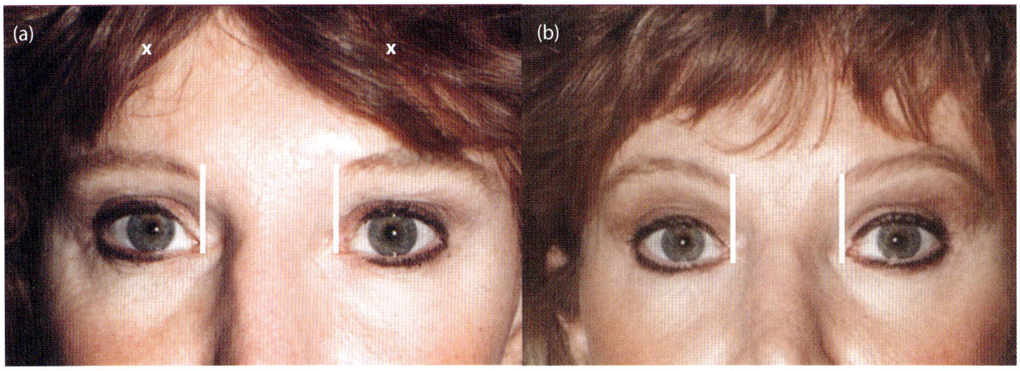

Figure 8.10 (a) Patient with a "mobile" glabella pretreatment with BoNT-A. (b) Several units of toxin were injected into the upper frontalis in the mid-pupillary line avoiding post-treatment splay.

The frontalis is actually comprised of paired flat muscles originating from the occipitofrontal-musculoaponeurotic system of the scalp in an angulated direction from lateral to a more medial insertion into the confluence of the glabellar complex and overlying dermis of the eyebrow. The dermal insertion is beneath the eyebrow in its medial and middle thirds, but extends for 0.5 cm inferior to the lateral brow. The frontalis glides easily over the frontal bone in its mimetic function due to the underlying galea, a thick fascia that is interposed between the posterior muscle and the underlying periosteum. Deposition of BoNT-A deeply into the forehead and under this fascia will result in diminished muscular response. It is therefore advisable to instill the toxin into the subdermal plane of the forehead, avoiding bruising from the underlying vasculature, and providing the same effect as intramuscular injection.[21] Most of the muscle's excursion is in its lower one-third just above the eyebrow (up to 2 cm) while the upper muscle is limited to around 8 mm of vertical movement. The subgaleal plane along the entire brow and to the lower limit of the forehead promontory has few significant vessels (periosteal branches of the supraorbital and supratrochelar vessels; the deep branch of the supraorbital artery which accompanies the nerve of the same name), and is a popular level for dissection in browlift surgery. Although the frontalis is considered to be a paired muscle with a midline aponeurotic gap and lateral extent to the temporal fusion line, occasional muscle fibers have been demonstrated both centrally as well as laterally beyond the temporal crest margin. The aesthetic injector should be wary of these variations in anatomy that are the culprit for post-toxin residual central furrowing or lateral "Spocking" of the brow (Figure 8.11).

The Beautiful Eyebrow and Botulinum Toxin

From its origin overlying the supraorbital ridge above the medial canthus, the beautiful female eyebrow slopes upward and laterally at an angle of 10–20 degrees. Male brows are classically flatter, extending laterally at 0–10 degrees. Ideal brow length in both genders should not exceed 1.618 of the intercanthal distance (ICD). The peak of the female brow is ideally located at the golden section of the brow length (0.618) which equals the intercanthal distance (Figure 8.6). The male eyebrow typically has a less pronounced peak located more laterally. The female tail of the eyebrow should be situated at a height equal to or higher than the medial segment.

The eyebrow is a floating structure whose position is determined by the opposing action of the frontalis muscle (elevator), and its antagonistic depressor muscles (procerus, corrugator and depressor supercilii, orbicularis oculi). Individualizing the dose and location of BoNT into these muscles can boost results beyond simple elevation to definitive brow-shaping. The authors contend that to raise a sagging brow is virtuous, but to contour it, divine.

Understanding the local anatomy while injecting botulinum toxin can deliver even greater aesthetic effects when the injector performs a more in-depth pre-injection assessment to determine those patients who may benefit from eyebrow positional changes. For instance, individuals with a pre-existing high lateral arch to the eyebrow may obtain an accentuated and exaggerated arch if injections more effectively reduce the caudal displacement effects of the lateral sub-brow orbicularis oculi muscle. This typically results in secondary lines above the lateral brow that disrupt the overall aesthetics. These individuals benefit from a more caudal placement of botulinum toxin to the lateral

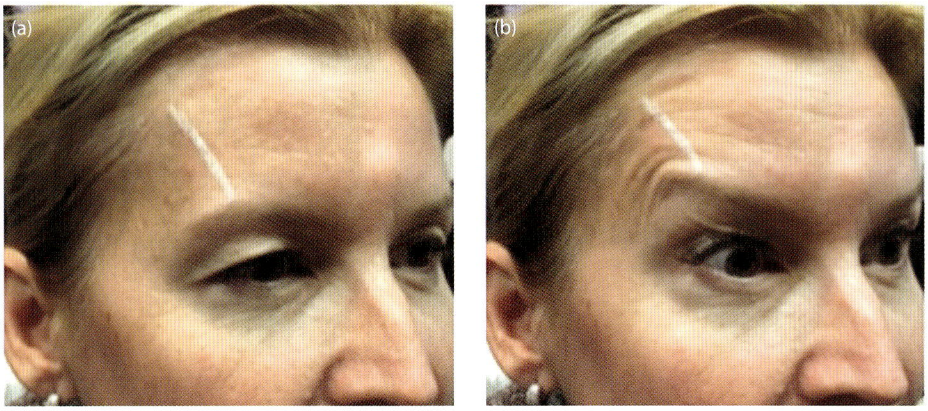

Figure 8.11 (a) Patient at rest after typical frontalis muscle chemomodulation with BoNT-A medial to the temporal crest (marked in white). (b) Same patient with attempted brow elevation displaying untreated frontalis fibers lateral to the crest ("Spocking").

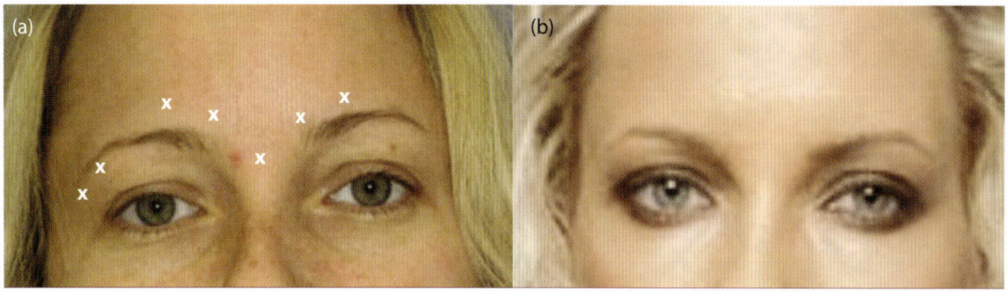

Figure 8.12 (a) Brow asymmetry pretreatment with BoNT-A. (b) Golden Ratio proportions of the eyebrows post-treatment.

periorbita and some may also benefit from the concurrent use of dermal fillers to the lateral forehead to pre-empt these secondary lines.

As previously mentioned, in most individuals, the frontalis muscle does not extend laterally beyond the temporal fusion line (temporal crest of the frontal bone). The outlying tail of the eyebrow beyond the temporal crest (in most foreheads) lies victim to gravity plus the downward pull of the vertical fibers of the orbicularis muscle. Like a cantilever, it must rely on the frontalis' upward pull on the adjacent middlebrow for vertical height. In patients who demonstrate a significant downward and medial pull on the outer brow with tight eye closure pretreatment, elevation of the tail is possible by decreasing the resting tone of the vertical superolateral fibers of the orbicularis with BoNT to the extent that an occasional "Spock" brow may occur. In those instances where depression of the tail of the brow is minimal with tight eye closure on pretreatment assessment, it may be necessary to simultaneously treat the central forehead with BoNT, thereby creating a partial hyperkinesis of the lateral frontalis.

Adjusting the individual doses and "patterning" injections into the frontalis according to the intended brow shape can allow this feature to approach *Phi* proportions (Figure 8.12), especially when combined with the synergy of appropriate sub-brow filler.

Surgical Anatomy Pearls: The sphincter muscle of the eye, the orbicularis oculi, is firmly anchored to bone at its medial aspect above and below the medial canthus. More laterally, there is a glide plane as the muscle slides over the sub-orbicularis oculi fat (SOOF) inferiorly and the retro-orbicularis oculi fat (ROOF) superiorly. Contraction of the orbicularis oculi is therefore more sphincteric than vertical, drawing the eyebrow inferomedially toward the nose. This explains why chemodenervation of the lateral vertical fibers very often results in an upward and lateral excursion of the tail of the brow.

The orbicularis oculi muscle is much more expansive than appears on the surface, extending superiorly and inferiorly beyond the orbital rim in an "aviator glasses" shape, and occasionally laterally as far as the temporal hairline. This sometimes necessitates a second row of toxin injections more lateral from the lateral orbital rim to have the desired effect.

NEUROMODULATORS AND THE BEAUTIFUL MIDFACE

Aging of the middle one-third of the face is the most apparent for deflation, deterioration, disproportion, and descent of the soft tissue envelope. The maxilla, including the pyriform region of the nose, recedes with age. The nose lengthens and the tip droops, with retraction of the columella, and alar base widening with superior excursion.

The periorbital complex typically shows signs of aging in the third decade of life with skin color and consistency changes. This early chronological senescence is not unexpected as the thin skin of the periorbital region is exposed to the stress of blinking an average of 1200 times per hour. Additionally, expansion of the inferolateral (middle age) and superomedial (advanced age) orbital rims, results in a volumetric increase of the bony orbit relative to its contents. Combined with a descent and stretching of the lateral canthal tendon and Lockwood's suspensory ligament, as well as orbital fat volume shifting due to pseudo-herniation of the orbital fat pads, this is hypothesized to be the cause of senile enophthalmos and loss of vertical palpebral aperture ("squintier" eyes in the elderly) (Figure 8.13).

Characteristically, volume "reflation" as well as laser and surgical skin-tightening procedures remain the workhorses of beautification and rejuvenation in the middle face. BoNT is typically relegated to softening of dynamic lines or unwanted tics and grimaces. However, the hallmark of "beyond the obvious" use of BoNT resides in the periorbital and nose regions, where a small difference in anatomy can lead to a big difference in appearance. Proper finesse of minute doses of toxin can sway the balance between agonist and antagonist muscles, creating more pleasing contours to the eyelid aperture or nasal profile.

Beautiful Eyes and Botulinum Toxin

The contribution of the eyes to overall facial attractiveness is overwhelming. Originally a Western tenet of beauty, large prominent eyes in the female is one of the most important determinants of facial beauty in Eastern cultures as well.[22,23] As mentioned previously,

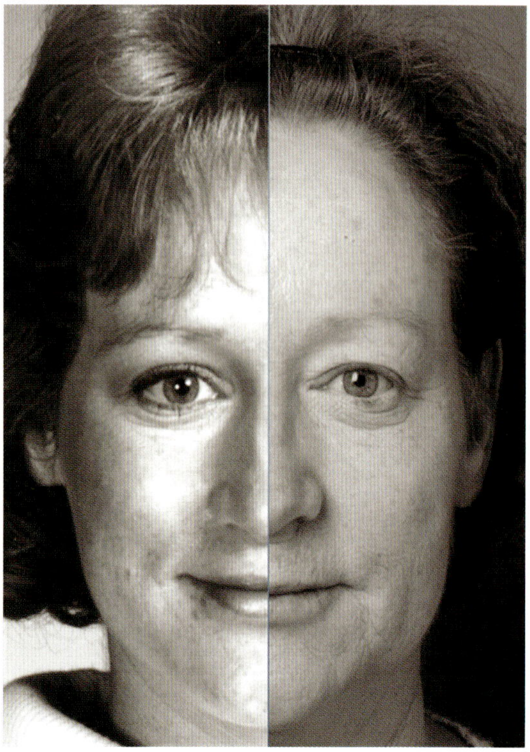

Figure 8.13 Hemi-face comparison of the decrease in eyelid fissure after 30 years.

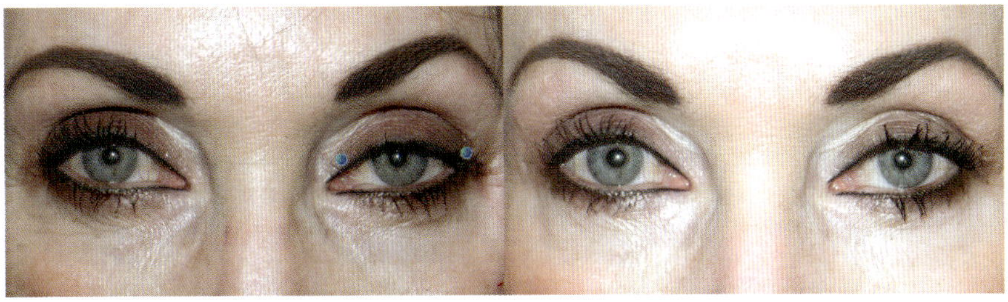

Figure 8.14 Figure showing the location of instillation of subdermal BoNT-A and its effect on increasing interlimbal aperture.

classical use of botulinum toxin to the upper face and particularly around the periorbita has been mostly for the improvement in the appearance of lateral canthal rhytids. While this has been quite effective for improving facial appearances and delivering a more restful persona, other effects, now quite evident, with toxin use in this region include the changes to the position of the lateral (tail of the) eyebrow as described above. Understanding the local anatomy while injecting botulinum toxin can deliver even greater aesthetic effects when the injector performs a more in-depth pre-injection assessment to determine eyelid fissure asymmetry.

The communicative potential of the subtle variations of eyelid position should not be underestimated. Sometimes, eyelid fissure asymmetries are unmasked after forehead botulinum toxin therapy has removed the contribution of the frontalis muscle compensation. Once eyelid fissure asymmetry has been brought to their attention, patients are often relieved to learn that improvement can be achieved through a nonsurgical treatment. They frequently relay that it had been evident in photographs but that they were unaware of noninvasive treatment options. The concepts of protagonist and antagonist relationships apply for eyelid position as they do for other areas of the face. The levator muscle and Muller's muscle are both upper lid elevators while the major lid depressors are certain regional components of the orbicularis oculi muscle. Local chemical effects can be seen with adrenergic agents such as naphazoline, antazoline, apraclonidine, and neo-synephrine all of which are topical aqueous (eye drops) agents. When instilled onto the ocular surface, they have adrenergic secondary effects on Muller's muscle and cause temporary contraction and upper eyelid elevation. Their utility has become common in some forms of "small eyes" including botulinum toxin-induced lid ptosis. Similarly, upper eyelid elevation with the creation of "round eyes" can be achieved by reducing the effective force of the upper eyelid depressors (orbicularis oculi) through precise chemodenervation.

Surgical Anatomy Pearls: There has also been confusion as to where the most effective placement is and what that dose should be. Again, understanding the details of the periorbital anatomy will shed light on this.[24] Since the periorbital (preseptal) orbicular muscle is a sphincteric like muscle that surrounds the upper and lower eyelids and lateral canthus, it is quite understandable that lateral contraction, in part, induces radial lines at the lateral canthus. The fibers of the orbicularis muscle at the lateral periorbita are more vertical hence contraction will cause the formation of "crow's feet" and lateral brow depression. Likewise, as the central horizontally oriented orbicularis muscle extends to the medial and lateral canthi, the fibers becomes more vertical in orientation, whereby their contraction pulls the upper lid downward. The most effective applications of BoNT would therefore reside at the extreme medial and lateral components of this muscle (Figure 8.14). Minute doses of 0.5–1.0 units of onabotulinum toxin are usually all that is required to improve upper lid posture while reducing the chance of lagophthalmos. Similar applications can be applied to those individuals with lower eyelid asymmetry with comparable dosing.

The Beautiful Nose and Botulinum Toxin

Nasal enhancement is one of today's most sought-after yet challenging cosmetic procedures. The intrinsic beauty of the nose can be found in its *Phi* proportions as well as the gentle transition between its aesthetic units. Almost exclusively the domain of dermal fillers, successful non-surgical nasal enhancement relies on the essential triad of understanding anatomy, *Phi* aesthetics, and injection principles. Of particular note is a pleasing nasal length from radix lash line to columella of 1.618 times the intercanthal distance (ICD); an ideal nasal tip height of 0.618 of the ICD; and tip defining points that are the most projecting aspect on profile (Figure 8.15).

The mimetic muscles of the nose lack well-defined fascia allowing for small bundles of each muscle to contract separately with separate synergistic and counteracting functions.[25] In cases of exaggerated nasal tip ptosis with animation, instillation of a small amount of BoNT into the tip depressors (inner fibers of the musculus myrtiformis (depressor septi nasi muscle and musculus digastricus septi nasi labialis muscle) located at the base of the columella can reduce unwanted tip depression creating a more open nasolabial angle.[26]

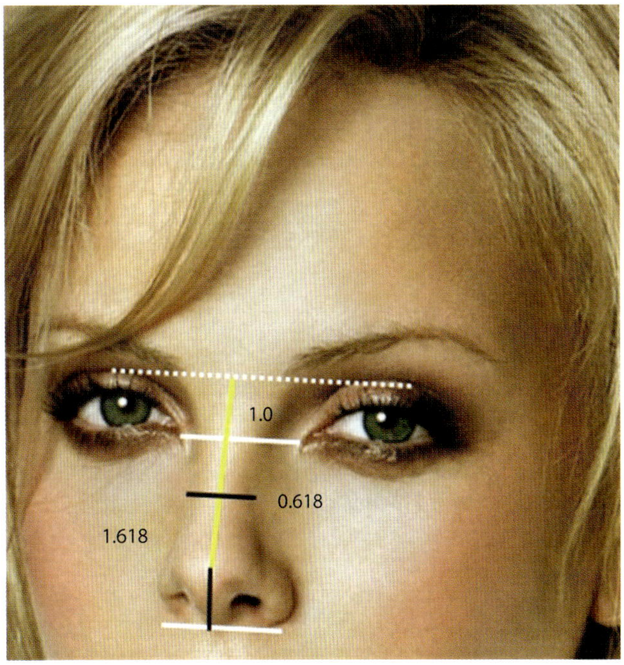

Figure 8.15 Ideal nasal proportions according to the Golden Ratio (see text).

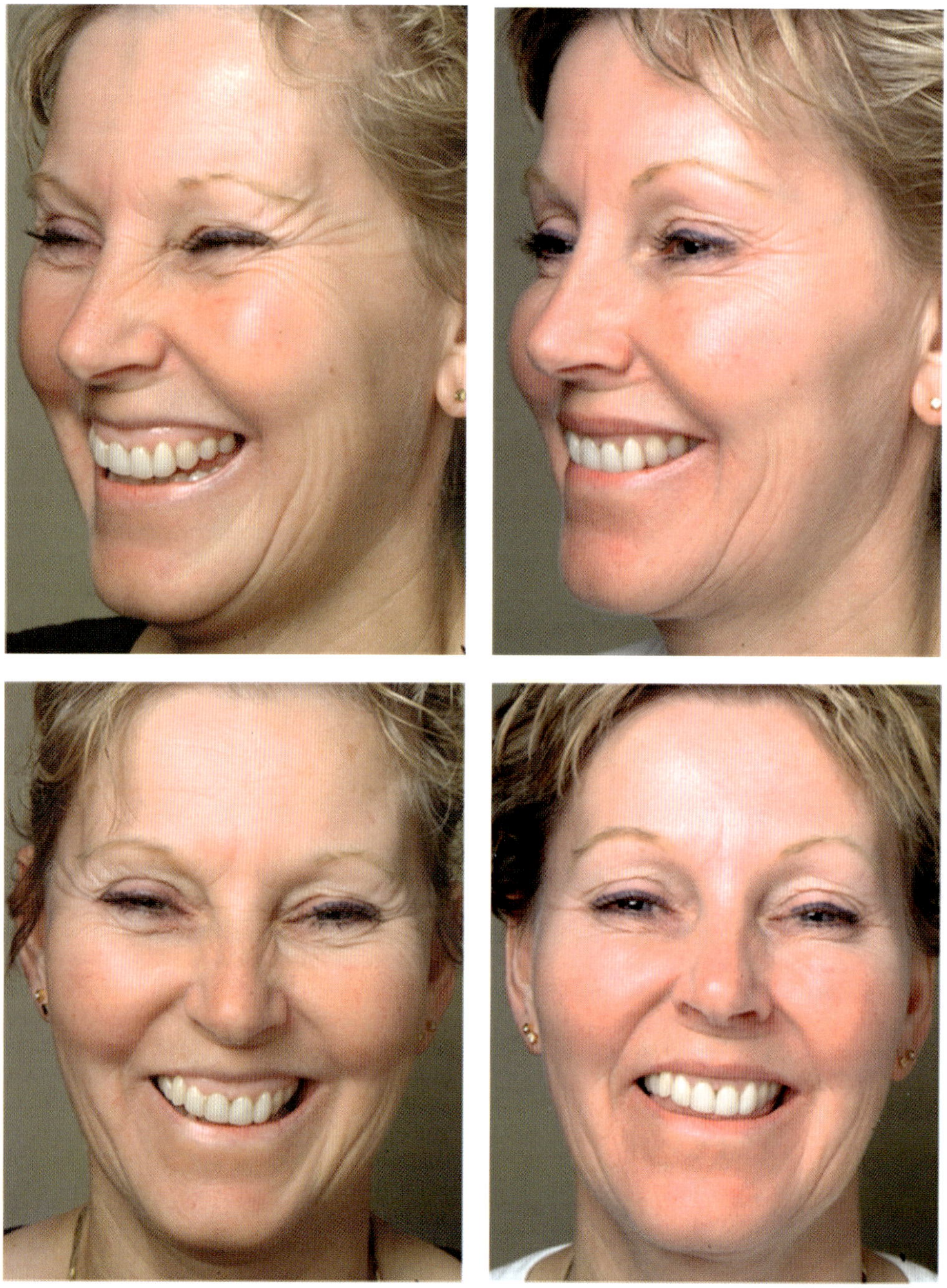

Figure 8.16 Panfacial BoNT-A demonstrating improved nasal proportions as a result of tip elevation (and nasal shortening) secondary to chemodenervation of the nasalis and tip depressor muscles as well as reduction in the gummy smile (photographs of patient aligned for head angle and tilt).

Surgical Anatomy Pearls: Further rotation and lift of the nasal lobule is possible with the concomitant chemodenervation of the upper fibers of the transversus nasalis muscle. This results in a hyperkinesis (similar to a Spock brow) of the alar portion of the transverse nasalis muscle (often referred to as the posterior dilator naris muscle) and lower lateral procerus, both of which elevate and rotate the drooping tip toward ideal Phi proprotions (Figure 8.16).

The arterial vasculature of the nose is expansive, but it is the authors' experience that the major arterial branches appear to be located under creases in the overlying skin. This concept of surface topography being related to underlying structures has been well established.[27–32] Deposition of toxin off the creases will limit untoward bruising when performing nasal injections of BoNT.

NEUROMODULATORS AND THE BEAUTIFUL LOWER FACE

Beautiful Lips and Botulinum Toxin

Gummy Smile and Lip Asymmetries

A gummy smile (greater than 2 mm of gingival show), in its mild form may be considered cute in the young, but can often be distracting in the adult. The perioral complex consists of interdigitating lip elevators and depressors with the orbicularis muscle, and as such is extremely diverse and confusing. Numerous anatomical variants of gummy smile have been described,[33–38] however, the authors have found that for the purposes of injection therapy, three basic types exist, as defined by the intended location of toxin injections: those that target the confluence of the levator labii superioris alaeque nasi (LLSAN) and zygomaticus minor muscles; those that target the orbicularis oris; and those that target both.

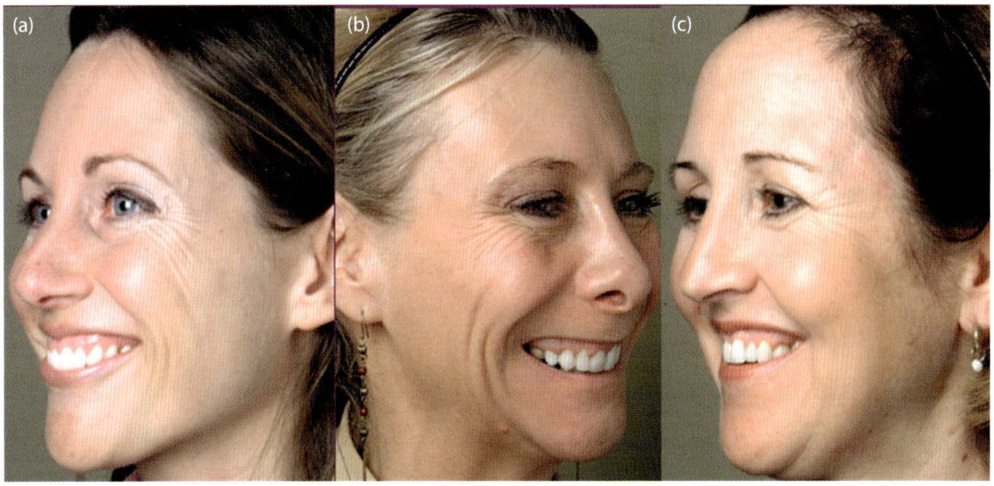

Figure 8.17 Variants of gummy smile according to muscle targeting with BoNT-A. (a) "Venetian blind" type (vermilion not inverted and shortening of ergotrid). (b) "Roll-up blind" type (vermilion inverted and no shortening of ergotrid). (c) Combination type.

Some patients with gummy smiles exhibit a vertical elevation of the upper lip without thinning of the vermilion, similar to a Venetian blind, with shortening of the ergotrid (white lip) (Figure 8.17). In these instances, deployment of small amounts of BoNT just lateral to the nasal alar base focusing on the LLSAN and zygomaticus minor muscles can produce a pleasing contour and position of the upper lip with spontaneous smiling. Other patients expose excessive gingiva by a rolling under of the upper lip vermilion with smiling, without a shortening of the ergotrid, resembling a roll-up blind. Chemodenervation in these instances should be directed symmetrically at the deeper fibers of the orbicularis oris muscle under the white roll of the upper lip (Figure 8.18).

Minute doses (typically 1 u of OnaBTX-A/IncoBTX-A or 2 u of AboBTX-A per injection) are indicated in the perioral region, as, contrary to glabellar treatment, the goal here is *moderation* not *obliteration* of movement. In those instances of both excessive elevation and curling under of the lip (combination type), BoNT treatment may be necessary at both regions described above (Figure 8.19). Lip and smile asymmetries secondary to uneven pull of mimetic muscles (e.g., post-Bell's palsy) can be similarly treated by targeting the muscle on the nonparetic side.

Surgical Anatomy Pearls: The LLSAN and zygomaticus minor muscles appear to insert in a confluence cephalad to the orbicularis muscle located 1 cm lateral to the nasal alar base, providing an ideal target for small doses of BoNT-A to have a significant effect on upper lip excessive retraction.

Additionally, the function of the orbicularis oris muscle appears to be somewhat stratified in that superficial fibers contribute more to pursing while deeper fibers more for lip position and support against the underlying dentition. This explains the rationale behind deeper injections when treating the "roll-up blind" form of gummy smile, with the caveat that the patient may experience some temporary (typically 1 day duration) minor difficulty with oral competence once the BoNT has taken effect. This can manifest as food gets trapped in the buccal-gingival sulcus that requires clearing with the tongue, or driveling when brushing the teeth.

Oral Commissure Position

A common request of patients seeking aesthetic facial improvement is to remove a sad or discontented look as a result of a depressed corner of the mouth. Carruthers and Carruthers originally described the application of botulinum toxin in the depressor anguli oris in 1998.

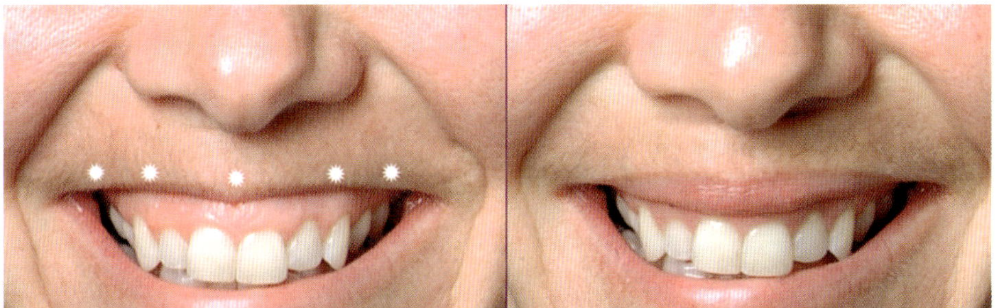

Figure 8.18 BoNT-A treatment of "roll-up" blind type of gummy smile.

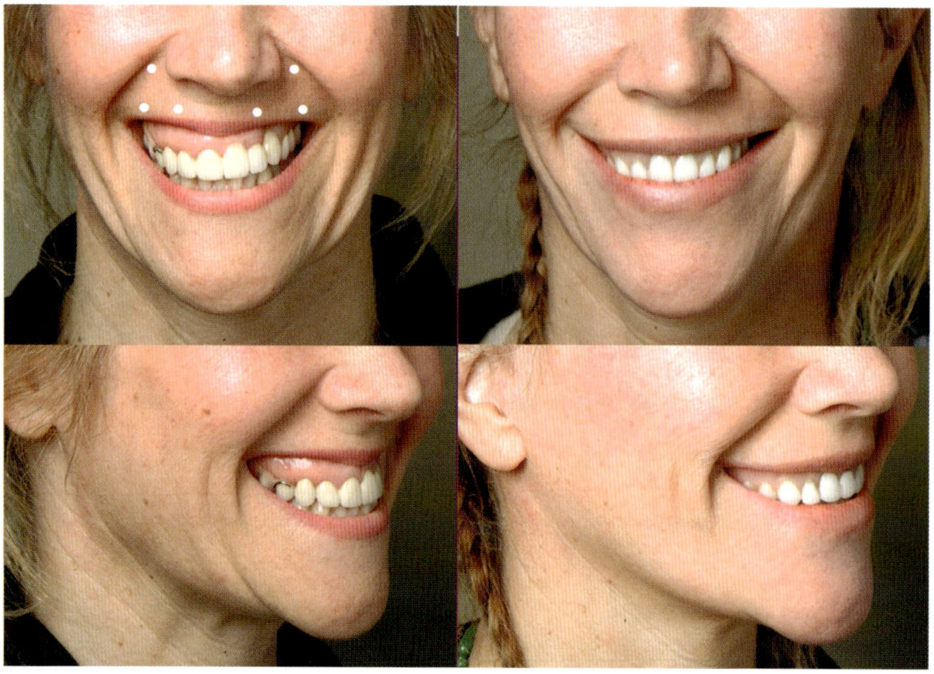

Figure 8.19 BoNT-A treatment of combination type of gummy smile.

While softening unsightly marionette lines, relaxing these depressor muscles leads to an elevation of the corner of the mouth through the anatagonistic action of the levator anguli oris and zygomaticus (major and minor) muscles.[39]

Beautifully proportioned lips exhibit horizontal vermilion show from commissure to commissure equal to the distance from medial pupil to medial pupil (*Phi* of the intercanthal distance) (Figure 8.20). Beyond the elimination of the dour look in the mature patient, restoring the corner of the mouth to the neutral position at rest with BoNT can further improve aesthetics by extending transcommissure width toward *Phi* proportions (Figure 8.21). The opposite should be avoided by excessive neuromodulation of the zygomaticus major in an attempt to eradicate upper cheek crow's feet lines.

Surgical Anatomy Pearls: The risorius muscle originates in a fan-like distribution from the anterior fascia of the masseter and parotid gland to insert horizontally in the modiolus of the periorbital region. In the majority of Asians, the modiolus is actually located below the level of the oral commissure.[40] With age, there is a dynamic discord as this muscle dominates the senescent tissue on which it is pulling, causing a widened smile with unsightly back molar show (Figure 8.22). The muscle has also displayed extreme sensitivity to inadvertent spread of BoNT in cases of masseter treatment for lower facial slimming. Nonetheless, moderating its activity with minute doses of BoNT (1–2 u of OnaBTX-A/IncoBTX-A and 3–4 u of AboBTX-A toxin) can be considered in cases of excessive grinning when smiling in the mature patient, or in cases of muscle hyperactivity of the contralateral hemiface in Bell's palsy. Injection is performed subdermally 1 cm below the intersection of a horizontal line drawn from the tragus to the commissure and a vertical line drawn along the anterior masseteric border (Figure 8.23).

The Beautiful Jaw Contour and Botulinum Toxin

The use of BoNT for lower facial slimming is discussed in greater detail in Chapter 17. The advantage of nonsurgical lower face contouring by reducing undesirable unilateral or bilateral masseter muscle hypertrophy is self-evident in its simplicity, predictability, and avoidance of the undesirable consequences of surgical intervention.[41–43] Although measured masticatory function is dramatically decreased over several months[44], patients do not report any difficulty chewing hard food, change in facial expression, or speech disturbances; and any initial asymmetries are easily corrected at a one-month follow-up visit. Of cautionary note is that instillation of toxin merely superficially can

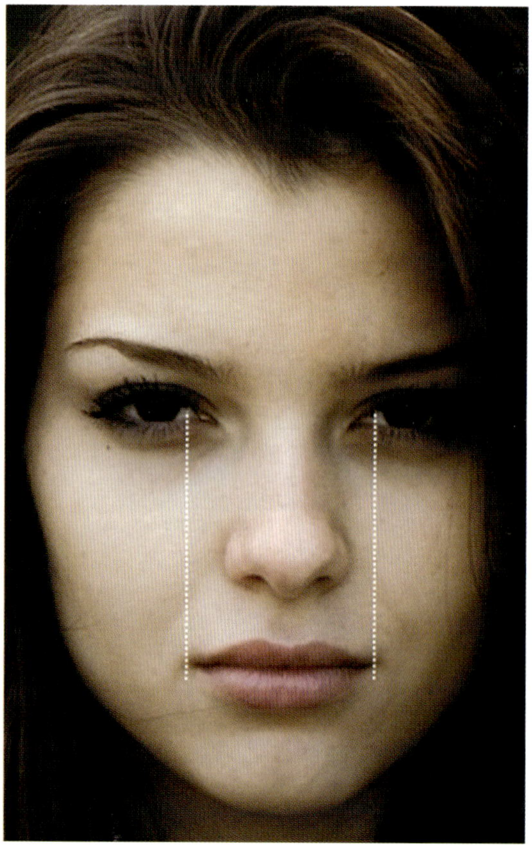

Figure 8.20 Ideal lip width in the female extends from medial iris to medial iris and is 1.618 times the intercanthal distance.

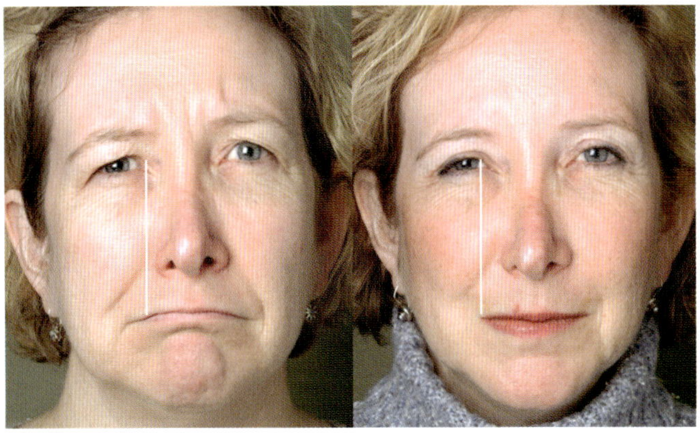

Figure 8.21 BoNT-A treatment of the depressor anguli oris muscles and mentalis allowing vermilion show to the oral commissures and medial iris. Both photographs were taken during exaggerated animation.

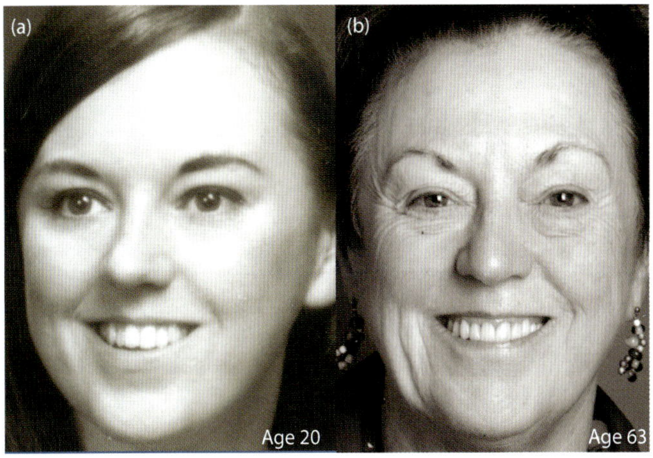

Figure 8.22 Dynamic discord. (a) The imbalance between risorius muscle pull and the resistance of the commissure on which it is acting often results in a "grinning caricature smile". (b) The patient at age 63 shows posterior dentition with a joker-like smile due to overpull of the risorius muscle.

lead to a disfiguring "herniation" of the deeper masseter through the chemodenervated outer muscle lamella. Furthermore, some laxity of the mandibular skin envelope due to loss of volume support can occur in the more mature patient with poor skin tone. Although several investigators have empirically noted compensatory temporalis hypertrophy, this has not borne out with cephalometric measurements post-treatment.

In cases of lower facial contouring, the injection specialist must appreciate that there must be an *aesthetic* endpoint for slimming—a so-called sweet spot beyond which further narrowing may actually detract away from beauty. Certainly, Liew's Angle of Beauty applies[45], and is the hallmark of the ideal vertical facial angle as seen in many noted beautiful faces globally. Additionally, the concepts of symmetry, balance, and harmony are nowhere more critical than in the lower face. Golden proportions in the female dictate that an attractive lower profile is typified by a transcommissure distance of 1.618 in ratio to 1 for the distance from the oral commissure to the ipsilateral mandibular outline (Figure 8.24).

Posterior cheek enlargement secondary to benign parotid gland hypertrophy, causing squaring of the lower face, can likewise be successfully treated with BoNT-A with excellent cosmetic results[46] (Figure 8.25). Clinical differentiation from masseter hypertrophy relies on both careful palpation during maximal bite and the presence of blunting of the gonial angle of the mandible by the tail of the gland. Parotid gland enlargement is a common finding in HIV-associated salivary gland disease, and carries with it significant cosmetic disfigurement and social stigmatization. Doses in the range of 25–30 units of OnaBTX-A/IncoBTX-A or 75 units of AboBTX-A toxin spread over 4–5 injection sites can cause temporary (6 month) glandular regression through pathways that have not yet been fully elucidated. Patients do not report any dry mouth adverse events, as has been confirmed by the medical use of BoNT in extreme cases of sialorrhea.

Contouring of a tight popply chin with BoNT can be accomplished through moderation of the corrugator-like dermal pull of the mentalis muscle. Targeting the deep origin in the midline just inferior to the labiomental crease, as well as symmetrical superficial injections of BoNT on either side of the midline over the point of the chin will avoid the adjacent depressors of the lower lip. As a three-dimensional structure, the chin's height, width, and projection should be addressed by the concomitant use of soft tissue filler (Figure 8.26).

Surgical Anatomy Pearls: The mentalis muscle extends from its mandibular origin deep beneath the mental crease upward in a cauliflower-like projection to insert into the dermis of the chin. Tight chins can be relaxed into more pleasing appearance both in profile and width by the relaxation of the offending muscle with BoNT. Simultaneous softening of a deep labiomental crease can be effected.

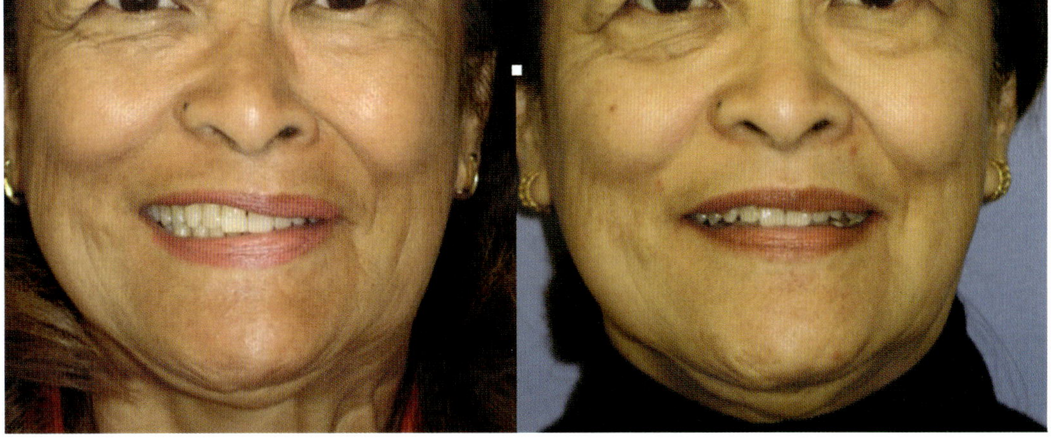

Figure 8.23 Bell's palsy asymmetric smile corrected by deposition of minute amounts of BoNT-A into the origin of the right risorius and zygomaticus major muscles (as well as into the body of the depressor right labii inferioris) (see text).

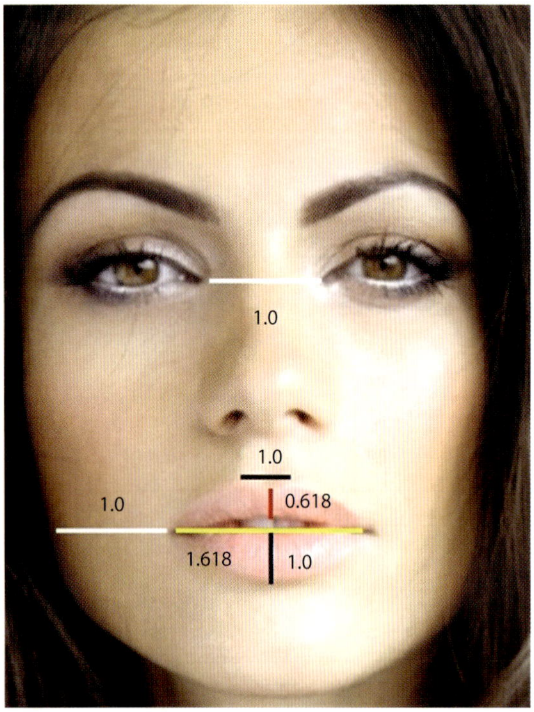

Figure 8.24 Golden proportions of the lower face.

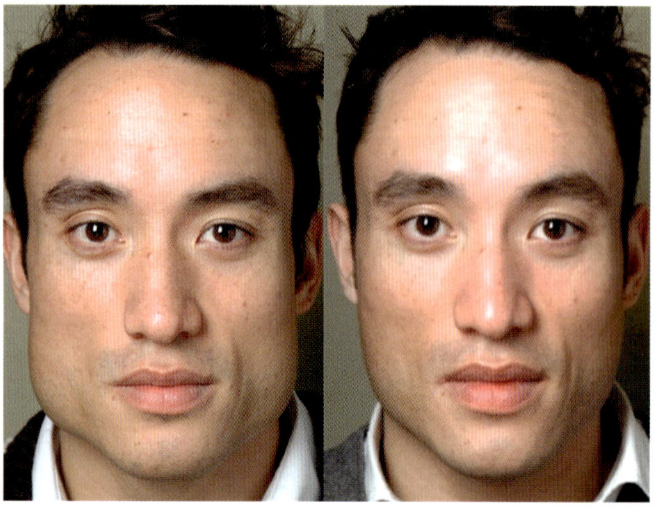

Figure 8.25 Lower facial slimming by BoNT-A treatment of both masseteric and parotid hypertrophy.

BOTULINUM TOXIN AND THE BEAUTIFUL NECK

It is well recognized that one of the most obvious clues to a women's age is the appearance of her neck. The second most obvious sign is "no appearance of the neck"—a more mature woman wearing a scarf or a turtleneck in the heat of summer implies she is self-conscious about the appearance of her neck.

It is important to understand for both the aesthetic physician and patient that the process of restoring the aging face and neck to a more youthful and attractive one is like restoring a painting, and requires a recipe of steps that needs to be performed in the right syntax of events. Botulinum toxin plays an important role in this process in simultaneously treating the depressor anguli oris muscles, the mentalis muscle, the submandibular and parotid glands (where indicated), the platysmal bands, and necklace lines.

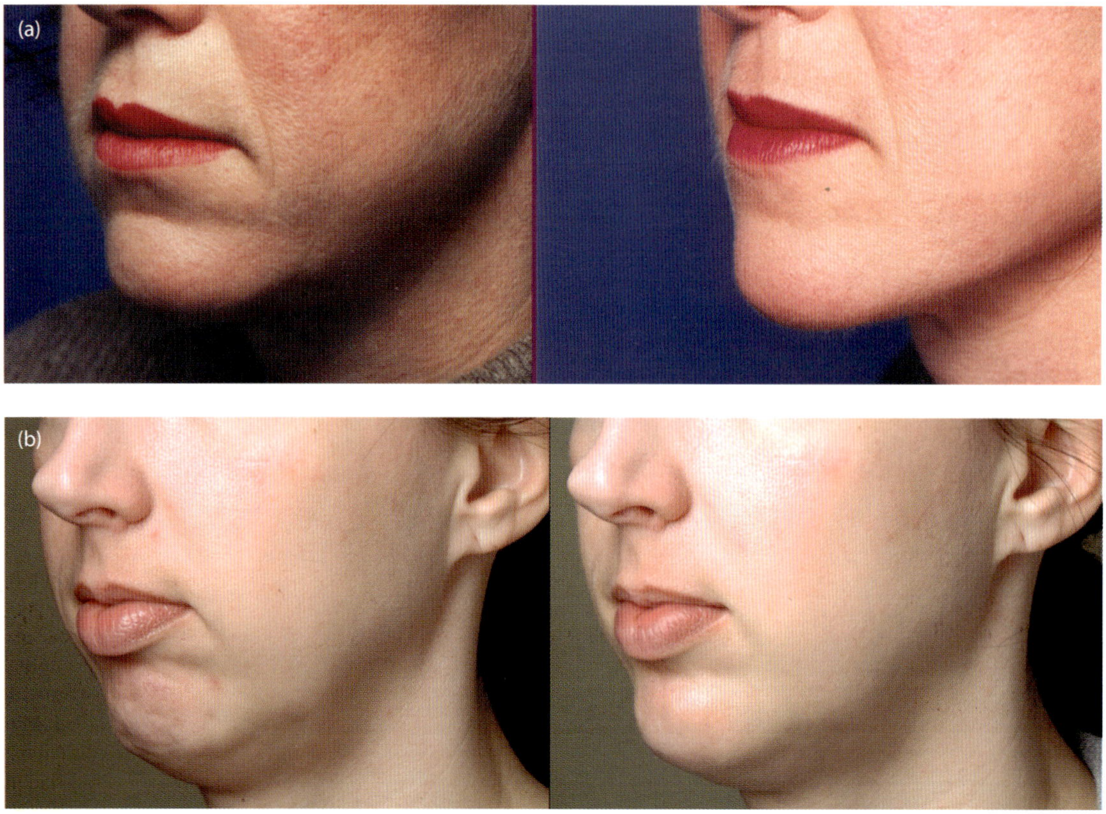

Figure 8.26 (a,b) Combination therapy of filler and BoNT-A for chin contouring.

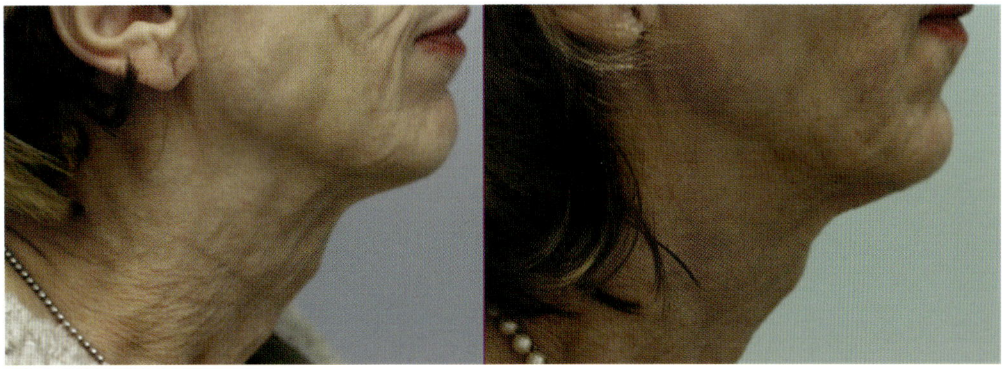

Figure 8.27 "Micro-Botox" treatment of the neck.

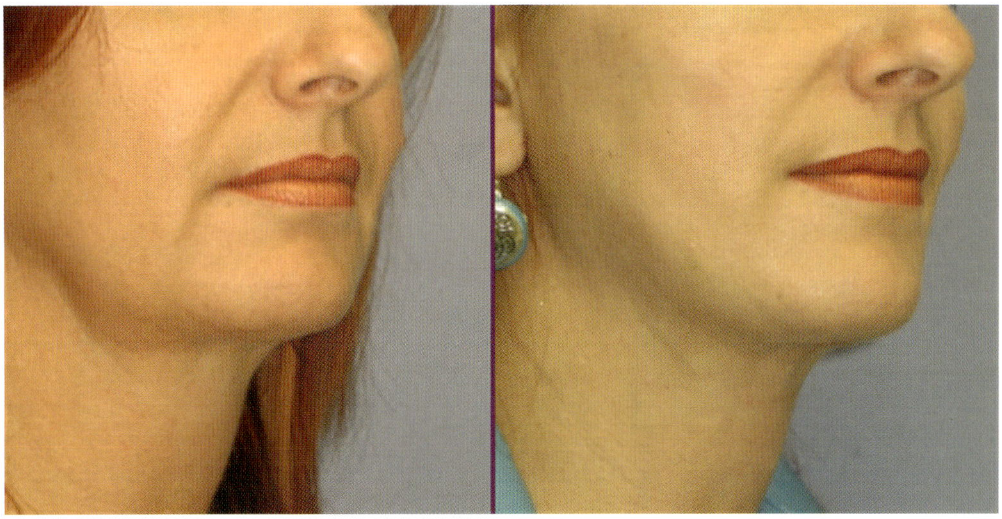

Figure 8.28 BoNT-A treatment of submandibular gland prominence.

Use of BoNT to reduce platysmal banding is well described in the literature. Levi modified its application across the upper neck in a procedure he coined the Nefertiti lift for redefining and accentuating the jawline.[47] Wu employs a "meso" technique of intradermal microdoses of BoNT-A spaced 1 cm apart to smooth neck contours and diminish skin crepiness[48] (Figure 8.27).

As with the parotid, unsightly submandibular gland hypertrophy can similarly be treated with BoNT providing a smooth jawline (Figure 8.28), whose ideal anterior angle lies at *Phi* (1.618 of the intercanthal distance) from the gonial angle (Figure 8.29). Typical doses range from 15–20 units of OnaBTX-A/IncoBTX-A or 50 units of AboBTX-A, with precise deposition into the gland necessary to avoid affecting the surrounding musculature of deglutition.

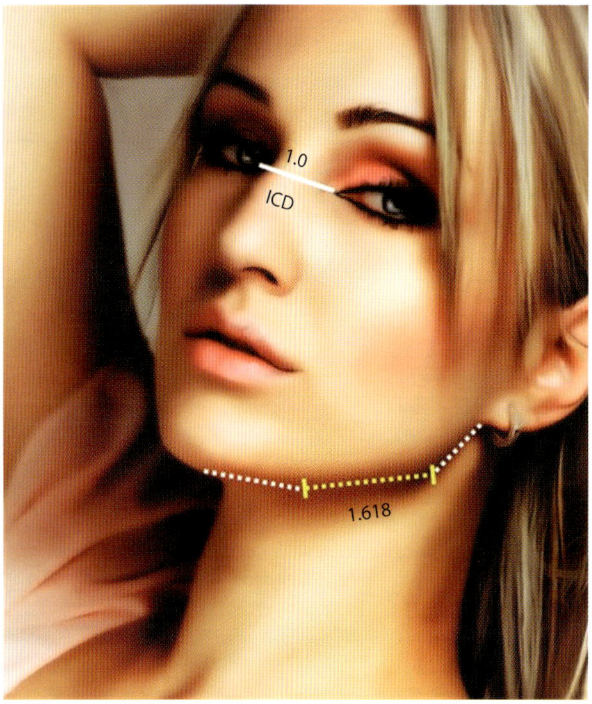

Figure 8.29 A youthful, golden proportioned jawline has its anterior angle lying *Phi* (1.618) of the intercanthal distance from the gonial angle.

BEYOND THE OBVIOUS—CONCLUSION

Aesthetic facial shaping with botulinum toxin relies on a comprehensive understanding of the facial muscular anatomy combined with a refined technique based on individual animation, appropriate dosing, and ideal aesthetics. Obsessive attention to detail is the key to creating great outcomes. Paying attention to the little changes that have made your patients lose their youthful proportioned appearance is critical—we have a tendency to see but not observe. Very often the most important issues are hiding in plain sight.

The role of botulinum toxin in the aesthetic arena has evolved dramatically since its original introduction for the treatment of dynamic glabellar lines. Today's aesthetic patient does not want to look good from their treatments—they expect to look fantastic. The primary goal of the aesthetic injection specialist should remain the creation of a "natural best version" of the patient while optimizing the procedural experience.

REFERENCES

1. Carruthers JDA, Carruthers JA. Treatment of glabellar frown lines with *C. botulinum*-A exotoxin. *J Dermatol Surg Oncol* 1992; 18: 17–21.
2. Swift A, Remington K. BeautiPHIcation™: A global approach to facial beauty. *Clinics in Plastic Surgery* 38(3): 347–77.
3. Slater A et al. Newborn infants prefer attractive faces. *Infant Behav Devel* 1998; 21: 345–54.
4. Langlois JH et al. Infant preferences for attractive faces: Rudiment of a stereotype? *Dev Psychol* 1987; 23: 363–9.
5. Langlois JH et al. Facial diversity and infant preferences for attractive faces. *Dev Psych* 1991; 27: 79–84.
6. Hammermesh DS, Biddle JE. Beauty and the labor market. *Am Econ Rev* 1994; 84: 1174–94.
7. Marlowe CM et al. Gender and attractiveness biases in hiring decisions: Are more experienced managers less biased? *J Appl Psycho* 1996; 81: 11–21.
8. Frieze IH et al. Perceived and actual discrimination in the salaries of male and female managers. *J Appl Soc Psychol* 1990; 20: 46–67.
9. Frieze IH et al. Attractiveness and income for men and women in management. *J Appl Soc Psychol* 1991; 21: 1039–57.
10. Jones DM, Hill K. Criteria for facial attractiveness in five populations. *Human Nat* 1993; 4: 271–96.
11. Cunningham M et al. Consistency and variability in the cross-cultural perception of female physical attractiveness. *J Personality Soc Psychol* 1995; 68: 261–79.
12. Perrett DI et al. Facial shape and judgments of female attractiveness. *Nature* 1994; 368: 239–42.
13. Rhee SC, Lee SH. Attractive composite faces of different races. *Aesthetic Plastic Surg* 2010; 34(6): 800–1.
14. Goodman GJ. The oval female facial shape—A study in beauty. *Derm Surg* 2015; 41(12): 1375–83.
15. Kane M. Commentary on the oval female facial shape—A study in beauty. *Derm Surg* 2015; 41(12): 1384–8.
16. Lee JY et al. Anatomical verification and designation of the superficial layer of the temporalis muscle. *Clin Anat* 2012; 25: 176–81.
17. Farella M et al. Masticatory muscle activity during deliberately performed oral tasks *Physiol. Meas* 2008; 29(12): 1397–410.
18. Jellinek NJ et al. Paramedian forehead flap: Advances, procedural nuances, and variations in technique. *Dermatol Surg* 2014; 40: S30–42.
19. Swift A. Anatomical study of the topographical landmarks of the supratrochlear artery, 2016. Submitted for publication.
20. Benedetto AV, Lahti JG. Measurement of the anatomic position of the Corrugator Supercilii. *Dermatol Surg* 2005; 31: 923–7.
21. Gordin EA et al. Subcutaneous vs. Intramuscular botulinum toxin split-face randomized study. *JAMA Facial Plast Surg* 2104; 16(3): 193–8.
22. McCurdy JA. Beautiful eyes: Characteristics and application to aesthetic surgery. *Facial Plast Surg* 2006; 22: 204–14.
23. Rhee SC et al. Biometric study of eyelid shape and dimensions of different races with respect to beauty. *Aesth Plast Surg* 2012; 36: 1236–45.
24. Fagien S. Temporary management of upper lid ptosis, lid malposition, and eyelid fissure asymmetry with botulinum toxin Type A. *Plas Recon Surg J* 2004; 114(7): 1892–902.
25. Figallo EE et al. Nose muscular dynamics: The tip trigonum. *Plast Recon Surg* 2001; 108(5): 1118–26.
26. Dayan SH. Treatment of the lower third of the nose and dynamic nasal tip ptosis with botox. *Plast Recon Surg* 2005; 115(6): 1783–4.
27. Kligman AM, Zheng P, Lavker RM. The anatomy and pathogenesis of wrinkles. *Br J Dermatol* 1985; 113: 37–42.
28. Hillebrand GG, Liang XY, Yoshii T. New wrinkles on wrinkling: an 8-year longitudinal study on the progression of expression lines into persistent wrinkles. *Br J Dermatol* 2010; 162: 1233–1241.
29. Tsugi T. Ultrastructure of deep wrinkles in the elderly. *J Cutan Pathol* 1987;14: 158–164.
30. Gambichhler T. Mid-dermal elastolysis revisited. *Arch Dermatol Res* 2010; 302(2): 85–93.
31. Tsuji T, Yorifuji T, Hayashi Y, Hamada T. Light and scanning electron microscopic studies on wrinkles in aged persons' skin. *Br J Dermatol* 1986; 114: 329–335.
32. Pessa, JE et al. The anatomical basis for wrinkles. *Aesthetic Surg J* 2014; 34(2): 227–234.
33. Rubin LR. The anatomy of a smile: Its importance in the treatment of facial paralysis. *Plast Reconstr Surg* 1974; 53: 384–7.
34. Mazzuco R, Hexsel D. Gummy smile and botulinum toxin: A new approach based on the gingival exposure area. *J Am Acad Dermatol* 2010; 63(6): 1042–51.
35. Suber JS et al. OnabotulinumtoxinA for the treatment of a "Gummy Smile". *Aesthetic Surg J* 2014; 34(3): 432–7.
36. Polo M. Botulinum toxin type A (Botox) for the neuromuscular correction of excessive gingival display on smiling (gummy smile). *Am J Orthod Dentofacial Orthop* 2008; 133(2): 195–203.
37. Sucupira E, Abramovitz A. A simplified method for smile enhancement: Botulinum toxin injection for gummy smile. *Plast Reconstr Surg* 2012; 130(3): 726–8.
38. Polo M. A simplified method for smile enhancement: Botulinum toxin injection for gummy smile. *Plast Reconstr Surg* 2013; 131(6): 934e–5e.
39. Goldman A, Wollina U. Elevation of the corner of the mouth using botulinum toxin Type A. *J Cutan Aesthet Surg* 2010; 3(3): 145–50.
40. Kim HS et al. An anatomical study of the risorius in Asians and its insertion at the modiolus. *Surg Radiol Anat* 2015; 37: 147–51.
41. Tartaro GT et al. Lower facial contouring with botulinum toxin Type A. *J Cran Fac Surg* 2008; 19(6): 1613–7.
42. Kim NH et al. The use of botulinum toxin Type A in aesthetic mandibular contouring. *Plas Recon Surg Journal* 2005; 115(3): 919–30.
43. Park MY et al. Botulinum toxin Type A treatment for contouring of the lower face. *Dermatol Surg* 2003; 29(5): 477–83.
44. Choong JL et al. Electrophysiologic change and facial contour following botulinum toxin A injection in square faces. *Plast Recon Surg Journal* 2007; 120(3): 769–78.
45. Liew S, Dart A. Nonsurgical reshaping of the lower face. *Aesth Surg Journal* 2008; 28(3): 251–7.
46. Shim WH et al. Effect of botulinum toxin Type A injection on lower facial contouring evaluated using a three-dimensional laser scan. *Dermatol Surg* 2010; 36: 2161–6.
47. Levi PM. The "Nefertiti Lift": A new technique for specific re-contouring of the Jawline. *J of Cosm & Laser Ther* 2007; 9(4): 249–52.
48. Wu WT. Microbotox of the lower face and neck—Evolution of a personal technique and its clinical effects. *Plast Reconstr Surg* 2015; 136: 92S–100S.

9 Botulinum toxin in the management of focal hyperhidrosis

David M. Pariser and DeeAnna Glaser

Hyperhidrosis (HH) is excessive sweating beyond that which is necessary for physiological thermoregulation and homeostasis. It is a common condition that has serious social, emotional, and professional consequences and adversely influences quality of life more than any other disease or disorder that dermatologists treat as measured by the Dermatology Life Quality Index. Although most commonly a chronic idiopathic condition that may involve one or more areas of the body such as the axillae, palms, soles, face, inframammary and inguinal folds, secondary medical conditions or medications as a cause for the excessive sweating should be excluded before making a diagnosis. When one area is involved, the term primary focal HH is used; if more than one area is affected, the term primary multifocal HH is appropriate. Botulinum toxins are one of the mainstays of treatments for primary focal and multifocal HH and will be the focus of discussion of this chapter.

SWEATING

Sweating is a normal physiological response to increased body temperature and is an important mechanism in releasing heat produced from endogenous as well as exogenous sources. The heat regulatory center is located within the hypothalamus, particularly involving the preoptic and anterior nuclei. Sweating is controlled by the sympathetic nervous system.[1] Nerve fibers exit the preoptic or anterior nuclei and descend ipsilaterally through the spinal cord until they reach the intermediolateral column, where they exit the cord and enter the sympathetic chain. Although the neurotransmitter for the sympathetic nervous system is generally norepinephrine, acetylcholine is the neurotransmitter mainly involved in the sweating response. Other chemical mediators found in periglandular nerves include vasoactive intestinal peptide (VIP), atrial natriuretic peptide (ANP), galanin, and calcitonin gene peptide (CGP).[2]

The eccrine glands, responsible for producing sweat, are distributed around the body, with high concentrations in areas such as the palms, soles, and forehead (Table 9.1). They are located at the junction of the dermis and subcutaneous fat and their function is to secrete water while conserving sodium chloride for electrolyte maintenance. Although they continually produce secretions, they are stimulated by heat, exercise, anxiety, and stress.[3,4] Under severe heat stress, up to 10 L of sweat can be produced in a day; however, the normal rate is 0.5–1.0 mL/min. While rates vary greatly among individuals, men generally sweat more than women.[5]

The apocrine glands open into the hair follicle and are located mostly in the axillae and perineum. They become functional around puberty and are not important for thermoregulation. The scant viscous secretions are thought to function as chemical attractants or signals, as an odor is produced when the secretions reach the skin surface and interact with bacteria.[1,3] The apocrine glands respond to adrenergic stimuli, epinephrine more than norepinephrine.

HYPERHIDROSIS

Hyperhidrosis simply describes excess sweating beyond that necessary for physiological thermoregulation and homeostasis.[6] Problems can occur within any portion of the system: from the hypothalamus to the sweat gland or duct.[2] The amount of sweat necessary to be considered "excessive" is not well-defined and is variable between individuals. Patients with HH do not demonstrate any histopathologic changes in their sweat glands, nor are there any changes in the numbers of sweat glands.[7]

HH may be generalized or focal, bilateral or unilateral, symmetric or asymmetric, primary or secondary in origin. Generalized HH affects the entire body whereas focal HH occurs in discrete sections of the body.[8] Generalized HH is usually secondary in nature, and the differential diagnosis is extensive (Table 9.2). Focal or localized HH may result from a secondary process including lesions or tumors of the central or peripheral nervous system.[9,10] Most commonly, however, it is idiopathic (primary) and may involve one area and be considered "focal" or may involve more than one area and be considered "multifocal." Usually, however, it is referred to simply as "hyperhidrosis." It is characterized by excessive sweating of small areas of the skin, usually the axilla, palms, soles, face, inframammary areas, or groin.[11] The onset is usually in adolescence to early adulthood but can

Table 9.1 Eccrine Sweat Glands: Area and Quantity

Area	Quantity (cm^2)
Sole of foot	620
Forehead	360
Palms	300
Axillae	300
Thigh	120
Scrotum	80
Back	65
Nail bed	None
Nipple	None
Inner preputial surface	None
Labia majora	None
Glans penis	None
Glans clitoris	None

Table 9.2 Etiologies of Generalized versus Focal/Localized Hyperhidrosis

Generalized	Focal/Localized
Fever	Primary focal hyperhidrosis[a]
Tumors	Intrathoracic tumors
Infections	Rheumatoid arthritis
Thyrotoxicosis	Spinal cord disease or injury
Pheochromocytoma	Stroke
Diabetes mellitus	Syringomyelia
Diabetes insipidus	Ross syndrome
Hypoglycemia	Atrioventricular fistula
Hypopituitarism	Gustatory hyperhidrosis (Frey's syndrome)
Endocarditis	Localized unilateral hyperhidrosis
Gout	Cold-induced hyperhidrosis
Medications	Eccrine nevus
Anxiety	Social anxiety disorder
Drug withdrawal	

[a]Most common.

Table 9.3 Criteria for Establishing the Diagnosis of Primary Focal Hyperhidrosis

Focal visible sweating of at least 6 months' duration; with no apparent cause; and at least two of the following characteristics:

- Bilateral and relatively symmetrical
- Age of onset <25 years
- Positive family history of focal hyperhidrosis
- Cessation of focal sweating during sleep
- Frequency of at least one episode per week
- Impairment of daily activities

Source: Hornberger J et al. *J Am Acad Dermatol* 2004; 51: 274–86.

begin in early childhood, especially the palmar-plantar variants[6,7] (Table 9.3). The differential diagnosis for excessive sweating is extensive, and an underlying cause must be considered, especially when the HH is generalized, asymmetrically distributed, or has an onset late in life.[6,12] A detailed history with comprehensive review of symptoms and thorough physical examination is the first step to identifying the type and cause of HH of a patient presenting with excessive sweating. The necessity for further testing is based on the findings from the history and physical exam.

This chapter will focus on primary focal hyperhidrosis henceforth identified simply as hyperhidrosis (HH). The prevalence of HH is reported to be 2.8% although it may be higher. It most commonly presents in the second or third decade of life and a family history has been reported in 30%–50% of patients.[13] The prevalence is similar for men and women, although interestingly, women are more likely to seek evaluation and treatment.[11] Patients may sweat on a continuous basis throughout the day, but more commonly, there are episodes of profuse sweating with a sudden onset. Trigger factors include emotional stress, stress at work or in the public, higher environmental temperatures, and stimulants such as caffeine and exercise. However, patients also often have episodes of HH without a known initiating factor or trigger when they are cool, comfortable, and calm.

HH has a negative impact on many aspects of patients' "daily living: physically, psychologically, and occupationally."[14–16] There is limited and mixed information on any real increase in cutaneous infections or other problems such as skin maceration with idiopathic HH.[17,18] The greatest impact of HH is the significant reduction in the quality of life and the alterations it has on daily functioning.[19] Patients report a lack of confidence, feeling depressed, refraining from meeting new people, and avoiding intimate activities. Work limitations are reported because of excessive sweating and patients describe having to change clothes during the day.

MEASURING HYPERHIDROSIS

The starch-iodine test is a simple way to detect the presence of sweat (Figures 9.1 and 9.2). The hyperhidrotic area to be treated is dried thoroughly, an iodine solution is painted over the area and when it has thoroughly dried, a starch powder such as corn starch is sprinkled on the surface. With the interaction of sweat, a purple to black color develops within minutes. Decolorized iodine solutions do not perform the colorimetric change properly and should not be used for this test. Many physicians today use iodine-containing surgical preparations such as Betadine™ solution or swabs to perform the iodine-starch test. Plain corn starch that is used for cooking is readily available and inexpensive. The starch may be applied with a brush, cotton ball, sifter, or loose gauze. The iodine-starch test is useful in localizing the areas of sweat production but is not a quantitative test. For iodine-sensitive patients, Alizarin or Ponceau red dye and starch can be used. The pink powder turns to a bright red color when wet. Ninhydrin is another variant, but regardless of which variant is used, they all achieve a colorimetric outline of the sweating area.[20–22]

Gravimetric testing measures the amount of sweat produced during a given time. It can be performed using a preweighed filter paper

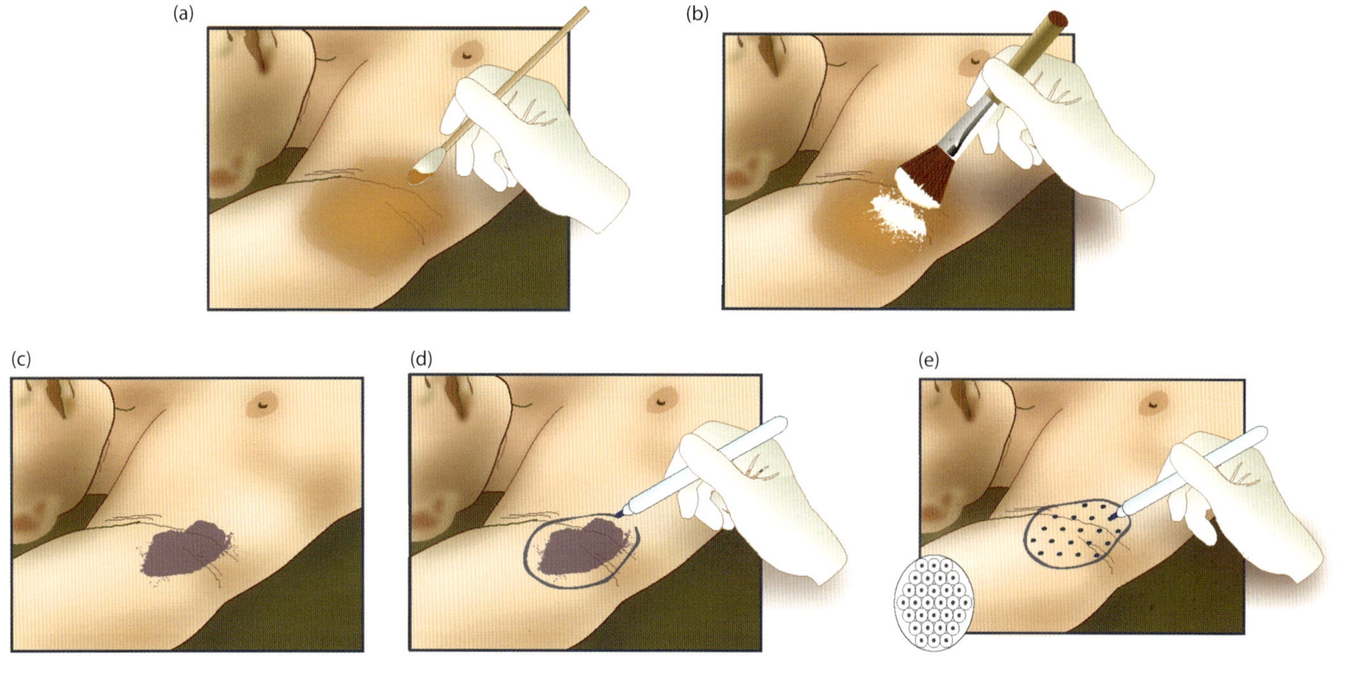

Figure 9.1 Starch-iodine test for detecting hyperhidrosis. (a) 1. Clean and dry the axilla thoroughly and completely. 2. Paint the entire underarm area with an iodine solution or povidone-iodine or with premoistened Betadine® swabs or swabsticks. (b) Evenly dust site with fine starch powder using sifter, gauze pad, or make-up brush. Wipe off any excess. (c) Wait several (10–15) minutes. Presence of sweat will cause mixture to turn dark blue-purple color, making location of sweat discernible. (d) With marker, outline areas of excessive sweating. May be a circle, oval, or "islands." Wipe off excess starch and iodine solution. (e) With marker, mark/identify regions of the sweating area with center points 1.5 cm apart. Do this in a zigzag or staggered pattern. You will have a grid. (By courtesy of Albert Ganss, International Hyperhidrosis Society).

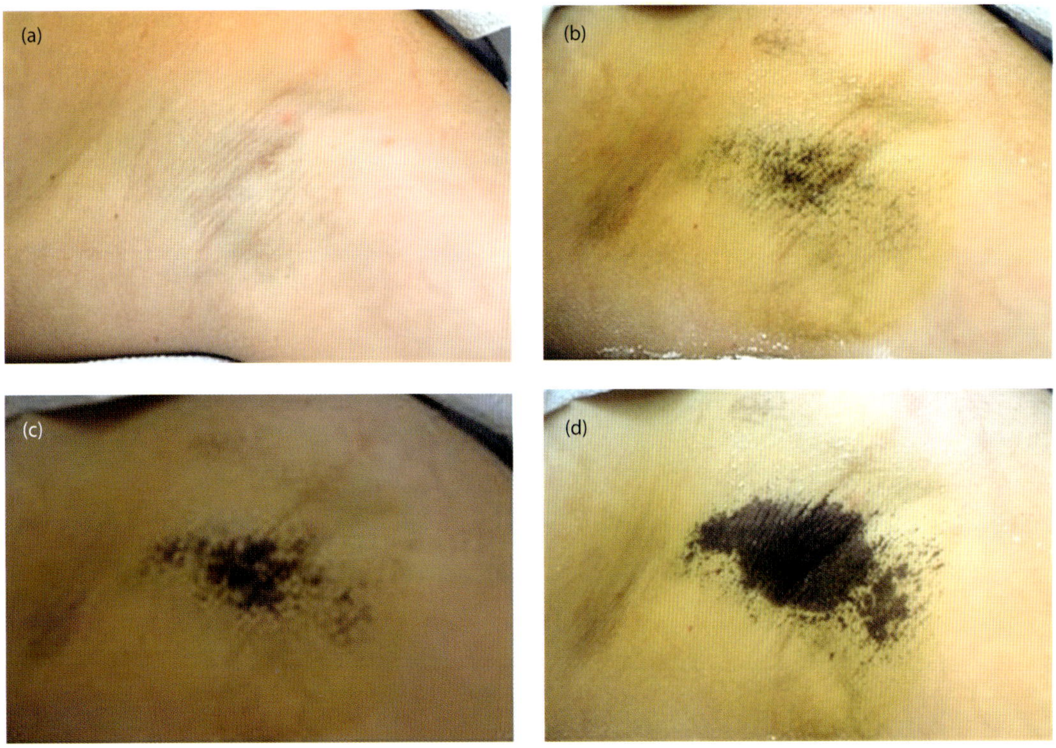

Figure 9.2 Starch-iodine test. (a–d) Over a period of 5 minutes, the area of sweating becomes visible and the area requiring treatment is clearly identified. (Courtesy of David Pariser.)

that is placed on the affected area (typically for 5 minutes) under occlusion and then reweighing the paper. Evaporation must be prevented. Another technique uses preweighed gauze pads held under the arms for a specific amount of time and then reweighed. There is no standard or validated quantity that separates HH from euhidrosis, although it can exceed 30 times that of normal nonhyperhidrotic individuals. Hund suggests a minimum of 100 mg/5 min for men and 50 mg/5 min for women will identify axillary HH.[5] A study of 60 patients demonstrated that the mean axillary sweat production was 346 mg/5 min for men and 186 mg/5 min for women with HH (healthy control subjects had values of 72 and 46, respectively). Likewise, the mean palmar gravimetric measurement was 300 mg/5 min.[23] Gravimetric evaluation is typically reserved for research purposes and is not routinely used in clinical practices.

A third method used to measure disease severity is with questionnaires and quality of life scales and patient-reported outcome measurements (PROs). Several such tools are available, including the Dermatology Life Quality Index (DLQI), the Hyperhidrosis Impact Questionnaire (HHIQ), and the Hyperhidrosis Disease Severity Scale (HDSS). The DLQI has 10 items that form six domains such that a total score of 0 is best and 30 indicates the worst quality of life. The HHIQ has items for a baseline evaluation and 10 items used to assess treatment follow-up. It too is most commonly used in clinical trials.[24] The HDSS is based on one question that the patient can answer in the office (Table 9.4). The HDSS is a simple tool to use in clinical setting and is responsive to treatment with a one-point HDSS improvement corresponding to approximately a 50% reduction in sweat. This validated scale can aid in selecting patients appropriate for therapy and for assessing effectiveness of treatment.[25]

Table 9.4 Hyperhidrosis Disease Severity Scale

Which best describes the impact of sweating on your daily activity?
1. My (underarm) sweating is never noticeable and never interferes with my daily activities.
2. My (underarm) sweating is tolerable but sometimes interferes with my daily activity
3. My (underarm) sweating is barely tolerable and frequently interferes with my daily activity.
4. My (underarm) sweating is intolerable and always interferes with my daily activity.
Source: Glaser DA, et al. *Presented at the Annual Meeting of the American Academy of Dermatology*, Washington, DC, 2004, with permission.

THERAPY

Many treatments are available for HH, and therapy should be tailored to the needs of the individual, based on factors such as age and health status, location of HH, extent and severity of the disease, occupation, lifestyle, and socioeconomic factors such as cost of the various treatments and insurance coverage considerations (Table 9.5). Antiperspirants are used as first-line therapy and function by decreasing sweat secretion through deposition of salts which block the distal eccrine ducts. Over-the-counter (OTC) products very rarely control patients with severe disease (HDSS 3 or 4).[7,11,26,27] Newer OTC products containing more complex aluminum-zirconium salts

Table 9.5 Most Commonly Used Treatments for Hyperhidrosis

Antiperspirants, over-the-counter products and prescription medicines
Iontophoresis
Oral medications
Botulinum neurotoxin
Microwave thermolysis
Local excision of eccrine glands
Liposuction with or without curettage
Endoscopic thoracic sympathectomy

Table 9.6 Anticholinergics Commonly Used to Treat Hyperhidrosis

Medication	Dosage
Glycopyrrolate topical preparations compounded as cream, lotion or wipes in 1%–4% concentrations	Apply daily to affected areas
Glycopyrrolate tablets	Starting dose 1 mg bid, escalate by one mg/day every 1–2 weeks until therapeutic success or development of side effects
Oxybutynin tablets	Starting dose 5 mg bid. Escalate by 5 mg mg/day every 1–2 weeks until therapeutic success or development of side effects
Propranolol	5–10 mg dose can be given 45 minutes before sweat-provoking event. Not for continuous use.
Propantheline bromide	15 mg bid gradually titrated
Benzotropine	1–2 mg/day not to exceed 6 mg/day

provide a better result for some patients. Prescription strength products containing higher concentrations of metal salts most commonly aluminum chloride may be more effective than OTC preparations.[28] Efficacy is still limited, and side effects are frequent with skin irritation, erythema, dryness, and pruritus. Several topical anticholinergic agents are currently in clinical trials and may offer an additional topical option on approval.

No systemic drugs are approved by the U.S. FDA for treatment of HH but several systemic anticholinergic drugs such as glycopyrrolate, atropine, or oxybutynin provide a generalized acetylcholine blockade and are widely used in clinical practice (Table 9.6).[26,29–31] The largest clinical trial of any anticholinergic was with oxybutynin. In this randomized placebo-controlled trial 50 patients received an initial dose of 2.5 mg daily increased over 3 weeks to 5 mg bid. Approximately 70% of the patients reported improvement in their axillary and palmar HH and 90% reported improvement in plantar sweating.[32] Adverse effects such as dry eyes, dry mouth, and urinary retention are frequently encountered at the doses required to achieve symptom relief. Additionally, the generalized reduction in sweat production can be dangerous in individuals who engage in exercise, sports, or work in hot environments.

Iontophoresis is a treatment that uses an electrical device to deliver direct current through tap water. The mechanism of action is unknown but may change the ability of the pores to secrete sweat, or physically block the release of sweat via ions that enter the ducts. It is most suited for treatment of the hands and feet. Anticholinergic agents can also be added to the tap water.[33] Side effects are relatively minimal but the treatment is relatively time-consuming and cumbersome, limiting its use for many patients (Figure 9.3).[33]

Local surgical excision and liposuction or curettage techniques can be used to remove eccrine units.[34] The outcome is highly technique-dependent and is typically limited to the axilla. Endoscopic thoracic sympathectomy (ETS) offers long-term improvement, more so for palmar than for axillary disease, but is not universally accepted. The sympathetic chain is interrupted at the T2, T3, and sometimes the T4 ganglion.[35,36] Success rates for palmar disease approximate 95% but is less for axillary HH. Surgical and anesthetic-related adverse events are relatively rare, but the major issue with ETS surgery for HH is the potential for patients to develop compensatory sweating (Figure 9.4).[37] The incidence varies, but approximately 60%–70% of patients seem to develop it, with its occurrence and severity being unpredictable.[35,38,39]

A relatively new addition to the treatment armamentarium for treatment of axillary HH only is the microwave thermolysis device (MiraDry®). It delivers microwave energy to the subcutaneous tissues which preferentially destroy eccrine glands (and to a lesser extent apocrine glands and hair follicles) due to the physical property of preferential absorption of the energy by tissues with high water content. The microwave energy induces rapid molecular

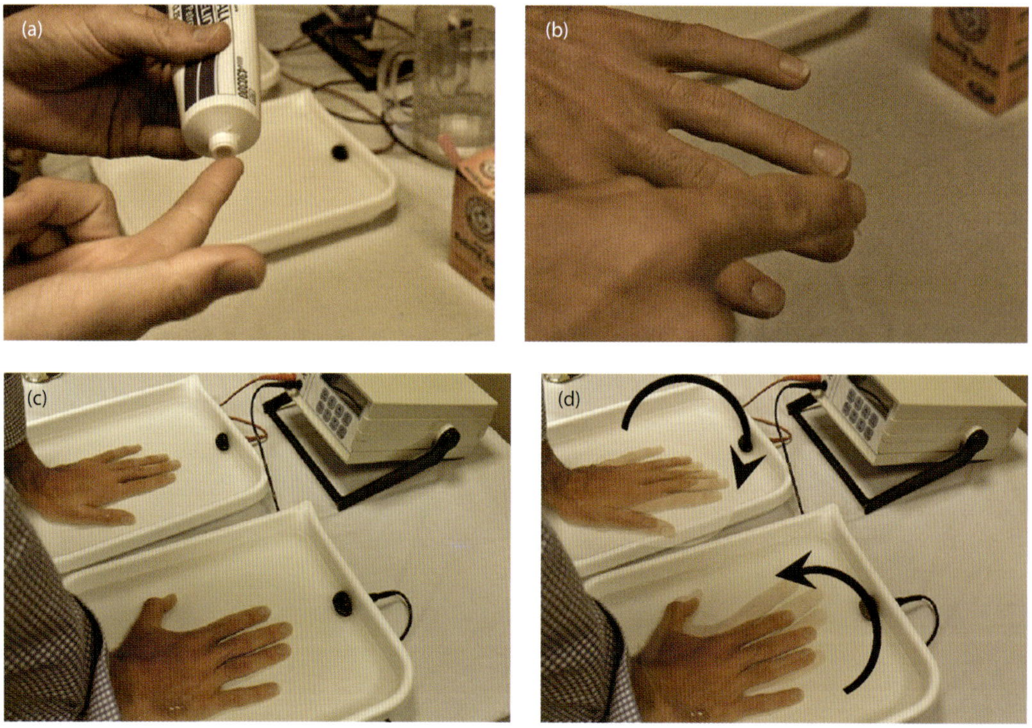

Figure 9.3 Iontophoresis. (a, b) cover any small cuts or abrasions or any disruptions in cuticles with petrolatum to avoid the feeling of a small but harmless electrical shock. (c) Immerse hands in trays filled with body-temperature tap water and operate the device according to directions. (d) Movement of hands from side to side in the water may relieve feeling of harmless electrical shock. (Courtesy of Albert Ganss, International Hyperhidrosis Society.)

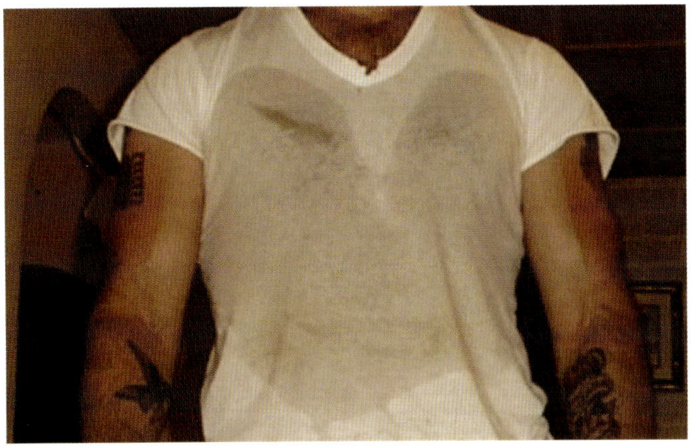

Figure 9.4 Compensatory hyperhidrosis following endoscopic thoracic sympathectomy. (Courtesy of Albert Ganss, International Hyperhidrosis Society.)

rotation generating heat and cellular thermolysis.[40,41] Microwave thermolysis is effective in reducing excessive eccrine sweating and may also improve axillary odor as noted by patients in one study.[42] Regarding eccrine sweat reduction, 94% of patients receiving microwave thermolysis achieved a 1-point decrease in the HDSS relative to baseline and 55%–83% achieved a 2-point reduction at 12 months after treatment.[40–42] Edema, redness from the vacuum suction employed in the procedure, and tenderness, pain, and swelling from the delivery of the microwave energy are usually mild to moderate and are expected adverse reactions which can be easily managed by postprocedure cooling with ice, nonsteroidal antiinflammatory agents during the first 24 hours, and analgesia as necessary. Numbness in the upper arm or axilla, blistering or burning in the treatment site, alopecia, and transient nerve injury are less common.[43]

BOTULINUM TOXIN THERAPY FOR HYPERHIDROSIS

Since sweating is mediated by acetylcholine, the use of botulinum toxin (BoNT) to treat focal HH is a logical choice. The chemodenervation is localized, reversible, and long-lasting although the therapeutic effect starts to decay over several months. One study documented an increase in the duration of efficacy of OnaBTX-A with repeated injections in patients with primary axillary HH.[44] OnaBTX-A (BOTOX®) has been most extensively studied, is widely used clinically, and is the only FDA approved agent in the United States to treat HH. AboBTX-A (Dysport®) and IncoBTX-A (Xeomin®) are not FDA approved for treating HH in the United States, have far less data for treating HH, and are not widely used for this indication. BoNT-B as RimaBTX-B (Myobloc®) in the United States and botulinum toxin type B (Neurobloc®) in other countries have been studied in small case series but are not used for HH due to incidence of systemic side effects and lack of FDA approval. The use of BoNT-B for treatment of HH is described later in this chapter.

The basic principle for using BoNTs to treat excessive sweating differs somewhat depending on the body area treated, but some basic principles apply to all areas. The area of sweating that needs to be treated should be identified using a colorimetric test such as the Minor's iodine-starch test (see Figures 9.1 and 9.2). Since the sweat glands are typically located at the junction of the dermis and subcutaneous fat, BoNT is usually placed as a deep intradermal injection. It is important to avoid injecting deeper structures such as muscle to prevent unwanted effects on the underlying muscles and for optimal BoNT interaction at the neuron–eccrine interface. Injections are generally placed 1–2 cm apart to allow for diffusion to the entire area. Although this basic technique can be used to treat many areas of the body, the more commonly treated sites will be described in more detail.

TREATMENT OF AXILLARY HYPERHIDROSIS WITH BOTULINUM TOXIN

No focal area of HH has been as extensively studied as the axilla[14,45–50] with numerous studies showing the benefit of BoNT-A, including large multicenter randomized, placebo-controlled trials in Europe and the United States. Naumann et al. reported on 320 patients with axillary HH that received 50 U of (BOTOX®) onabotulinumtoxinA (OnaBTX-A) per axilla or placebo.[49] At 4 weeks, 94% of the OnaBTX-A group had responded compared with 36% of the placebo group as measured by 50% reduction of sweat production from baseline. By 16 weeks, the response rates were 82% and 21%, respectively. Repeated injections with OnaBTX-A over 16 months continued to produce similar results.[45] The mean duration between OnaBTX-A treatments was approximately 7 months and patient satisfaction was high. Similar results were published in a large phase 3 double-blind trial in North America.[50] Subjects with axillary HH were randomized to receive placebo, 50 U, or 75 U of OnaBTX-A into each axilla. The HDSS was the primary efficacy parameter in this study with gravimetric measurements being secondary. Successful response, defined as $\geq$2 point reduction in HDSS, was seen in 75% of patients in both treatment groups compared with 25% in the placebo group while 80%–85% of the treated subjects had >75% reduction in sweat production. No significant differences were noted between the two doses of OnaBTX-A and the durability of therapy was approximately 7 months for both. A 3-year open label extension study revealed continued effectiveness and with similar duration of results.[51] Specifically, the researchers were able to show a significant sustained improvement in the quality of life of subjects. The DLQI showed significant improvement in overall quality of life and occupation and work-specific improvements were noted as well.

Although the U.S. FDA labeling is for patients aged 18 and older, an open-label study was conducted in 141 adolescents ages 12–17 years with severe primary axillary HH. The majority (79.4%–93.2%) had a 75% or greater reduction in sweat production at week 4. The median duration of effect for responders ranged from 134 to 152 days. These results were similar to the previously reported outcomes for adults. No unexpected safety signals were observed and neutralizing antibodies to OnaBTX-A did not develop.[52]

Although studies have consistently shown that 50 U OnaBTX-A per axilla provides safe and durable results (averaging ~7 months), there is some debate whether higher doses of OnaBTX-A can provide prolonged efficacy.[53,54] One small open label study of 200 U OnaBTX-A per axilla in 47 patients found prolonged results (over 19 months) in half of the patients, although the methodology was very different from other studies; starch iodine testing and telephone calls were used to assess patients.[53] Likewise, 250 U of OnaBTX-A[41] in each axilla resulted in prolonged benefit in a small study of 12 patients. Half remained symptom-free for 12 months and 9 months free of symptoms was achieved for 25% of the subjects.[54] Currently the standard dose in the United States, and that listed in the package insert for OnaBTX-A, is 50 U per axilla. This achieves excellent results, high patient satisfaction, and helps to keep costs down. There is no dosing consensus with BoNTs other than OnaBTX-A.

The efficacy of Dysport® (abobotulinumtoxinA) (AboBTX-A) for treatment of HH has been demonstrated in several studies. A multicenter trial of 145 subjects was performed with 200 U AboBTX-A in one axilla while the contralateral axilla was injected with placebo.[54] After 2 weeks, the placebo-treated axilla was injected with 100 U AboBTX-A. Axillary sweating decreased within 2 weeks in both treatment sides and results were maintained for 6 months. There were no significant differences gravimetrically between the two doses used. Therapy was well-tolerated and 98% of subjects said they would recommend the therapy to others. In a comparative study of AboBTX-A versus OnaBTX-A in 8 patients each subject received one agent in one palm and the other agent in the other palm. The authors concluded that the efficacy was similar for both agents although the AboBTX-A-treated palm showed better improvement than OnaBTX-A at 3 weeks postinjection, but at 8 weeks there was no difference.[54] Lecouflet et al. retrospectively tabulated the duration of effect of repeated injections of AboBTX-A. They concluded that there was an increase in the duration of efficacy after repeated treatments.[55] In a comparative study of OnaBTX-A and INCO, each subject received one agent in one palm and the other agent in the other palm. The authors concluded that OnaBTX-A and INCO were comparable in terms of anhidrotic effect in the short term as well as long-term efficacy, safety (as measured by muscle strength reduction), pain of injections, and patient treatment satisfaction.[55]

TECHNIQUE OF AXILLARY INJECTION OF BOTULINUM TOXIN

To optimize treatment, the area of axillary involvement should be identified before treatment by a Minor's iodine-starch test (as previously described) so that the BoNT can be concentrated into the affected area. Although it is true that the majority of the eccrine glands in the axilla are located in the hair-bearing area of skin, often the problematic areas extend beyond the visible hair-bearing area and if these ectopic areas of eccrine glands are missed, the results of treatment may be suboptimal. The key to performing a high-quality iodine-starch test is to thoroughly dry the region before beginning the test (see Figures 9.1 and 9.2). The axilla does not need to be shaved prior to performing an iodine-starch test or to injecting BoNT.

Although the package insert describes the use of unpreserved saline to reconstitute BoNT, many physicians have found that the use of preserved saline reduces pain without altering efficacy.[56,57] Typically, the 100-unit vial of OnaBTX-A is reconstituted with 4.0 mL of saline for axillary injections.

Approximately 2 units of OnaBTX-A or equivalent in one of the other toxins are injected into the deep dermis at the dermal subcutaneous level in doses placed 1.5–2 cm apart. Because the axillary skin is thin, a wheal should be seen with each injection. An average of 10–15 injections per axilla is required, but will depend on the size of the axilla and hyperhidrotic area.[58] In the event that an iodine-starch test cannot be performed prior to treatment or is equivocal, the physician should treat the hair-bearing areas as described above (Figure 9.5). Should symptoms fail to be alleviated within 2 weeks, the patient can return to the office and an iodine-starch test performed to identify any "active" eccrine glands. The skin in these "active" areas should be injected with 3–5 U of OnaBTX-A or equivalent of one of the other forms of BoNT for each 1 cm surface area identified.

Pain is minimal and the procedure is well tolerated. The use of 2% lidocaine to reconstitute BoNT has been reported in one small study to be less painful than the use of unpreserved saline when injecting axillary HH and with equal efficacy.[59] Side effects noted in studies include pain, hematoma, bruising, headache, muscle soreness, increased facial sweating, perceived compensatory sweating, and axillary pruritus.

Treatment intervals are determined by the duration of the patient's treatment response but will average every 6–9 months. Some clinicians have advocated that patients use a topical therapy twice a week when the sweating starts to return to try to extend the time interval between injections and help to reduce costs.[60]

PALMAR HYPERHIDROSIS

BoNT injections are useful in the treatment of palmar HH. No large-scale studies have been published but multiple small-scale studies and case series have demonstrated the ability of BoNT to establish clinical improvement in patients' symptoms.[23,61,62] Several challenges exist when treating the hands such as choosing optimal dose of BoNT, control of pain during injection, and side effects which include muscle weakness.[23,63–67]

The optimum dose of BoNT to control palmar HH is unknown and the issue is complicated by large variations in hand size (Figure 9.6). Typically, OnaBTX-A is reconstituted with 4 mL of preserved saline for palmar injections. Published data report doses as low as 50 U of OnaBTX-A per hand and as high as 200 U of OnaBTX-A per hand.[62,68] Doses of AboBTX-A have ranged from 120 U per hand to 500 U per hand.[22,61,68] Some authors have suggested using a defined dose per

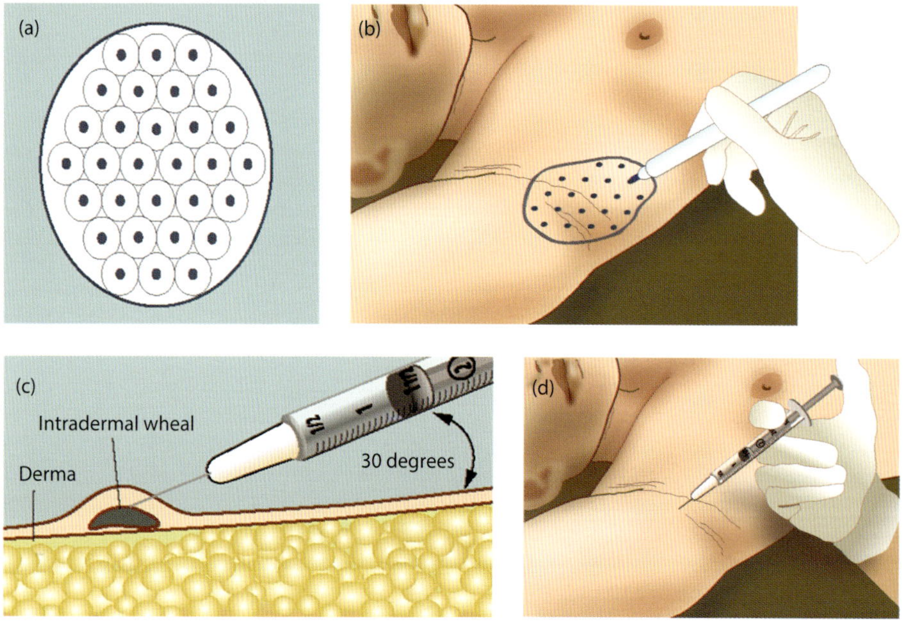

Figure 9.5 Technique of axillary botulinum toxin injections. (a, b) Diffusion diagram; (c, d) when injecting BOTOX for hyperhidrosis, physicians should try to obtain a visible wheal that confirms the placement of the drug in the proper plane of the skin. (Courtesy of Albert Ganss, International Hyperhidrosis Society.)

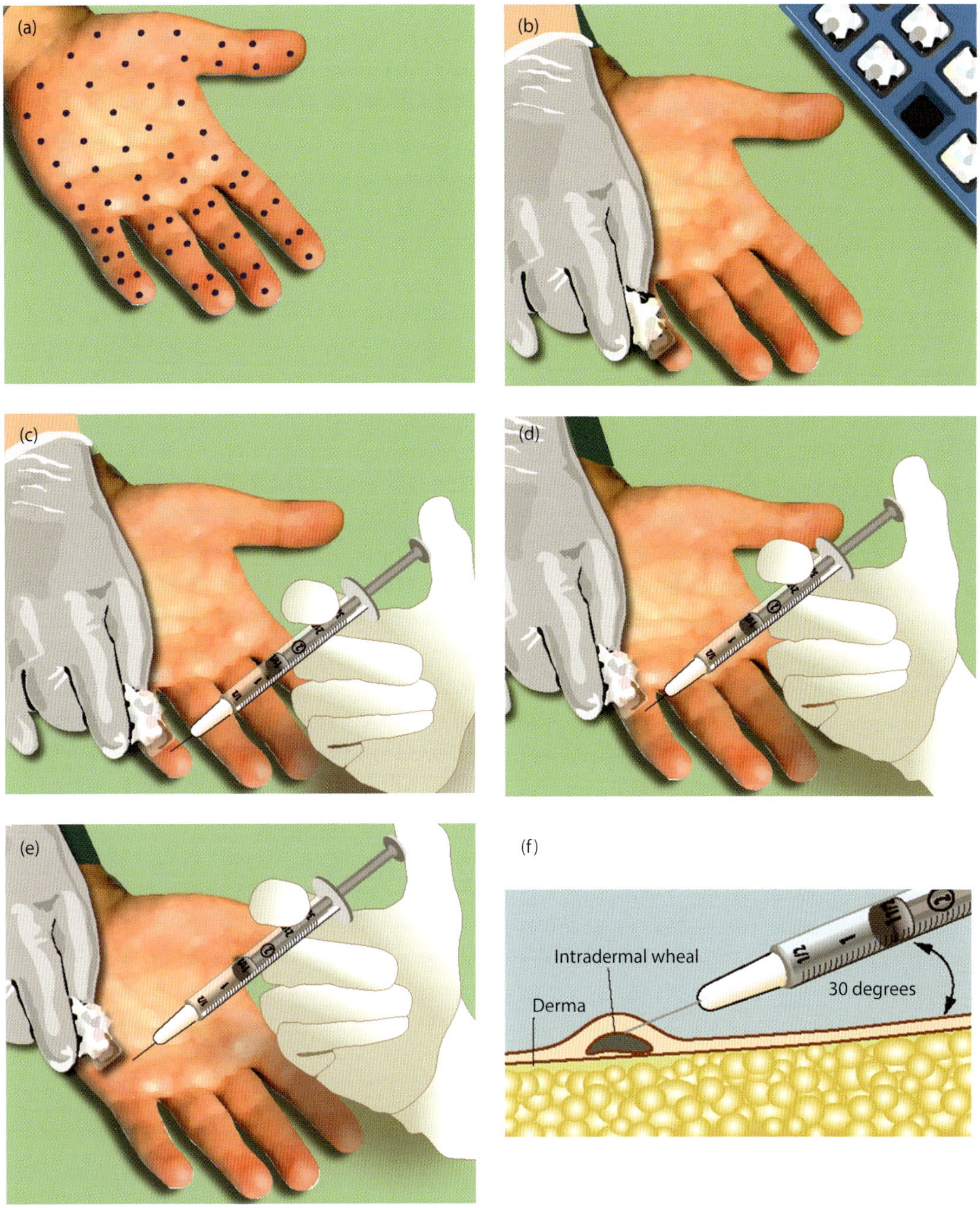

Figure 9.6 Technique of palmar injections of botulinum toxin. (a) Injection sites should be evenly spaced with 45–50 injection sites per palm. (b) A simple ice cube can ease discomfort. Freeze gauze pads in ice for easier handling. (c) Ice each site for 7–10 seconds using firm pressure. (d) Inject immediately and move ice to next site. (e) Progress in this manner for entire affected area. (f) When injecting BOTOX for hyperhidrosis, physicians should try to obtain a visible wheal that confirms the placement of the drug in the proper plane of the skin. (Courtesy of Albert Ganss, International Hyperhidrosis Society.)

injection, with Swirling's group using 0.8 U/cm^2, and Naumann's group using 2 U OnaBTX-A injected every 1.5 cm on the palm with three injections per fingertip and two injections over each of the middle and proximal phalanx using 1–2 U per injection[62,69](Figure 9.7). The Canadian Advisory Committee recommends 1.5–2 U/cm^2 with a mean dose of 100 U OnaBTX-A per palm.[7] It is unclear whether larger doses add to the duration of symptom relief or increase the risk of developing muscle weakness. When Wollina used 200 U of OnaBTX-A per hand in 10 patients, his relapse time varied from 3–22 months.[59] Saadia studied 24 patients: 11 received 50 U OnaBTX-A per hand and 13 received 100 U/hand. There was higher patient satisfaction reported in the high-dose group, but no difference in terms of duration (measured as a percentage of the palm area sweating) for the two doses. There were more patients with hand and finger weakness in the high-dose treatment group.[54] Until larger studies are available to address this issue, 75–100 U OnaBTX-A or equivalent of other BoNTs per hand is a good starting point with adjustments being made as needed based on the size of the hand and past responses.[27]

Another challenge with palmar BoNT therapy is an apparent shorter duration of response when compared with axillary injections.[55] Responses range from 3 to 12 months.[62] Aghaei found that anhidrosis lasted up to 5 months for his patients treated with 500 U AboBTX-A per hand,[70] although he observed HH lasting an average of 10 months.[70] The reason for this shorter duration is unknown but may be[71] related to a smaller diffusion radius in the thicker palm skin and compartmentalized areas of the phalanges, a higher number of

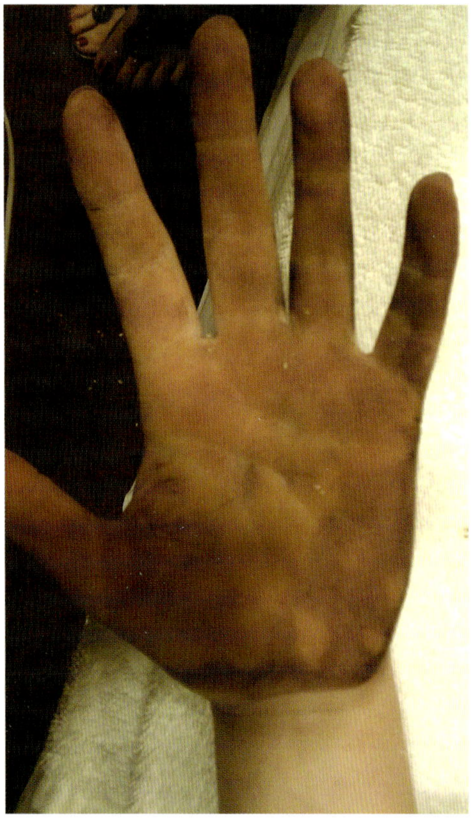

Figure 9.7 Starch-iodine test showing "skipped" areas following suboptimal palmar injections. The "skipped" areas may be improved with "touch-up" injections. (Courtesy of David Pariser.)

cholinergic nerve endings or a differential recovery rate of the nerves in the hands compared with the axilla. Backflow of the BoNT solution on injection can be an issue with palmar injections and perhaps this plays a role as well.[72]

Injection of the hand can be quite painful due to the density of nerve receptors and the large number of injections that are required. Pain during injection of the palm has been rated an average 68.1 ± 31.8 compared to 29.9 ± 24.5 for axillary treatment (using a visual analogue scale of 1–100).[15] Several methods of pain control have been tried (Table 9.7), although a rare patient will not require anesthesia. Topical anesthetic containing lidocaine and cold packs tend not to provide adequate pain control. More intensive cold exposure can be helpful: the use of dichlorotetrafluoroethane or liquid nitrogen, submersion of the hand in an ice bath, direct exposure of an ice cube or ice pack.[73,74] Machines that emit chilled air or utilize a chilled tip can be beneficial but are more expensive and can cause freezing of the BoNT in the needle during injection. Kreyden describes a technique of iontophoresis with 2% lidocaine for 30 minutes, followed by a light spray of liquid nitrogen just prior to inserting the needle to inject BoNTA.[75] The use of a dermojet to inject BoNTA was found to be less painful than standard needle injections, but was much less effective in controlling the sweating and thus not recommended as a useful tool to treat the palms.[76] Benohanian has described the use of a pressure unit to inject lidocaine into the palms and soles without the use of needles, before injecting BoNTA.[77] The Med-JetMBX II (MIT Canada)[78] device system consists of a CO_2-powered variable dose injector to which a 12-cc disposable syringe is attached containing lidocaine. When the trigger is pulled, a volume of 0.02–0.3 cc anesthesia is injected to the targeted depth within the skin. The starting pressure is typically around 130 psi (with a range of 1–350 psi) depending on the epidermal thickness. The device is approved by Health Canada and the European Union. After the anesthetic wheals appear, BoNT can be administered with a standard needle system.

Table 9.7 Pain Control Techniques Used for Palmar and Plantar Injections

Topical anesthesia
Nerve blocks
Tetrafluoroethane
Liquid nitrogen
Machine-assisted cold air
Intravenous regional anesthesia (Bier's block)
Conscious sedation
General anesthesia
Vibratory anesthesia[a]
Ice and pressure[a]

[a] Authors' preferences for most cases.

Nerve blocks are effective and can be performed in the office[69,79–81]; however, with the much simpler technique of ice and pressure described below, nerve blocks are not often used. The palm is innervated by three nerves, median, ulnar, and radial nerves. All can be anesthetized at the level of the wrist using 1% or 2% lidocaine (Figure 9.8). Risks of a nerve block include infiltration of the nerve with subsequent nerve injury and vascular puncture. In addition, temporary hand weakness after the nerve blocks may limit the patients' activities and ability to have both hands treated at one session. A 30 G 0.5-inch needle should be used to minimize any nerve trauma. Approximately 2 cc of 1% or 2% lidocaine is injected around each of the nerves. If the patient feels any unusual tingling or sensation during the injection, the needle should be withdrawn slightly. Twenty minutes or more may be necessary for the full effect to develop. If the anesthesia is not complete, other techniques may also be used (Table 9.7).

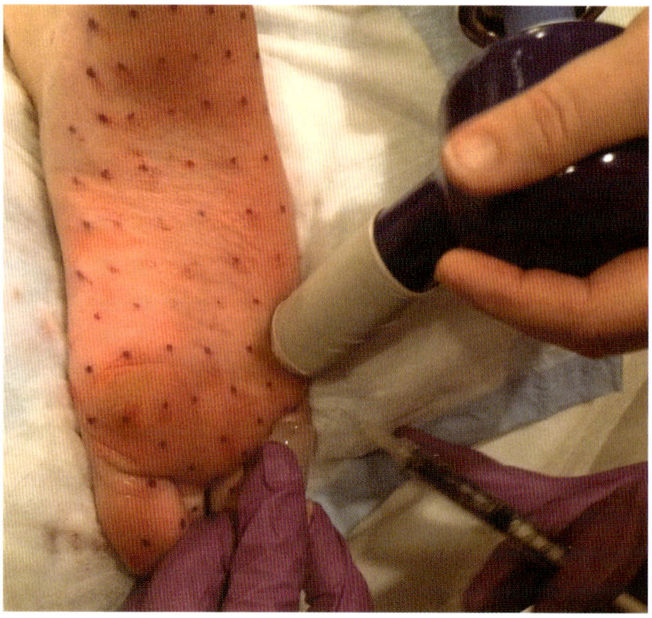

Figure 9.8 Injection pattern and technique for plantar injection using both ice and pressure as well as vibratory anesthesia. The ice is held with firm pressure for 7–10 seconds. Just as the ice is removed, the vibrator is applied and the injection performed simultaneously. This is the authors' preferred method of pain control for plantar injections. (Courtesy of Albert Ganss, International Hyperhidrosis Society.)

Intravenous regional anesthesia (IVRA), also known as a Bier's block, is effective anesthetic.[82,83] An anesthetic such as prilocaine is injected intravenously following the application of a tourniquet cuff on the forearm. Exsanguination of the extremity is performed and an electronic double cuff is applied. Complete anesthesia is obtained in 20 minutes using 40–60 mL of 0.5% prilocaine. The total tourniquet time for IVRA ranges from 50 to 80 minutes and is well-tolerated. Due to the risk of toxic cardiovascular and central nervous system reactions, blood pressure and electrocardiogram are monitored during the IVRA and for about 30 minutes after the procedure.

Vibratory anesthesia is another useful method for the palms and soles.[84] The theory is that the nervous system is unable to perceive fully two different types of sensory inputs simultaneously. A handheld vibrator is applied to the volar and dorsal surface of the hand near the site of BoNTA injection. This requires an assistant and there is some movement of the patient's hand, which can make injections challenging. The use of one vibrator to the volar aspect does not diminish pain as much as the use of two vibrators, one on the dorsal and other on the volar (personal experience). Neither technique results in a pain-free injection, but rather a diminishment of perceived pain. A study by Sherer found that pain threshold is significantly higher during vibration compare to pre- or postvibration, and that vibration applied distal to the site of pain provided better analgesia than vibration applied proximal to the site of pain.[85]

The authors most commonly use ice with pressure for palmar injections. An ice cube is pressed firmly to the planned injection site for 7–10 seconds (see Figure 9.8). If the patient requires additional pain control, a combination of ice and vibration may be used. Ice is applied firmly to the area for 7–10 seconds and then the vibrator is firmly applied immediately adjacent to the injection site simultaneous to the injection (no more than 2–3 seconds). This technique requires an assistant and coordinated timing to optimize pain control. A 30 G 0.5-inch needle with a luer lock syringe or insulin type syringe is especially helpful because of the thicker skin of the palm and higher pressures needed to inject the palm. Injections should be placed every 1–1.5 cm but the digits will usually need two to three injection sites per phalangeal unit (see Figure 9.8).

Bruising is common with injections into the palm, but it is temporary. Weakness of the hand or fingers is possible but is usually minor and of limited duration. The incidence varies in published series, but ranges from 0% to 77%.[23,63,64,86] The most commonly affected area of weakness is the thenar eminence and can be measured in the thumb-index finger pinch, whereas gross strength or grip strength of the hand is not usually affected.[62,65] Rarely, patients report numbness, tingling, or decreased dexterity. Injections of BoNTA should be in the dermal layer, especially superficial over the thenar eminence to limit the chance that the drug will come in contact with the muscle layer. Subepidermal injections may increase the incidence of hematoma.[64] There is one report of atrophy of the intrinsic musculature of the hands with "debilitating" weakness associated with BoNTA injections for palmar HH, after five treatment sessions using 500 U AboBTX-A per palmar basin every nine months.[87] Patients should be adequately counseled on the risks of weakness, which is usually mild and transient.

In an attempt to prevent muscle weakness, Zaiac advocates the use of the ADG® needle, a device designed for the injection of collagen.[88] He found the average depth of the eccrine glands in 10 consecutive palmar biopsies to be 2.6 mm. By adjusting the needle to a length of 2.6 mm and using a total of 60–70 U OnaBTX-A per palm, he had no weakness in a series of 10 patients. Likewise, Almeida uses an adapter to shorten her 7 mm 30 G needle to measure 2.5–3.0 mm for palmar injections.[67,89]

Children with palmar HH can be treated with BoNTs but pain control remains the biggest challenge. Less is known about the dosing, duration, and adverse events associated with pediatric use. Coutinho dos Santos published a series of nine children aged 6.5–11 years with palmar HH successfully treated with OnaBTX-A. Nerve blocks were used for pain control and doses of 75–150 units were given per palm.[90]

Starch-iodine testing is usually not necessary prior to palmar and plantar injections, but can be useful in the event that a patient reports less than satisfactory results. In this case, a starch iodine test can detect missed or skipped areas which can be "touched up."

PLANTAR HYPERHIDROSIS

BoNTs can be useful in treating plantar HH, but very little has been published on BoNT therapy for plantar HH. Like the palms, there is no consensus on the optimal dose, the duration is variable, and the injections are painful. Typically, OnaBTX-A is reconstituted with 4.0 mL of preserved saline. Naumann used 42 and 48 units of OnaBTX-A to treat two soles by injecting 3 U OnaBTX-A (0.15 mL) into each 2 × 2 cm squares.[91] Blaheta's group used 100 U OnaBTX-A per sole (100 U/5 mL saline) in a study of eight patients with severe plantar hyperhidrosis.[92] Campanati studied 10 patients with plantar hyperhidrosis using 100 U OnaBTX-A per foot. All patients had an improvement in symptoms and a "significant decrease of Minor's test" for 12 weeks without significant side effects.[93]

An iodine-starch test may help to delineate the hyperhidrotic area, which can extend up the sides and onto the dorsum of the foot. BoNTA should be evenly distributed every 1–2 cm using small gauge needles and should be injected into the deep dermis. Injections of the plantar surface can be technically more challenging due to the thickness of the stratum corneum in some areas, especially if calloused. The physician must adjust for the variation in depth to accurately place BoNT into the appropriate cutaneous level.

The need for pain control has to be addressed as with palmar injections. IVRA can provide sufficient anesthesia for the sole and has been reported to be effective when administering BoNTA. In a small series of eight patients, IVRA was found to be more effective than nerve blocks in reducing the pain of BoNTA injections.[94] However, nerve blocks can also be used and are generally performed at the level of the ankle. The tibial and sural nerves need to be blocked, and if the dorsum of the foot must be injected, the superficial peroneal nerve can be anesthetized.[91] A 30 G 0.5-inch needle should be used to minimize any nerve trauma. Approximately 2 cc of 1% or 2% lidocaine is injected around each of the nerves. If the patient feels any unusual tingling or sensation during the injection, the needle should be withdrawn slightly. Twenty minutes or more may be necessary for the full effect to develop. If the anesthesia is not complete another technique may also be used. Vadoud-Seyedi reported on using the Dermojet® to inject BoNTA for plantar HH. Ten patients were treated with 50 U OnaBTX-A/5 mL saline per foot. Fifteen to 20 points were injected per foot and no analgesia was used. The injections were tolerated well by all patients, although one developed a localized hematoma. The duration of benefit lasted 3–6 months; however, 20% of patients reported the treatment had no effect on their condition.[95]

At this time, the authors' preferred method of pain control for plantar injections is ice and pressure combined with vibration as described earlier (see Figure 9.8). Doses of 100–200 U OnaBTX-A per foot are typically required.

Bruising and pain with injection are the most common side effects. In the published literature, one patient reported weakness of plantar flexor muscles in both feet following BoNTA injections, with resolution in 10 days.[96]

CRANIOFACIAL HYPERHIDROSIS

Primary craniofacial HH has several patterns, but most commonly involves the forehead plus or minus the scalp. Patients with craniofacial HH may present with involvement of the forehead, scalp perimeter, entire scalp, cheeks, nose, upper lip, chin, or a combination of the areas. Gustatory sweating (Frey's syndrome) is a relatively common complication after surgery or injury in the region of the parotid gland and will be discussed later in the chapter. All forms of facial HH can respond to BoNT, with gustatory sweating responding for very long periods of time.

There is a paucity of literature published on craniofacial HH. It is the authors' practice to use a less diluted concentration of OnaBTX-A for craniofacial injections since delivering the same number of units in a smaller volume may cause less diffusion into underlying musculature. Typically, the 100 unit vial of OnaBTX-A is reconstituted with 2.0 mL of preserved saline for craniofacial injections.

Kinkelin's group injected a mean of 86 U OnaBTX-A (3 U OnaBTX-A per injection site) over the forehead at equidistant locations (1–1.5 cm) in 10 men with frontal hyperhidrosis.[97] The intradermal injections were kept 1 cm superior to the eyebrow to help prevent drooping of the eyelid. Five of 10 patients had partial disability in frowning of the forehead, but this was limited to a maximum of 8 weeks. There was no ptosis noted and satisfaction was good or excellent in 90% of the subjects. The benefits were maintained for 5 months in 90% of patients. Similarly, Tan and Solish report that symptoms return on average of 4–12 months after treatment of the forehead.[15]

Böger treated 12 men suffering from bilateral craniofacial hyperhidrosis with AboBTX-A 0.1 ng per injection.[98] Half of the forehead was treated using a total of 2.5–4 ng injected equidistantly with a total of 25–40 injections given. Decreased sweating was seen within 1–7 days after injection and lasted a minimum of 3 months, but one patient experienced anhidrosis for 27 months. Side effects were limited to temporary weakness of the frontalis muscle (100%) and brow asymmetry that lasted 1–12 months in 17% of subjects.

It is the observation of the authors that patients typically present with forehead sweating that may be combined with scalp sweating in a diffuse pattern or in an ophiasis pattern. OnaBTX-A injections are performed with approximately 2 units every 1–2 cm, avoiding the inferior 1–2 cm of the forehead to reduce the risk of brow ptosis[90] (Figure 9.9). The forehead can be treated more inferiorly if the response is not sufficient and if the patient is willing to accept the possibility of brow ptosis. Doses range from 50 U (forehead) to 250–300 U for the forehead and entire scalp.[99]

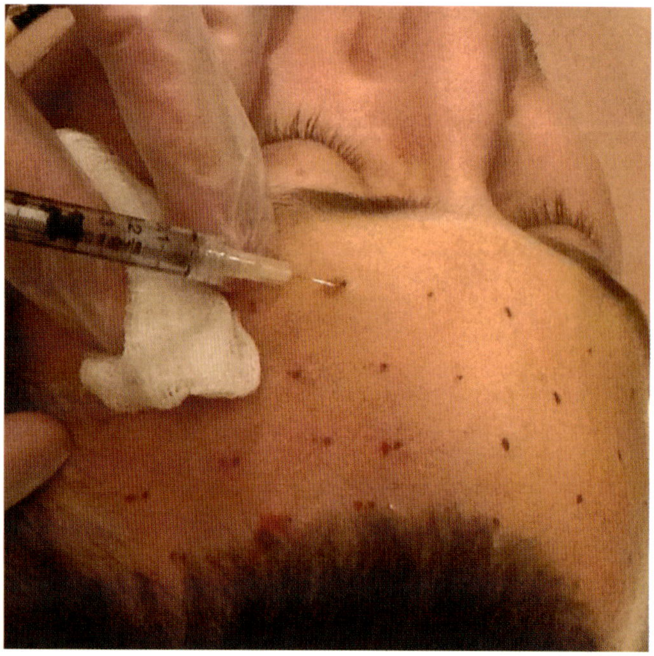

Figure 9.9 Injection pattern and technique for craniofacial injections. Craniofacial injections, particularly on the forehead or over any facial muscles, should be placed as superficially as possible in order to attempt to minimize diffusion into underling muscles. Approximately 2 units of botulinum toxin are injected into each site about 1.5–2 cm apart. Note that the injection is superficial and is raising a wheal. (Courtesy of Albert Ganss, International Hyperhidrosis Society.)

INGUINAL AND SUBMAMMARY HYPERHIDROSIS

Although traditionally inguinal HH has been thought to affect 2%–10% of individuals with primary HH,[14] a recent unpublished survey of nearly 2000 HH sufferers by the International Hyperhidrosis Society shows that both inguinal and submammary HH are more frequent and are commonly associated with HH in other body areas and present as primary multifocal HH. Inguinal and submammary HH usually develops in adolescence. Intradermal injections of BoNTA can control symptoms for 6 months or more. Identifying the surface areas that need injection by the iodine-starch test can be technically challenging due to the body location, but is valuable. Similarly to the technique for axillary injections, OnaBTX-A is reconstituted with 4 mL of preserved saline in a 100-unit vial and 2–2.5 units OnaBTX-A are injected every 1.5–2 cm within the affected area (Figure 9.10). Typical doses range from 60 to 100 U per side depending on the extent of the involved area.[100]

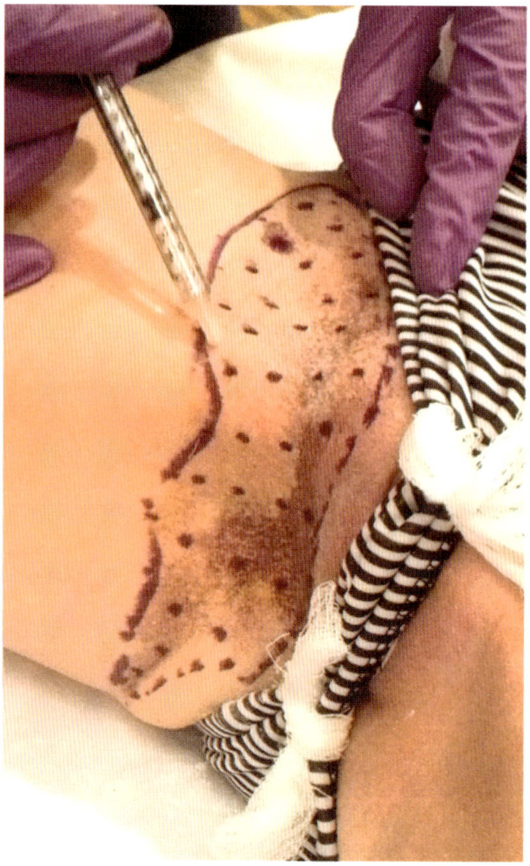

Figure 9.10 Inguinal injection. Using technique much the same for axillary injections, the treatment area is identified with the starch-iodine technique and injections of 2.0–2.5 units of botulinum toxin are placed in a grid pattern every 1.5–2 cm apart. (Courtesy of Albert Ganss, International Hyperhidrosis Society.)

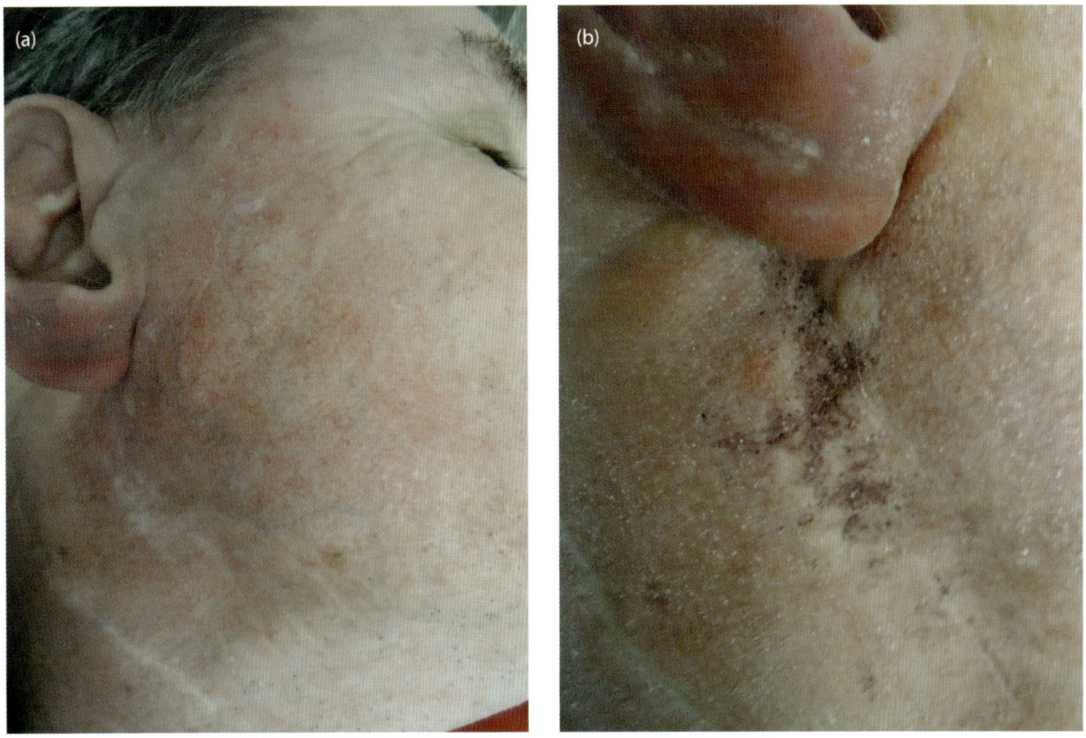

Figure 9.11 Gustatory hyperhidrosis (Frey's syndrome). (a) Facial redness and flushing, followed by (b) a localized area of sweating, occurs during or after eating due to injury and inappropriate regeneration of the auriculotemporal nerve following parotid gland or other facial surgery.

GUSTATORY SWEATING (FREY'S SYNDROME)

The main symptoms of Frey's syndrome are undesirable sweating and flushing occurring on the cheek, temple, jawline, or behind the ears after eating certain foods, or even just the anticipation of eating certain foods, especially those that produce a strong salivary response. It usually results from misdirection of autonomic nerve fibers after surgery and can also be observed in diseases of the parotid gland and in diabetes.

BoNT is a highly effective treatment option for gustatory sweating as shown by several uncontrolled studies.[101–105] In a large open study of 45 patients, there was a significant reduction of local facial sweating after injection of OnaBTX-A using a mean dose of 21 U (range 5–72 U) and no recurrence of sweating was observed during the follow-up period of 6 months. A marked long-lasting benefit of 11–36 months was also observed in three other open studies.[93–95] Thus, BoNT appears to have a particularly long-lasting effect on gustatory sweating. See Figure 9.11.

In clinical practice, the Minor's iodine-starch test should be performed before injection to visualize the affected area that needs to be injected. After the iodine and starch have been applied to the area, the patient should chew on a piece of candy or food to stimulate the facial sweating. Injections with 2–3 U OnaBTX-A or 8 U AboBTX-A are given intradermally at sites 2.0–2.5 cm apart and evenly distributed over the affected area. Specific side effects of the injection of BoNT include pain on injection, local hematomas, and local muscle weakness due to diffusion of the toxin to adjacent muscles (particularly the zygomatic muscle).

OTHER SWEATING DISORDERS WHERE BOTULINUM TOXIN THERAPY MAY BE HELPFUL

Compensatory Sweating

Compensatory sweating is the most common complication of endoscopic transthoracic sympathectomy (ETS), ranging from 44% to 91%.[106] Treatment has been particularly difficult but a few reports have noted success using BoNTA. Huh used 300 U OnaBTX-A to treat the chest and abdomen after identifying the area with an iodine-starch test.[106] He diluted each 100 U of OnaBTX-A with 10 mL saline and injected 0.1 mL into each square centimeter. The effects gradually reduced but were reported to remain for 8 months. Belin and Polo reported good results treating the upper abdomen with OnaBTX-A, but unfortunately their patient's compensatory sweating was from the nipple line down to his knees and the entire area was not treated.[37] Kim and colleagues reported on 17 patients with severe compensatory hyperhidrosis being treated with BoNTA.[98] One hundred to 500 units of OnaBTX-A were used, administering 2 units every 1.5 cm. The injections were well-tolerated, but the authors noted incomplete resolution of the sweating due to insufficient dosing, and the duration lasted only 4 months.[107] The major drawback of treating compensatory HH with BoNT is the quantity of drug that needs to be administered.

Chromhidrosis

Chromhidrosis is a rare disorder characterized by the excretion of colored or pigmented sweat. It is most commonly confined to the face or axilla but has been noted elsewhere on the body. Matarasso used 15 U OnaBTX-A into the affected area of each cheek which measured 3 cm in diameter. Within 48 hours, the patient had a marked reduction in the amount of discharged black sweat.[108]

Ross Syndrome

Ross syndrome was first described by the neurologist Alexander Ross in 1958.[109] It is characterized by the triad of unilateral tonic pupils, generalized areflexia (Holmes–Adie syndrome), and progressive segmental anhidrosis with a compensatory band of excessive perspiration. Patients suffering from Ross syndrome usually do not perceive the HH; instead, it is the compensatory segmental HH that is bothersome. In addition, many patients suffer from several symptoms of vegetative dysfunction, such as palpitation, stenocardia, orthostatic

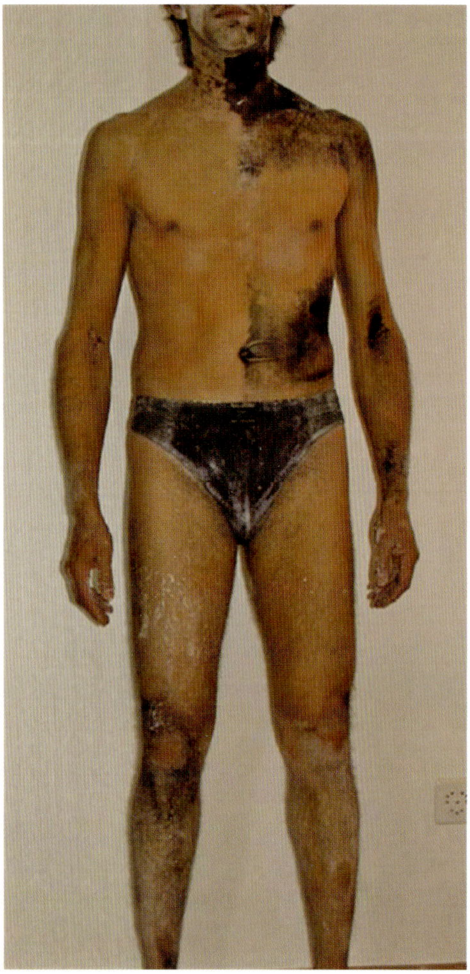

Figure 9.12 Patient with Ross syndrome characterized by progressive segmental anhidrosis with a compensatory band of excessive perspiration leading the patient to the physician. This is the very same patient 11 years after Itin et al.[111] first published their case study, showing extensive progression of the disease (unpublished data). (From Kreyden OP. *Botulinum Toxin in Clinical Dermatology*. Boca Raton, FL: Taylor & Francis Group; 2006; Chapter 10: 281–285. With permission.)

hypotonia, and irritable colon.[110] The pathogenesis of Ross syndrome is unknown. Multiple neuropathies of the autonomic nervous system or a failure in the synthesis or release of neurotransmitters have been suggested as possible causes.[109] There is no histologic evidence of nerve fiber destruction. Therefore, Ross postulated a defect in acetylcholine cholinesterase activity, rather than the degeneration of sweat glands. The progression of Ross syndrome is very slow. There is no therapy for the segmental progressive anhidrosis. The bothersome compensatory HH can be improved, however, with systemic antimuscarinic drugs or with injections of BoNTA into the affected areas, usually the face. In 1992, Itin et al.[111] presented a case study of a patient suffering from Ross syndrome with a defined area of anhidrosis in the right hand, the right axilla, and the right side of the face. In follow-up, after 11 years, the patient presented with additional anhidrotic areas in the right hemithorax and the underside of the left arm (Figure 9.12). Unfortunately, the patient refused treatment with BoNT, even though the HH was so severe that electrolyte replacement was necessary (unpublished data).

Localized Unilateral Hyperhidrosis

Localized unilateral hyperhidrosis (LUH) is a rare form of idiopathic localized HH and is defined as a confined area of HH of less than 10 × 10 cm, mainly found on the forehead or the forearm, whose

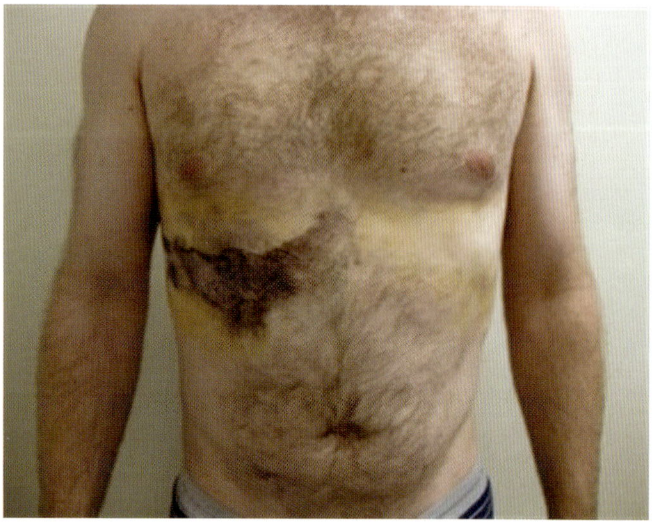

Figure 9.13 Segmental hyperhidrosis. This patient had a dermatomal band of hyperhidrosis as identified here with starch-iodine testing. Neurologic evaluation failed to detect a cause and he was successfully treated with botulinum toxin after which he was lost to follow-up. (Courtesy of David Pariser.)

pathogenesis is unknown. Beside the unusual localization, the major difference from essential HH is that LUH has no typical triggering factor and occurs even while patients are asleep. The etiology of LUH is unknown but may be due to a misdirected reconnection of the sympathetic nerve fiber network after injury, similar to Frey's syndrome.[103] Before BoNT, no treatment was available for this distinctive but enigmatic skin disorder. However, excellent results have been experienced following injection of 30 U OnaBTX-A in a patient suffering from LUH.[112]

Segmental Hyperhidrosis

Segmental hyperhidrosis (Figure 9.13) is an uncommon finding which is usually associated with irritation or infiltration of preganglionic sympathetic fibers or the sympathetic chain. Shultz et al. report two cases of segmental HH with striking clinical features. In one case, a mesothelioma produced ipsilateral simultaneous underactivity and overactivity of sympathetic outflow and in the other case a thoracic central disc herniation was probably responsible for a band of sweating which clearly extended beyond the segmental level of injury. The authors conclude that segmental HH should trigger a search for structural disease in the spinal and paraspinal region.[113]

Residual Limb Hyperhidrosis Following Amputation

HH in patients following limb amputations can present problems with the wearing of prostheses and can significantly impair quality of life. Several small case series have demonstrated the efficacy of BoNTs for this indication.[114,115] The dilution and injection technique and dosing is similar to that for other anatomic areas. After identifying the hyperhidrotic area using the Minor's iodine-starch test, approximately 2 units of OnaBTX-A or equivalent of one of the other toxins are injected into the deep dermis at the dermal subcutaneous level in doses placed 1.5–2 cm apart.

USE OF BOTULINUM TOXIN TYPE B FOR HYPERHIDROSIS

Botulinum toxin type B (BoNT-B) use has been primarily limited to treatment of cervical dystonia, but there are a few reports of its use for treating HH. Injection of BoNT-B can induce focal anhidrosis in a dose-dependent fashion. Birklein found that a threshold dose of 8 U Neurobloc®/Myobloc® (RimaBTX-B)

(RimaBTX-B) led to anhidrotic skin areas greater than 4 cm after 3 weeks. The duration was prolonged for 3 months when 15 U BoNT-B were injected, and for 6 months when 125 U were injected.[116]

Despite its ability to induce anhidrosis, the use of BoNT-B is limited by the occurrence of systemic adverse events.[117] Dressler reported that 100 U OnaBTX-A, 2000 U RimaBTX-B, and 4000 U RimaBTX-B were equally effective in blocking axillary sweating when studying 19 HH patients.[118] The extent of improvement was similar (16 weeks) in all groups, but the onset of action was earlier with the RimaBTX-B and there was greater discomfort with the RimaBTX-B compared with OnaBTX-A. One patient developed severe dryness of the mouth starting 1 week after injection, lasting 5 weeks, as well as accommodation difficulties and conjunctival irritation that lasted 3 weeks. Likewise, patients treated with 5000 U RimaBTX-B in each axilla achieved excellent reduction in sweating, but the incidence of side effects was high and included dry mouth, headache, and sensory motor symptoms of the hand.[119]

A patient treated with 2500 U BoNTB to each palm for HH developed bilateral blurred vision, indigestion, dry sore throat, and dysphagia.[120] The largest published study to date on BoNT-B to treat palmar HH included 20 subjects that used 5000 U per palm.[121] Adverse events were common: dry mouth or throat (90%), indigestion (60%), excessively dry hands (60%), muscle weakness (60%), and decreased grip strength (50%).

Lower dosing may be the key to reducing the high incidence of side effects.[122] However, because of the incidence of systemic side effects using BoNT-B and the high safety profile using BoNT-A to treat focal HH, to date, BoNT-A is the botulinum toxin of choice.

FUTURE DIRECTIONS

Since its widespread introduction for treatment of HH a dozen years ago, botulinum toxins have revolutionized the treatment of HH and other secretory disorders and significantly improved the quality of life for the many patients who have been treated with it. Compared with other treatments, BoNTs are unmatched in efficacy, ease of administration, and patient satisfaction. Development of quick, safe, and effective pain control is needed for the treatment of more tender areas such as the palms and soles. New delivery devices are already being researched to help provide the most comfortable and efficient therapy. Kavanagh and colleagues have successfully used a small iontophoresis machine to deliver BoNT-A to two patients with severe palmar HH, sparing them the injections.[123] Glogau demonstrated that OnaBTX-A can be successfully delivered into the axillary skin when combined with a proprietary transport peptide molecule (see Chapter 4).[124] Other forms of topically applied BoNTs are being investigated. See Clinical Trials.gov. for a list of current studies with topical forms of BoNT. Research is ongoing, looking at the clinical applications of different BoNT serotypes. Another area of potential research is with combination therapy. For the present, BoNT therapy is a valuable, well-tolerated therapy and can provide meaningful improvement in the quality of life of patients with HH and other secretory disorders.

REFERENCES

1. Goldsmith L. Biology of eccrine and apocrine sweat glands. In: Freedberg I, Eisen A, Wolff K, Goldsmith L, Katz S, Fitzpatrick T (eds). *Fitzpatrick's Dermatology in General Medicine*. New York: McGraw-Hill; 1999: 157–164.
2. Goldsmith L. Goldsmith disorders of the eccrine sweat gland. In: Freedberg I, Eisen A, Wolff K, Goldsmith L, Katz SI, Fitzpatrick T (eds). *Fitzpatrick's Dermatology in General Medicine*. New York: McGraw-Hill; 1999: 800–809.
3. Stenn K, Bhawan J. The normal histology of the skin. In: Farmer E, Hood A (eds). *Pathology of the Skin*. New York: McGraw-Hill; 2000: 3-29.
4. Glogau R. Botulinum A neurotoxin for axillary hyperhidrosis: No sweat Botox. *Dermatol Surg* 1998; 24: 817–19.
5. Hund M, Kinkelin I, Naumann M, Hamm H. Definition of axillary hyperhidrosis by gravimetric assessment. *Arch Dermatol* 2002; 138: 539–41.
6. Hornberger J, Grimes K, Naumann M et al. Recognition, diagnosis, and treatment of primary focal hyperhidrosis. *J Am Acad Dermatol* 2004; 51: 274–86.
7. Solish N, Bertucci V, Dansereau A et al. A comprehensive approach to the recognition, diagnosis, and severity-based treatment of focal hyperhidrosis: Recommendations of the Canadian Hyperhidrosis Advisory Committee. *Dermatol Surg* 2007; 33: 908–23.
8. Kreyden O, Scheidegger E. Anatomy of the sweat glands, pharmacology of botulinum toxin, and distinctive syndromes associated with hyperhidrosis. *Clin Dermatol* 2004; 22: 40–4.
9. Cheshire W, Freeman R. Disorders of sweating. *Semin Neurol* 2003; 23(4): 399–406.
10. Grazziotin T, Buffon R, Manzoni A, Libis A, Weber M. Treatment of granulosis rubra nasi with botulinum toxin type A. *Dermatol Surg* 2009; 35: 1298–9.
11. Lear W, Kessler E, Solish N, Glaser D. An epidermiological study of hyperhidrosis. *Dermatol Surg* 2007; 33: S69–75.
12. Seline P, Jaskierny D. Cutaneous metastases from a chondroblastoma initially presenting as unilateral palmar hyperhidrosis. *J Am Acad Dermatol* 1999; 40: 325–7.
13. Strutton D, Kowalski J, Glaser D, Stang P. US Prevalence of hyperhidrosis and impact on individuals with axillary hyperhidrosis: Results from a national survey. *J Am Acad Dermatol* 2004; 51: 241–8.
14. Naumann M, Hamm H, Lowe NJ. Effect of botulinum toxin type A on quality of life measures in patients with excessive axillary sweating: A randomized controlled trial. *Br J Dermatol* 2002; 147: 1218–26.
15. Tan S, Solish N. Long-term efficacy and quality of life in the treatment of focal hyperhidrosis with botulinum toxin A. *Dermatol Surg* 2002; 28: 495–9.
16. Kowalski J, Ravelo A, Glaser D, Lowe NJ. Quality-of-life effect of botulinum toxin type A on patients with primary axillary hyperhidrosis: Results from a North American clinical study population. P196. *American Academy of Dermatology Annual Meeting*. San Francisco, California, March 21–26, 2003.
17. Walling H. Primary hyperhidrosis increases the risk of cutaneous infection: A case–control study of 387 patients. *J Am Acad Dermatol* 2009; 61(2): 242–6.
18. Ingordo V, Naldi L, Fracchiolla S, Colecchia B. Prevalence and risk factors for superficial fungal infections among Italian Navy Cadets. *Dermatology* 2004; 209(3): 190–6.
19. Hamm H, Naumann M, Kowalski J et al. Primary focal hyperhidrosis: Disease characteristics and functional impairment. *Dermatology* 2006; 212: 343–53.
20. Bushara K, Park D. Botulinum toxin and sweating. *J Neurol Neuros Psy* 1994; 57(11): 1437–8.
21. Tugnoli A, Ragona R, Eleopra R, De Grandis D, Montecucco C. Treatment of Frey syndrome with botulinum toxin type F. *Arch Otolaryngol Head Neck Surg* 2001; 127: 339–40.
22. Schnider P, Binder M, Auff E et al. Double-blind trial of botulinum A toxin for the treatment of focal hyperhidrosis of the palms. *Br J Dermatol* 1997; 136: 548–52.
23. Lowe N, Yamauchi P, Lask G, Patnaik R, Iyer S. Efficacy and safety of botulinum toxin type a in the treatment of palmar

hyperhidrosis: A double-blind, randomized, placebo-controlled study. *Dermatol Surg* 2002; 28: 822–7.
24. Swartling C, Naver H, Lindberg M. Botulinum A toxin improves life quality in severe primary focal hyperhidrosis. *Eur J Neurol* 2001; 8(3): 247–52.
25. Glaser DA, Kowalski J, Eadie N et al. Hyperhidrosis disease severity scale (HDSS): Validity and reliability results from three studies. *Presented at the Annual Meeting of the American Academy of Dermatology*, Washington, DC, 2004.
26. Stolman L. Treatment of hyperhidrosis. *Dermatol Clin* 1998; 16(4): 863–9.
27. Glaser D, Hebert A, Pariser D, Solish N. Palmar and plantar hyperhidrosis: Best practice recommendations and special considerations. *Cutis* 2007; 79(Suppl 5): 18–28.
28. Benohanian A, Dansereau A, Bolduc C, Bloom E. Localized hyperhidrosis treated with aluminum chloride in a salicylic acid gel base. *Int J Dermatol* 1998; 37: 701–3.
29. Praharaj SK, Arora M. Paroxetine useful for palmar-plantar hyperhidrosis. *Ann Pharmacother* 2006; 40: 1884–6.
30. Bajaj V, Langtry JAA. Use of oral glycopyrronium bromide in hyperhidrosis. *Br J Dermatol* 2007; 157: 118–21.
31. Klaber M, Catterall M. Treating hyperhidrosis: Anticholinergic drugs were not mentioned. *BMJ* 2000; 3217262: 703.
32. Wolosker N, de Campos JR, Kaufman P et al. A randomized placebo-controlled trial of oxybutynin for the initial ttreatment of palmar and axillary hyperhidrosis. *J Vasc Surg* 2012; 55(6): 1696–1700.
33. Stolman L. Treatment of excess sweating of the palms by iontophoresis. *Arch Dermatol* 1987; 123: 893–6.
34. Swinehart J. Treatment of axillary hyperhidrosis: Combination of the starch-iodine test with the tumescent liposuction technique. *Dermatol Surg* 2000; 26: 392–6.
35. Gossot D, Galetta D, Pascal A et al. Long-term results of endoscopic thoracic sympathectomy for upper limb hyperhidrosis. *Ann Thoracic Surg* 2003; 75: 1075–9.
36. Kim B, Oh B, Park Y et al. Microinvasive video-assisted thoracoscopic sympathicotomy for primary palmar hyperhidrosis. *Am J Surg* 2001; 181(6): 540–2.
37. Belin E, Polo J. Treatment of compensatory hyperhidrosis with botulinum toxin type A. *Cutis* 2003; 71: 68–70.
38. Andrews B, Rennie J. Predicting changes in the distribution of sweating following thoracoscopic sympathectomy. *Br J Surg* 1997; 84(12): 1702–4.
39. Kao M, Chen Y, Lin J, Hsieh C, Tsai J. Endoscopic sympathectomy treatment for craniofacial hyperhidrosis. *Arch Surg* 1996; 131(10): 1091–4.
40. Johnson JE, O'Shaughnessy KF, Kim S. Microwave thermolysis of sweat glands. *Lasers Surg Med* 2012; 44(1): 20–25.
41. Chin-Ho Hong H, Lupin M, O'Shaughnessy KF. Clinical evaluation of a microwave device for treating axillary hyperhidrosis. *Dermatol Surg* 2012; 38(5): 726–735.
42. Lee SJ, Chang KY, Suh DH et al. The efficacy of a microwave device for treating axillary hyperhidrosis and osmidrosis in Asians: A preliminary study. *J Cosmet Laser Ther* 2013; 15(5): 255–259.
43. Glaser DA, Coleman W, Fan LK et al. A randomized blinded clinical evaluation of a novel microwave device for treating axillary hyperhidrosis. *Dermatol Surg* 2012; 38(2): 185–191.
44. Lecouflet M, Leux C, Fenot M et al. Duration of efficacy increases with the repetition of botulinum toxin A injections in primary axillary hyperhidrosis: A study in 83 patients. *J Am Acad Dermatol* 2013; 69(6): 960–4.
45. Naumann M, Lowe N, Kumar C, Hamm H. Botulinum toxin type A is a safe and effective treatment for axillary hyperhidrosis over 16 months: A prospective study. *Arch Dermatol* 2003; 139(6): 731–6.
46. Heckmann M, Ceballos-Baumann A, Plewig G. Botulinum toxin A for axillary hyperhidrosis (excessive sweating). *N Eng J Med* 2001; 344(7): 488–93.
47. Heckmann M, Breit S, Ceballos-Baumann A, Schaller M, Plewig G. Side-controlled intradermal injection of botulinum toxin A in recalcitrant axillary hyperhidrosis. *J Am Acad Dermatol* 1999; 41: 987–90.
48. Schnider P, Binder M, Kittler P et al. A randomized, double-blind, placebo-controlled trial of botulinum A toxin for severe axillary hyperhidrosis. *Br J Dermatol* 1999; 140: 677–80.
49. Naumann M, Lowe NJ. Botulinum toxin type A in treatment of bilateral primary axillary hyperhidrosis: Randomised, parallel group, double blind, placebo controlled trial. *Br Med J* 2001; 323: 596–9.
50. Lowe N, Glaser D, Eadie N et al. Botulinum toxin type A in the treatment of primary axillary hyperhidrosis: A 52-week multi-center double-blind, randomized, placebo-controlled study of efficacy and safety. *J Am Acad Dermatol* 2007; 56: 604–11.
51. Glaser D, Kowalski J, Ravelo A, Weng EY, Beddingfield F. Functional and dermatology-specific quality of life benefits with repeated botulinum toxin type A treatment of primary axillary hyperhidrosis. *Presented at the Annual Meeting of the American Academy of Dermatology*, San Francisco, 2006.
52. Glaser DA, Pariser DM, Hebert AA, Landells I, Somogyi C, Weng E, Brin MF, Beddingfield F. A prospective, nonrandomized, open-label study of the efficacy and safety of onabotulinumtoxinA in adolescents with primary axillary hyperhidrosis. *Pediatr Dermatol.* 2015; 32(5): 609–17. doi:10.1111/pde.12620.
53. Wollina U, Karamfilov T, Konrad H. High-dose botulinum toxin type A therapy for axillary hyperhidrosis markedly prolongs the relapse-free interval. *J Am Acad Dermatol* 2002; 46: 536–40.
54. Lecouflet M, Leux C, Fenot M et al. Duration of efficacy increases with the repetition of botulinum toxin A injections in primary axillary hyperhidrosis: A study in 83 patients. *J Am Acad Dermatol* 2013; 69(6): 960–4.
55. El Kahky HM, Diab HM, Aly DG et al. Efficacy of onabotulinum toxin a (Botox) versus abobotulinum toxin a (Dysport) using a conversion factor of 1:2.5 in treatment of primary palmar hyperhidrosis. *Dermatol Res Pract* 2013; 2012: 686329.
56. Alam M, Dover J, Arndt K. Pain associated with injection of botulinum A exotoxin reconstituted using isotonic sodium chloride with and without preservative: A double-blind, randomized controlled trial. *Arch Dermatol* 2002; 138: 510–4.
57. Sarifakioglu N, Sarifakioglu E. Evaluating effects of preservative-containing saline solution on pain perception during botulinum toxin type-A injections at different locations: A prospective, single-blinded, randomized controlled trial. *Aesth Plast Surg* 2005; 29: 113–5.
58. Glaser D. Treatment of axillary hyperhidrosis by chemodenervation of sweat glands using botulinum toxin type A. *J Drugs Dermatol* 2004; 3: 627–31.
59. Vadoud-Seyedi J, Simonart T. Treatment of axillary hyperhidrosis with botulinum toxin type A reconstituted in lidocaine or in normal saline: A randomized, side-by-side, double-blind study. *Br J Dermatol* 2007; 156: 986–9.

60. Lowe N, Campanati A, Bodokh I et al. The place of botulinum toxin type A in the treatment of focal hyperhidrosis. *Br J Dermatol* 2004; 151: 1115–22.
61. Moreau M, Cauhepe C, Magues J, Senard J. Therapeutics: A double-blind, randomized, comparative study of Dysport vs. Botox in primary palmar hyperhidrosis. *Br J Dermatol* 2002; 149: 1041–5.
62. Saadia D, Voustianiouk A, Wang A, Kaufmann H. Botulinum toxin type A in primary palmar hyperhidrosis: Randomized, single-blind, two-dose study. *Neurology* 2001; 57: 2095–9.
63. Naver H, Swartling C, Aquilonius S. Treatment of focal hyperhidrosis with botulinum toxin type A. Brief overview of methodology and 2 years' experience. *Eur J Neurol* 1999; 6(4): S117–120.
64. Vadoud-Seyedi J, Heenen M, Simonart T. Treatment of idiopathic palmar hyperhidrosis with botulinum toxin. *Dermatology* 2001; 203: 318–21.
65. Glaser D, Kokoska M, Kardesch C. Botulinum toxin type A in the treatment of palmar hyperhidrosis: the effect of dilution and number of injection sites. *American Academy of Dermatology Annual Meeting*, Poster. Washington, DC, March 2–7, 2001.
66. Baumann L, Frankel S, Esperanza W, Halem M. Cryoanalgesia with dichlorotetrafluoroethane lessens the pain of botulinum toxin injections for the treatment of palmar hyperhidrosis. *Dermatol Surg* 2003; 29(10): 1057–62.
67. Trindade de Almeida A, Kadunc B, Martins de Oliveira E. Improving botulinum toxin therapy for palmar hyperhidrosis: Wrist block and technical considerations. *Dermatol Surg* 2001; 27: 34–6.
68. Wollina U, Karamfilov T. Botulinum toxin A for palmar hyperhidrosis. *J Eur Acad Dermatol Venereol* 2001; 15: 555–8.
69. Hund M, Rickert S, Kinkelin I, Naumann M, Hamm H. Does wrist nerve block influence the result of botulinum toxin A treatment in palmar hyperhidrosis. *J Am Acad Dermatol* 2004; 50: 61–2.
70. Aghaei S. Botulinum toxin therapy for palmar hyperhidrosis: Experience in an Iranian population. *Int J Dermatol* 2007; 46: 212–4.
71. Perez BA, Avalos-Peralta P, Moreno-Ramirez D, Camacho F. Treatment of palmar hyperhidrosis with botulinum toxin type A: 44 months of experience. *J Cosmetic Dermatol* 2005; 4: 163–6.
72. Glogau R. Treatment of hyperhidrosis with botulinum toxin. *Dermatologic Clinics* 2004; 22: 177–85.
73. Kontochristopoulos G, Gregoriou S, Zakopoulou N, Rigopoulos D. Cryoanalgesia with dichlorotetrafluoroethane spray versus ice packs in patients treated with botulinum toxin A for palmar hyperhidrosis: Self-controlled study. *Dermatol Surg* 2006; 32(6): 873–4.
74. Smith K, Comite SL, Storwick GS. Ice minimizes discomfort associated with injection of botulinum toxin type A for the treatment of palmar and plantar hyperhidrosis. *Dermatol Surg* 2007; 33: S88–91.
75. Kreyden OP. Botulinum toxin in the management of focal hyperhidrosis. In: Benedetto, AV (ed). *Botulinum Toxin in Clinical Dermatology*. Boca Raton, FL: Taylor & Francis; 2006; Chapter 10: 281–285.
76. Naumann M, Bergmann I, Hofmann U, Hamm H, Reiners K. Botulinum toxin for focal hyperhidrosis: Technical considerations and improvements in application. *Br J Dermatol* 1998; 139: 1123–4.
77. Benohanian A. Needle-free anaesthesia prior to botulinum toxin type A injection treatment of palmar and plantar hyperhidrosis. *Br J Dermatol* 2007; 156(3): 593–6.
78. Benohanian A. What stands in the way of treating palmar hyperhidrosis as effectively as axillary hyperhidrosis with botulinum toxin type A. *Dermatol Online J* 2009; 15(4): 12.
79. Trindade de Almeida AR, Kandunc BV, Martins de Oliveira EM. Improving botulinum toxin therapy for palmar hyperhidrosis. *Derm Surg* 2001; 27: 34–36.
80. Hayton MJ, Stanley JK, Lowe, NJ. A review of peripheral nerve blockade as local anaesthesia in the treatment of palmar hyperhidrosis. *Br J Dermatol* 2003; 149: 447–451.
81. Campanati A, Lagalla G, Penna L, Gesuita R, Offidani A. Local neural block at the wrist for treatment of palmar hyperhidrosis with botulinum toxin: Technical improvements. *JAAD* 2004; 51(3): 345–348.
82. Vollert B, Blaheta H, Moehrle E, Juenger M, Rassner G. Intravenous regional anaesthesia for treatment of palmar hyperhidrosis with botulinum toxin type A. *Br J Dermatol* 2001; 144: 632–3.
83. Ponce-Olivera RM, Tirado-Sanchez A, Arellano-Mendoza MI, Leon-Dorantes G, Kassian-Rank S. Palmar hyperhidrosis. Safety efficacy of two anaesthetic techniques for botulinum toxin therapy. *Dermatology Online J* 2006; 12(2): 9.
84. Reed M. Surgical pearl: Mechanoanesthesia to reduce the pain of local injections. *J Am Acad Dermatol* 2001; 44: 671–2.
85. Scherer C, Clelland J, O'Sullivan P, Doleys D, Canan B. The effect of two sites of high frequency vibration on cutaneous pain threshold. *Pain* 1986; 25(1): 133–8.
86. Solomon B, Hayman R. Botulinum toxin type A therapy for palmar and digital hyperhidrosis. *J Am Acad Dermatol* 2000; 42: 1026–9.
87. Glass GE, Hussain M, Fleming AN, Powell BW. Atrophy of the intrinsic musculature of the hands associated with the use of botulinum toxin-A injections for hyperhidrosis: A case report and review of the literature. *J Plastic Reconstr Aesthetic Surg* 2009; 62(8): 274–6.
88. Zaiac M, Weiss E, Elgart G. Botulinum toxin therapy for palmar hyperhidrosis with ADG needle. *Dermatol Surg* 2000; 26: 230.
89. Trindade de Almeida A, Boraso R. Palmar hyperhidrosis. In: Trindade de Almeida A, Hexsel D (eds). *Hyperhidrosis and Botulinum Toxin*. Sao Paulo: Know-how Editorial Ltd, 2004; 155–62.
90. Coutinho dos Santos C, Gomes A, Giraldi S, Abagge K, Marinoni L. Palmar hyperhidrosis: Long-term follow-up of nine children and adolescents treated with botulinum toxin type A. *Pediatr Dermatol* 2009; 26(4): 439–44.
91. Naumann M, Hofmann U, Bergmann I et al. Focal hyperhidrosis: Effective treatment with intracutaneous botulinum toxin. *Arch Dermatol* 1998; 134(3): 301–4.
92. Blaheta H, Deusch H, Rasner G, Vollert B. Intravenous regional anesthesia (Bier's block) is superior to a peripheral nerve block for painless treatment of plantar hyperhidrosis with botulinum toxin. *J Am Acad Dermatol* 2003; 48(2): 302–4.
93. Campanati A, Bernardini M, Gesuita R, Offidani A. Plantar focal idiopathic hyperhidrosis and botulinum toxin: A pilot study. *Eur J Dermatol* 2007; 17(1): 52–4.
94. Blaheta H, Deusch H, Rassner G, Vollert B. Intravenous regional anesthesia (Bier's block) is superior to a peripheral nerve block for painless treatment of plantar hyperhidrosis. *J Am Acad Dermatol* 2003; 48(2): 301–3.
95. Vadoud-Seyedi J. Treatment of plantar hyperhidrosis with botulinum toxin type A. *Int J Dermatol* 2004; 43: 969–71.
96. Sevim S, Dogu O, Kaleagasi H. Botulinum toxin-A therapy for palmar and plantar hyperhidrosis. *Acta Neurol Belg* 2002; 102: 167–70.
97. Kinkelin I, Hund M, Naumann M, Hamm H. Effective treatment of frontal hyperhidrosis with botulinum toxin A. *Br J Dermatol* 2000; 143: 824–7.

98. Boger A, Herath H, Rompel R, Ferbert A. Botulinum toxin for treatment of craniofacial hyperhidrosis. *J Neurol* 2000; 247(11): 857–61.
99. Glaser DA, Herbert AA, Pariser DM, Solish N. Facial hyperhidrosis: Best practice recommendations and special considerations. *Cutis* 2007; 79(5 Suppl): 29–32.
100. Hexsel D, Dal'forno T, Hexsel C. Inguinal, or Hexsel's hyperhidrosis. *Clin Dermatol* 2004; 22(1): 53–9.
101. Drobik C, Laskawi R. Frey's syndrome: Treatment with botulinum toxin. *Acta Otolaryngol (Stockh)* 1995; 115: 459–61.
102. Naumann M, Zellner M, Toyka K, Reiners K. Treatment of gustatory sweating with botulinum toxin. *Ann Neurol* 1997; 42(6): 973–75.
103. Bjerkhoel A, Trobbe O. Frey's syndrome: Treatment with botulinum toxin. *J Laryngol Otol* 1997; 111(9): 839–44.
104. Laskawi R, Drobik C, Schonebeck C. Up-to-date report of botulinum toxin type A treatment in patients with gustatory sweating (Frey's syndrome). *Laryngoscope* 1998; 108: 381–4.
105. Laccourreye O, Akl E, Gutierrez-Fonseca R et al. Recurrent gustatory sweating (Frey's syndrome) after intracutaneous injection of botulinum toxin type A: Incidence, management, and outcome. *Arch Otolaryngol Head Neck Surg* 1999; 125: 283–6.
106. Huh C, Han K, Deo K, Eun H. Botulinum toxin treatment for compensatory hyperhidrosis subsequent to an upper thoracic sympathectomy. *J Dermatol Treat* 2002; 13: 91–3.
107. Kim W, Kil H, Yoon K, Noh K. Botulinum toxin: A treatment for compensatory hyperhidrosis in the trunk. *Dermatol Surg* 2009; 35(5): 833–8.
108. Matarasso S. Treatment of facial chromhidrosis with botulinum toxin type A. *J Am Acad Dermatol* 2005; 52(1): 89–91.
109. Ross AT. Progressive selective sudomotor denervation; a case with coexisting Adie's syndrome. *Neurology* 1958; 8: 808–17.
110. Kreyden OP. Rare forms of hyperhidrosis. In: Kreyden OP et al. (eds). *Hyperhidrosis and Botulinum Toxin in Dermatology*. Basel: Karger; 2002; 30: 178–87.
111. Itin P, Hirsbrunner P, Rufli T et al. Das Ross-Syndrom. *Hautarzt* 1992; 43: 359–60.
112. Kreyden OP, Schmid-Grendelmeier P, Burg G. Idiopathic localized unilateral hyperhidrosis. Case report of successful treatment with botulinum toxin type A and review of the literature. *Arch Dermatology* 2001; 137: 1622–5.
113. Schulz V, Ward D, Moulin DE. Segmental hyperhidrosis as a manifestation of spinal and paraspinal disease. *Can J Neurol Sci* 1998; 25(4): 325–7.
114. Charrow A, DiFazio M, Foster L et al. Intradermal botulinum toxin type A injection effectively reduces residual limb hyperhidrosis in amputees: A case series. *Arch Phys Med Rehabil* 2008; 89; 1407–9.
115. Gratrix M, Hivnor C. Botulinum toxin A treatment for hyperhidrosis in patients with prosthetic limbs. *Arch Dermatol* 2010; 145: 1314–5.
116. Birklein F, Eisenbarth G, Erbguth F, Winterholler M. Botulinum toxin type B blocks sudomotor function effectively: A 6 month follow up. *J Invest Dermatol* 2003; 121(6): 1312–6.
117. Schlereth T, Mouka I, Eisenbarth G, Winterholler M, Birklein F. Botulinum toxin A (Botox) and sweating-dose efficacy and comparison to other BoNT preparations. *Autonom Neurosci* 2005; 117: 120–6.
118. Dressler D, Abid Saberi F, Benecke R. Botulinum toxin type B for treatment of axillary hyperhidrosis. *J Neurol* 2002; 249: 1729–32.
119. Nelson L, Bachoo P, Holmes J. Botulinum toxin type B: A new therapy for axillary hyperhidrosis. *Br J Plastic Surg* 2005; 58: 228–32.
120. Baumann L, Halem M. Systemic adverse effects after botulinum toxin type B (myobloc) injections for the treatment of palmar hyperhidrosis. *Arch Dermatol* 2003; 139: 226–7.
121. Baumann L, Slezinger A, Halem M et al. Double-blind, randomized placebo-controlled pilot study of the safety and efficacy of myobloc (botulinum toxin type B) for the treatment of palmar hyperhidrosis. *Dermatol Surg* 2005; 31: 263–70.
122. Hecht M, Birklein F, Winterholler M. Successful treatment of axillary hyperhidrosis with very low doses of botulinum toxin B: A pilot study. *Arch Dermatol* 2003; 295: 318–9.
123. Kavanagh G, Oh C, Shams K. BOTOX delivery by iontophoresis. *Br J Dermatol* 2004; 151: 1093–5.
124. Glogau R. Topically applied botulinum toxin type A for the treatment of primary axillary hyperhidrosis: Results of a randomized, blinded, vehicle-controlled study. *Dermatol Surg* 2007; 33: S76–80.

10 Botulinum toxin type A treatment for depression, Raynaud's phenomenon, and other novel dermatologic therapeutic applications

Irèn Kossintseva, Benjamin Barankin, and Kevin Smith

INTRODUCTION

This chapter will discuss the use of botulinum toxin type A (BoNT-A) in dermatology for the treatment of painful conditions including Raynaud's phenomenon, postherpetic neuralgia, headache, reflex sympathetic dystrophy (or complex regional pain syndrome), depression, and a variety of other conditions. The use of BoNT-A to improve upper thoracic posture and thus improve the appearance and presentation of female breasts also will be discussed. An approach to the management of acute overdoses of BoNT-A will be described. The more modern and more accurate term "neuromodulator" is preferred over the original term "neurotoxin." Members of the botulinum family (notably types A and B) are used in clinical practice as neuromodulators, and never as "toxins."

Since BoNT-A was first reported to be useful for the reduction in the pain of spasmodic torticollis in 1985,[1] the number of references in PubMed Central to "botulinum" and "pain" has been growing at an increasing rate, and by January 2016 there were over 3000 publications.[2] The list of painful conditions reported to respond well to BoNT-A is also growing, and now includes some dermatologic conditions, and other conditions like headache which are treated by some dermatologists who have expertise in the use of BoNT-A.[3,4]

It is important to note that the BoNT-A used by the authors in the management of these conditions was BOTOX®, and the doses described in this chapter refer to BOTOX®. Because the diffusion characteristics and dosing of other forms of BoNT-A differ from BOTOX®, it is not possible to establish a simple ratio for the conversion of BOTOX® doses to other formulations of BoNT-A, or to other botulinum neuromodulator serotypes, for example, BoNT-B or BoNT-E (see Chapter 1). To reduce the risk of confusion, the recently designated generic instead of the trade name of the BoNT-A actually injected will be used throughout this chapter which is OnaBTX-A for BOTOX®; AboBTX-A for Dysport®; and IncoBTX-A for Xeomin®. The term BoNT-A will be used to refer to the general class of neuromodulator.

BoNT-A TREATMENT FOR DEPRESSION

Three prospective, randomized, double-blind studies have now shown that OnaBTX-A[5–7] injection to the corrugator and procerus forehead muscles can improve the symptoms of major depression.

In a fascinating review, Reichenberg et al.[8] de-identified the data from the above three studies,[5–7] scored the severity of the frown lines at baseline, and found that:

1. More severe frown lines at baseline were not predictive of reduced symptoms of depression in response to BoNT-A.
2. More severe frown lines at baseline were not predictive of having worse depression at baseline.
3. There was no significant association between visible improvement in frown scores and improvement in depression scores.

These findings suggest that the mechanism of action of BoNT-A in depression is related neither to cosmetic effect perceived by the patient, nor is it related to a cosmetic effect that might affect the way other people relate to the patient.

Finzi et al.[5] have reported that patients who do not have frown lines at baseline can have remission of depression after BoNT-A.

Magid et al.[6] have observed that improvement in depression after treatment with BoNT-A outlasts the cosmetic effects.

Wollmer et al.[7] reported that even subjects who dislike the cosmetic effects of BoNT-A had improvement in depression after treatment with BoNT-A.

There is growing support for the hypothesis that decreased glabellar complex activation reduces afferent nerve signals back to the brain, and so reduces "negative emotional feedback." This is supported by magnetic resonance imaging studies which have shown that BoNT-A treatment of corrugators impacts brain areas involved with emotion-processing by decreasing afferent signals from facial muscles.[9]

Patients who received BoNT-A in crow's feet (i.e., suppressing "smile muscles") were noted in one abstract to have worsening depression scores.[10]

In April 2017, the results of a proof of concept Phase 2, multicenter, randomized, double-blind, placebo-controlled, 30 or 50 unit cohort parallel group study of 258 women using OnaBTX-A to the glabellar complex for the treatment of moderate to severe depression, were released.[11] The 30 unit dose was superior to the 50 unit dose, but the overall effects were equivocal. The data were sufficient for Allergan to announce that it was proceeding to a Phase 3 clinical trial of OnaBTX-A for the treatment of depression.

One author (KCS) has cared for many individuals who return specifically for treatment of the glabellar complex with BoNT-A when they are sad and/or distressed, for example, during a marriage breakdown, or the illness or death of a pet or of a loved one. Improvement and/or long-term control of depression or subclinical depression may be part of the reason why some cosmetic patients are motivated to return for treatment with BoNT-A. This phenomenon may also help to motivate headache patients who also have an element of depression to return on a very regular basis for treatment with BoNT-A.

BoNT-A TREATMENT IN RAYNAUD'S

Raynaud's phenomenon is defined as an episodic digital asphyxia caused by vasospasm of the digital arteries triggered by cold exposure or stress. It is either idiopathic and known as Raynaud's disease, or secondary to diseases such as scleroderma, lupus, rheumatoid arthritis, and occlusive arterial disease and called Raynaud's phenomenon. Its symptoms include a progression from digital blanching and cyanosis to reactive hyperemia, to pain and dysthesias, which if prolonged can result in severe digital vascular compromise, ulceration, digital infarction, and may even necessitate amputation. The etiology of Raynaud's disease is complex, but both vasospasm and nociception appear to play a major role. The inhibitory effects of BoNT-A on somatic and autonomic neurotransmission are well documented. BoNT-A inhibits norepinephrine (NE)-mediated sympathetic vasoconstriction, thus improving perfusion of digits by opening the vasculature and allowing for better oxygenation. It concurrently inhibits pain-mediating neuropeptides (substance P (SP), neuropeptide-Y (NPY), vasoactive intestinal peptide (VIP), calcitonin gene-related peptide (CGRP), and glutamate) thus interfering with nociception, both peripheral and central sensitization, and decreasing swelling and inflammation.

BoNT-A is successfully used in Raynaud's phenomenon as a safer and easier alternative to surgical sympathectomy.[12] It essentially produces a chemical sympathectomy that lasts for months and effectively improves hand temperature within 1–2 days as well as shortens warm-up time after exposure to cold,[13] controls rest pain, shortens and reduces frequency and severity of attacks[14] including stiffness, numbness, acute pain, color change, and swelling,[15] prevents impending infarction of digits, and successfully heals ischemic ulcerations caused by profound vasospasm in the majority of patients.[1] These favorable changes of improved perfusion are quantified using a Visual Analogue Scale (VAS) and confirmed by digital surface temperature readings,[1,2] imaging studies with laser Doppler interferometry,[3] intravascular arteriography or high-resolution digital magnetic resonance angiography.[1] The adverse events reported are rare and include mild and temporary hand weakness. Amelioration of pain improves hand function despite occasional muscle weakness.[1]

PHYSIOLOGICAL BASIS OF BoNT-A FOR RAYNAUD'S PHENOMENON

Autonomic: Vasodilator and Vasoconstrictor

In addition to the widely recognized inhibitory effects on the release of acetylcholine (Ach) from neurons innervating striated muscle and sweat glands, BoNT-A has been shown to produce a neuromodulating effect on autonomic nerves.[16] Cutaneous vasoconstriction and vasodilation are regulated by modulation of sympathetic and parasympathetic neuronal inputs and the complex actions of released Ach, NE, peptides like NPY, and small molecules such as nitric oxide on vascular smooth muscle.

In an animal model of significantly constricted uterine arteries, BoNT-A has been shown to reduce the amplitude of sympathetic NE-mediated vasoconstriction by 80%.[17] Likewise, isometric contractions of venae cavae mediated by NE acting on alpha-adrenoceptors are substantially reduced by BoNT-A administration.[18] Concurrently, in parasympathetic neurons, BoNT-A is found to significantly reduce the autocrine acetylcholine-mediated inhibition of vascular relaxation and also to reduce the slow component of neurogenic vasodilation mediated by the peptides VIP and CGRP.[11] Thus, a differential effect of BoNT-A on different classes of neurotransmitters is observed, whereby it may reduce neurotransmitter and botulinum toxin release from vasoconstrictor and vasodilator neurons depending on various regulatory mechanisms.

Local BoNT-A injection consistently shows an ability to improve perfusion of the injected tissue by both substantial opening of the vascular bed and an increase in aerobic metabolism. BoNT-A inhibits the neurogenic contractions of tumor vessels by blocking NE, thus improving tumor perfusion and oxygenation and thus aiding in delivery of cancer therapy.[19,20] In inflammatory muscle states due to decreased microcirculation, such as in lateral epicondylitis secondary to low intramuscular blood flow in extensor carpi radialis brevis, BoNT-A injection allows for muscle relaxation, a shift toward aerobic metabolism, and a decrease in lactate production, restoration in intramuscular blood flow, decreased pain, and improved muscle strength and function.[21]

BoNT-A Has Antiinflammatory and Antinociceptive Effects

BoNT-A also acts on the nociceptive portion of the sensory system to reduce pain and neurogenic inflammation by attenuating the peripheral release of neuroactive compounds such as SP and glutamate from C-fibers, as well as reducing central sensitization.[6] BoNT-A does not directly decrease excitability of nociceptors, but acts by reducing inflammatory pain,[22] and thus pathological pain.[23]

Substance P

BoNT-A inhibits substance P (SP), a peptide released both peripherally and centrally by nociceptive primary afferent C-fibers, thus producing the analgesic effect seen in treating primary headache disorders.[24] It markedly inhibits SP secretion in dorsal root ganglia neurons[25] within hours and lasts for at least 2 weeks. Local inflammation sensitizes peripheral nociceptive neurons, and as the increase in peripheral pain input causes increased release of SP in the spinal cord, it induces central sensitization.[6] BoNT-A thus attenuates both the peripheral and central sensitization by its inhibition of SP.

CGRP

BoNT-A inhibits the release of calcitonin gene-related peptide (CGRP), an inflammatory neuropeptide found on its own as well as co-localized with SP in sensory ganglia neurons, when pain stimulus is present, but not basally. It reduces bladder pain response by 62% through inhibition of CGRP release from afferent nerve terminals,[26] and in trigeminal nerves,[27] explaining the observed efficacy of BoNT-A in migraine and cluster headache therapy. Curiously, CGRP released during inflammation causes vasodilation, thus BoNT-A's analgesic effect in migraines may be secondary to vasoconstriction of the meningeal vasculature.

Glutamate

BoNT-A dose-dependently inhibits inflammatory pain by decreasing glutamate release. Glutamate is a stimulant of local nociceptive neurons through activation of receptors on primary afferents.[28] Peripheral glutamate release results in edema, pain, and inflammation,[29] which is abolished by local BoNT-A injection at doses below ones that would elicit muscle paralysis.[15]

PRACTICAL TIPS

Assessment

Assessment of disability caused by Raynaud's phenomenon or disease should be performed prior to and after the BoNT-A treatment at 1 week, 1 month, and then routine follow-up. This is done by asking patients to evaluate the level of their (a) pain and (b) hand function using the 10-point VAS, as well as the Dermatology Quality of Life Scale. If digital ulcerations are present, a photographic record is useful.

Injection Parameters

There is no consensus of how many injection sites should be administered per affected hand, and whether the entire hand should be treated or just the most affected digits. The clinical decision will be based on the extent and severity of the patient's Raynaud's phenomenon/disease, with consideration given to the pharmacoeconomics of using BoNT-A and also consideration of how best to avoid causing unwanted muscle weakness in the treated hand.

The authors consider that it is reasonable to administer up to 100 units of BOTOX® per hand being treated, reconstituted in 3–6 cc of normal saline/100 U vial.[1,4] This relatively high reconstitution volume is presently preferred as the increased volume may facilitate spread of the injected BoNT-A from the injection point to the vessels we wish to relax. The trend is to inject the palm and all fingers at their base, except for the thumb unless it is specifically symptomatic (since thumb ischemia is uncommon in Raynaud's). Targeted anatomy includes the superficial palmar arch, common digital arteries and proper digital arteries, with injections being just adjacent to the targeted vasculature (to avoid injury to vessels) and needle tip perpendicular to the palm and deep to the palmar fascia[1] (Figure 10.1). A 30-, 31-, or 32-gauge needle is used to infiltrate the soft tissues, with 10–40 injection sites spaced approximately 1 cm apart, of equally distributed volume of reconstituted 100 U of BOTOX®.[1,4] This is followed by a massage of

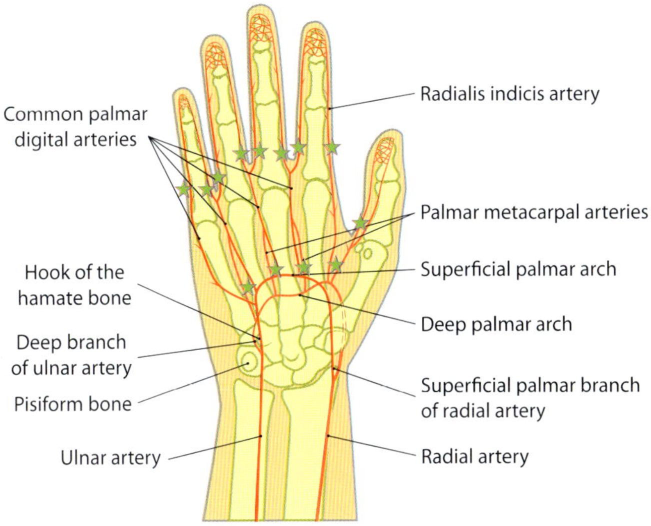

Figure 10.1 Typical injection points (starred) when BoNT-A is administered to control Raynaud's phenomenon. Each subcutaneous dose of OnaBTX-A is 5–10 units.

the injected tissues to help distribute the medication throughout the region. Due to the discomfort associated with palmar injections, sufficient anesthesia (e.g., ice, vibration, or nerve blocks) is necessary to make the procedure tolerable (see Chapter 9). To minimize weakness of the thumb, it is important to avoid injection into the thenar muscle group on the radial side of the proximal part of the palm (flexor, extensor and abductor pollicis longus, and extensor pollicis brevis).

OTHER NOVEL DERMATOLOGIC USES OF BoNT-A

Targeting Hypersecretion

Based on the positive results seen with treatment of hyperhydrosis using BoNT-A injections, BoNT-A has been found to be helpful for other conditions made worse by increased sweating. These conditions include persistent facial flushing with or without localized sweating, gustatory sweating (Frey's syndrome), localized unilateral hyperhydrosis, Ross' syndrome,[30] familial benign pemphigus (Hailey–Hailey disease), and dishydrotic eczema[31] (See Chapter 9).

Frey's syndrome is facial hyperhidrosis in the preauricular region from gustatory stimulus, observed commonly after parotidectomy. A small amount of BoNT-A, on average 40 units of BOTOX®, effectively alleviates the symptoms within days after injection and remission has been reported to persist for 15–18 months.[32] Other glandular hypersecretory disorders, including sialorrhea, excessive lacrimation, chronic rhinitis,[33,34] and parotid fistulas[35–37] also have been reported to respond to treatment with BoNT-A.

Hailey–Hailey disease is an autosomal-dominant acantholytic blistering disease affecting the intertriginous skin, and is exacerbated by heat, sweat, moisture, friction, and infection. Intertriginous injection of BoNT-A has been reported to induce significant improvement within two weeks[38] and improvement can be maintained for many months.[39] Dyshidrotic hand eczema (pompholyx) is a chronic, relapsing inflammatory vesiculobullous disease also aggravated by hyperhidrosis.[40] The addition of BoNT-A injection to topical steroid therapy has shown significant benefit in managing pompholyx eruptions and the associated symptoms of pruritus.[41,42] Inverse psoriasis is exacerbated by maceration, secondary infection, and inflammatory pain; BoNT-A injections to affected intertriginous regions also improve the symptoms and eruptions of inverse psoriasis.[43]

Targeting Pain

BoNT-A's antinociceptive properties have been used in the treatment of multiple cutaneous piloleiomyomas, with effective rapid and sustained resolution of pain.[44] It has also shown substantial benefit in the treatment of notalgia paresthetica.[45]

BoNT-A enters neurons by binding to the synaptic vesicle protein SV2 receptor (isoforms A, B, and C).[46] SV2 is transiently exposed when synaptic vesicles fuse with the presynaptic membrane to discharge neurotransmitter into the synaptic junction (Figure 10.2). This is the physiological basis for the important clinical observation that generally the most effective and efficient way to administer BoNT-A for painful conditions is to inject BoNT-A in the points and areas of maximum discomfort indicated by the patient because

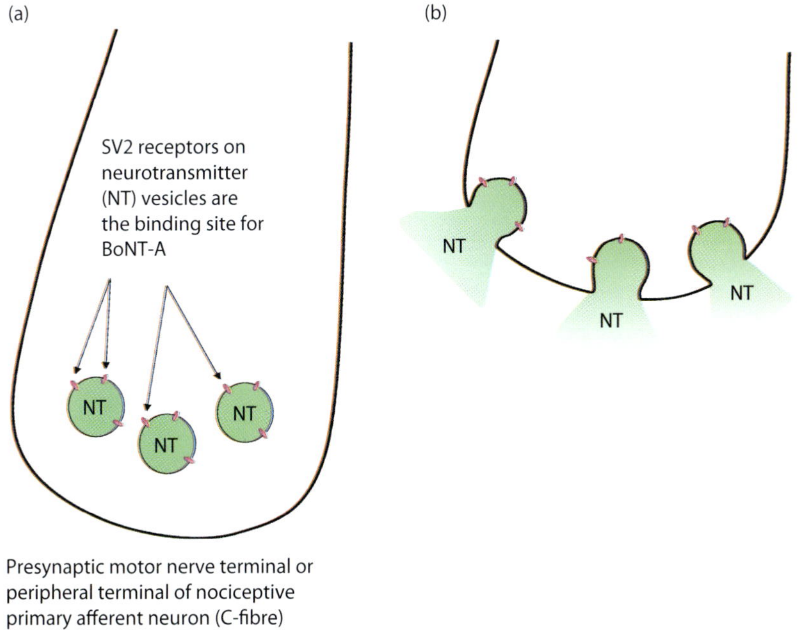

Figure 10.2 (a) SV2 receptors for the binding domain (i.e., heavy chain) of BoNT-A are exposed when the contents of vesicles of neurotransmitter are released at the presynaptic membrane. (b) After stimulation of the nerve terminal, vesicles containing NT (e.g., actylcholine) fuse with the neuronal membrane (via the SNARE complex), releasing NT and exposing SV2 receptors to BoNT-A.

it is in these areas that there is maximum discharge of pain mediating neurotransmitter and thus maximal exposure of the SV2 protein which mediates uptake of BoNT-A. This method of administration of BoNT-A is commonly referred to as the "follow the pain" approach. Clinical trials of BoNT-A for painful conditions sometimes use a rigid protocol of doses and injection sites rather than the "follow the pain" approach, which customizes the treatment to the needs of each individual patient, and this difference may explain why some clinical trials (in particular for headache) do not obtain the degree of improvement that is commonly achieved in clinical practice.[47–50]

BoNT-A for Postherpetic Neuralgia

Perhaps the first to use OnaBTX-A for the treatment of postherpetic neuralgia (PHN) were Dr. Arnold Klein,[51] and later Drs. Mariusz Sapijaszko and Richard Glogau (personal communications) who used OnaBTX-A to treat PHN on the trunk. Their informal oral reports, together with a consideration of the well-established role of SP in the pathogenesis of PHN, and considering reports that BoNT-A blocked the release of SP from vesicles in nerve terminals, provided the rationale for additional trials of treatment with BoNT-A for severe, intractable PHN.[52] One author (KCS) has found OnaBTX-A to be a very reliable treatment for PHN on the face and scalp, but has had only treatment failures when attempting to use OnaBTX-A to treat PHN on the trunk and extremities. The reason for this difference in responses is not known, and additional investigations are warranted.

It is important clinically for communication with other physicians and with third-party payers, and in terms of pharmacoeconomics, to objectively quantify a patient's conditions at baseline and in response to therapy. The four tools that are helpful include:

1. Likert pain scale and global assessment (Figure 10.3).
2. Physician's global assessment (Figure 10.4).
3. Number of doses of pain medication taken in the 7 days preceding evaluation, and the number of doses taken since the last visit.
4. Marking and photographing the boundaries of the area or areas of PHN before treatment and then marking and photographing the involved areas at every subsequent visit (Figure 10.5).

Patients are advised to continue their usual pain medications, and only to reduce the dose of pain medication as they respond to their BoNT-A treatment.

The patient identifies the area or areas of involvement. The boundaries of the areas of involvement are marked with washable pink fluorescent marker, photographed (Figure 10.5), then injected with OnaBTX-A intradermally or subdermally at doses ranging from 2.5 to 5 units per injection site, with the injections spaced 2–3 cm apart. The total dose of BOTOX® is generally in the range of 1–2 units per cm or cm^2.

BoNT-A is reconstituted using normal saline with benzyl alcohol preservative (which has local anesthetic properties and reduces injection discomfort). A reconstitution volume of 1 mL per 100 units of OnaBTX-A is used by the author (KCS), but the reconstitution volume does not seem to influence efficacy—the only thing that matters is how many units of BoNT-A are administered.[53] Because there is commonly hyperalgesia in areas of PHN, it is best to use Becton-Dickinson BD-II 0.3 mL diabetic syringes with attached 31-gauge needles. It is not usually necessary to pretreat patients with topical anesthetics like EMLA®, but this could be used in cases where there is a likelihood of intolerable injection discomfort.

Patients should be informed that there will very likely be some unwanted relaxation of muscles in the treated area. Injecting BoNT-A intradermally can minimize muscle weakness. Injections for the pain of PHN seem to be equally effective whether given intradermally, subdermally, or intramuscularly.

The maximum analgesic effect of BoNT-A treatment for PHN often occurs at around 3–4 weeks. For this reason, patients are asked to return for reassessment and possibly additional treatment every 3–4 weeks until they are pain free.

Last Name ________ First Name ________ Chart # ________ Date ________

Patient's rating scale:

Please circle the number which best describes the amount of pain you are having today in the involved area:

When you are not touching the area:

NO Pain 0 1 2 3 4 5 6 7 8 9 10 WORST possible pain

When the area is touched or rubbed:

NO Pain 0 1 2 3 4 5 6 7 8 9 10 WORST possible pain

Please circle the number which best describes your PAIN in the involved area is BETTER or WORSE compared to how it was at your last visit:

BETTER 5 4 3 2 1 0 1 2 3 4 5 WORSE

Please circle the number which best describes your OVERALL impression of how you are doing, compared to the previous visit:

BETTER 5 4 3 2 1 0 1 2 3 4 5 WORSE

Figure 10.3 Visual analog scale used to measure patients' perception of their pain and of their global well-being.

Last Name ______ First Name ______ Chart # ______ Date ______

Patient's rating scale:

Please circle the number which best describes the amount of pain the patient appears to be having today in the involved area:

When the area is not touched:

NO Pain 0 1 2 3 4 5 6 7 8 9 10 WORST possible pain

When the area is touched or rubbed:

NO Pain 0 1 2 3 4 5 6 7 8 9 10 WORST possible pain

Please circle the number which best describes whether the patient's pain in the involved area appears to be BETTER or WORSE compared to how it was at the patient's last visit:

BETTER 5 4 3 2 1 0 1 2 3 4 5 WORSE

Please circle the number which best describes your OVERALL impression of how this patient is doing, compared to the previous visit:

BETTER 5 4 3 2 1 0 1 2 3 4 5 WORSE

Figure 10.4 Visual analog scale used to measure the physician's assessment of the patient's pain and of the patient's global well-being.

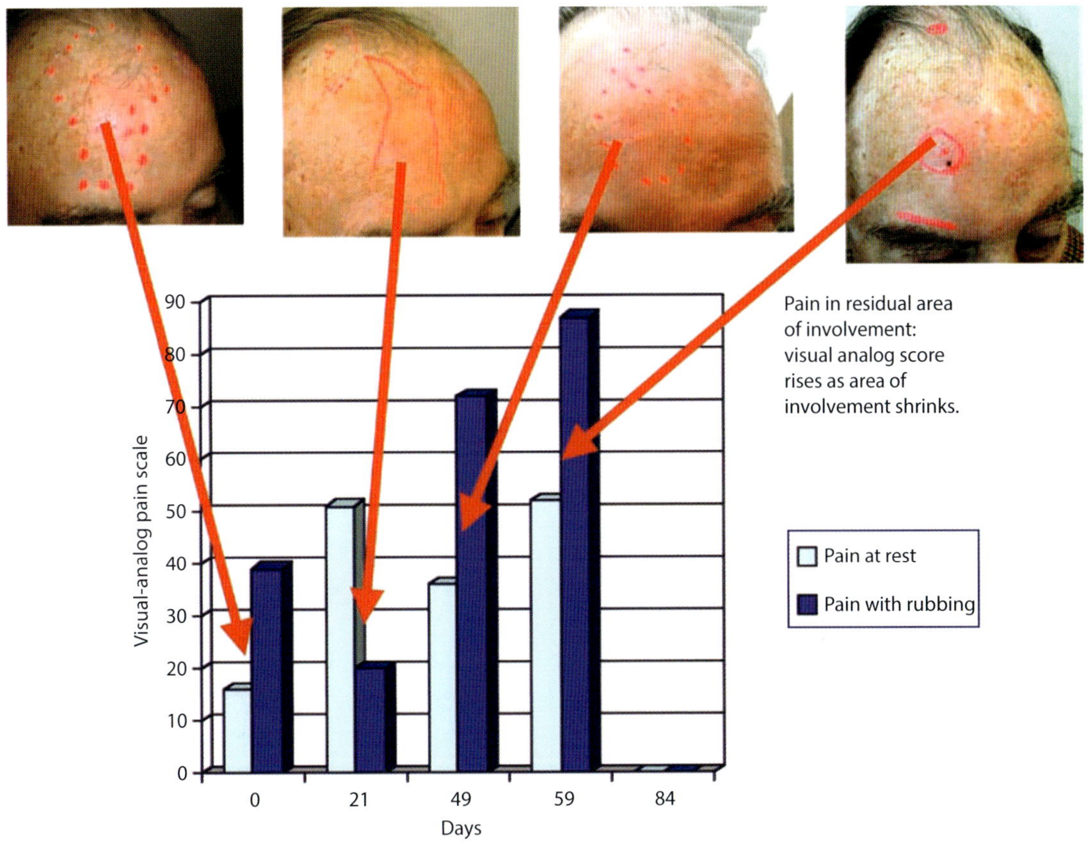

Figure 10.5 The area identified by the patient is marked and photographed, the patient completes a visual analog pain score (Figure 10.3), and then the painful area is injected with OnaBTX-A.

While the occasional patient will respond in a dramatic manner to a single session of treatment with BoNT-A, it is more typical for patients to improve in a stepwise manner. Patients generally need between one and four treatment sessions to become pain free. Objective quantification of the area of involvement, medication intake, Likert pain score, and patient's and physician's global assessment will help both the patient and the physician to determine whether additional treatment is justified. The author (KCS) has only had success treating PHN on the face and scalp with BoNT-A, and has not found BoNT-A useful for the treatment of PHN on the trunk or extremities. The reasons for treatment failure on the trunk and extremities are not known, and further studies are warranted.

Usually, serial photographs of the involved area demonstrate progressive reduction of the surface area (Figure 10.5). Patients find this encouraging. There is often a paradoxical increase in the patient's Likert pain score as the total area of involvement shrinks. The reason for this phenomenon is not well understood. It could be that the mildest areas of PHN resolve first, with the result that because of "averaging" by the patient, the pain score in the residual area of involvement would tend to rise.

When the patient with PHN has been rendered pain-free by treatment with BoNT-A, there is usually a long-term drug-free remission of pain.

BoNT-A IN THE MANAGEMENT OF PAINFUL SCARS

Immunohistochemistry has demonstrated substantial numbers of nerves staining for SP and CGRP in some scars.[54] This observation, together with successful experience treating PHN, formed the rationale for offering a trial of treatment with injections of BoNT-A to patients suffering from chronic intractable painful scars. Objective quantification of the patient's pain is of great importance in the management of painful scars. Tools that are useful for this purpose are essentially the same as those used in the assessment of patients who have PHN:

1. Likert pain scale and global assessment (Figure 10.3).
2. Physician's global assessment (Figure 10.4).
3. Marking the boundaries of the area or areas of pain prior to treatment and then marking and photographing the involved areas at every subsequent visit (Figure 10.6).

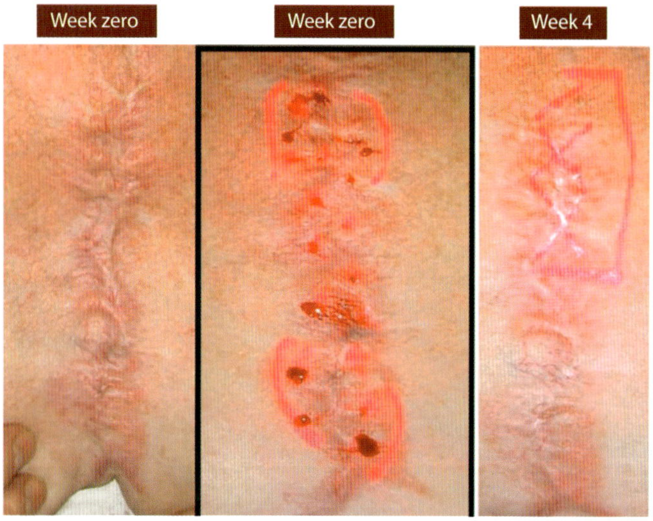

Figure 10.6 Keloid scar on the chest of a woman who had, 8 years previously, a coronary artery bypass grafting procedure, and whose pain had not responded adequately for surgical resection of the keloid, or to injections of triamcinolone acetonide, or to the application of silicone gel.

Injections are usually performed using a 30-gauge 1-inch needle, or a BD-II 0.3 mL diabetic syringe with 31 g needle, inserted into the scar. In the case of a thick scar (e.g., a keloid on the central chest after thoracotomy) (Figure 10.6), the patient may indicate or advise whether the pain is deep or superficial and the injection can be adjusted to take this into account. Application of ice for 30–60 seconds, or injection of lidocaine around and below the scar, is generally not necessary but could be used in a very sensitive patient to reduce the pain of injection. KCS has successfully used injections of BoNT-A to treat pain associated with keloid scarring, hypertrophic scarring, and normal scarring.

The author (KCS) uses a reconstitution of 1 mL in 100 units of OnaBTX-A. The amount of OnaBTX-A administered in each treatment has ranged from 10 to 50 units per mL of scar tissue.

As with the treatment of PHN, the antinociceptive effect of BoNT-A for painful scars seems to reach a maximum at around 3 weeks, so it is advisable to have patients return for reassessment and retreatment every 3–4 weeks until the patient is pain-free. The required number of treatments has ranged from one to four. As with PHN, the visual analog or Likert pain score may rise in residual areas of involvement even as the patient globally improves (Figure 10.7), and patients typically remain pain-free for a long time once they have been rendered pain-free by treatment with BoNT-A. In one case, there have been partial relapses at 6–12 month intervals, and these have responded within 5–10 days to additional injections of BoNT-A.

There has been no clinically significant improvement in the appearance (assessed by serial photography) of the scars injected by the author (KCS) with OnaBTX-A, but one hypertrophic scar on the breast (Figure 10.8) seemed much softer 6 months after two injections with OnaBTX-A. Because SP and CGRP interact with some of the cytokines involved in collagen remodeling and collagen deposition[55–57] it is conceivable that treatment with BoNT-A could affect the physical properties of some scars, perhaps with repeated treatments or after longer follow-up.

BoNT-A in the Management of Reflex Sympathetic Dystrophy (Complex Regional Pain Syndrome)

Reflex sympathetic dystrophy syndrome (RSDS) is characterized by constant burning pain and hyperesthesia in an extremity. Swelling, sweating, vasomotor instability, and sometimes trophic changes often accompany pain. There is often a history of injury or other trauma. Muscle spasms, myoclonus, or focal dystonia may occur.

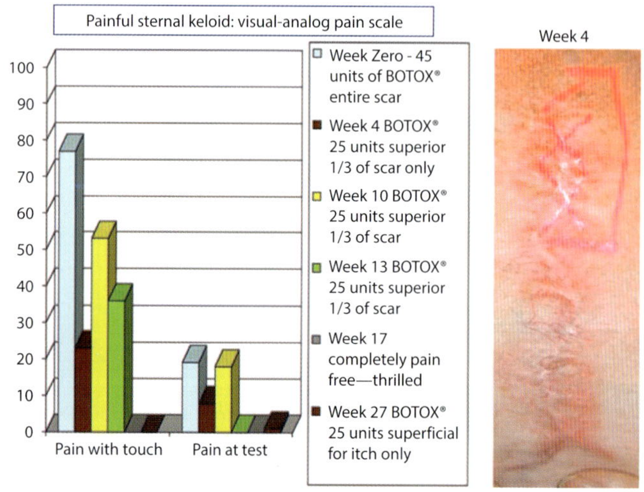

Figure 10.7 Chart illustrating gradual reduction in visual analog pain scores in response to injection of painful areas in the keloid scar with OnaBTX-A.

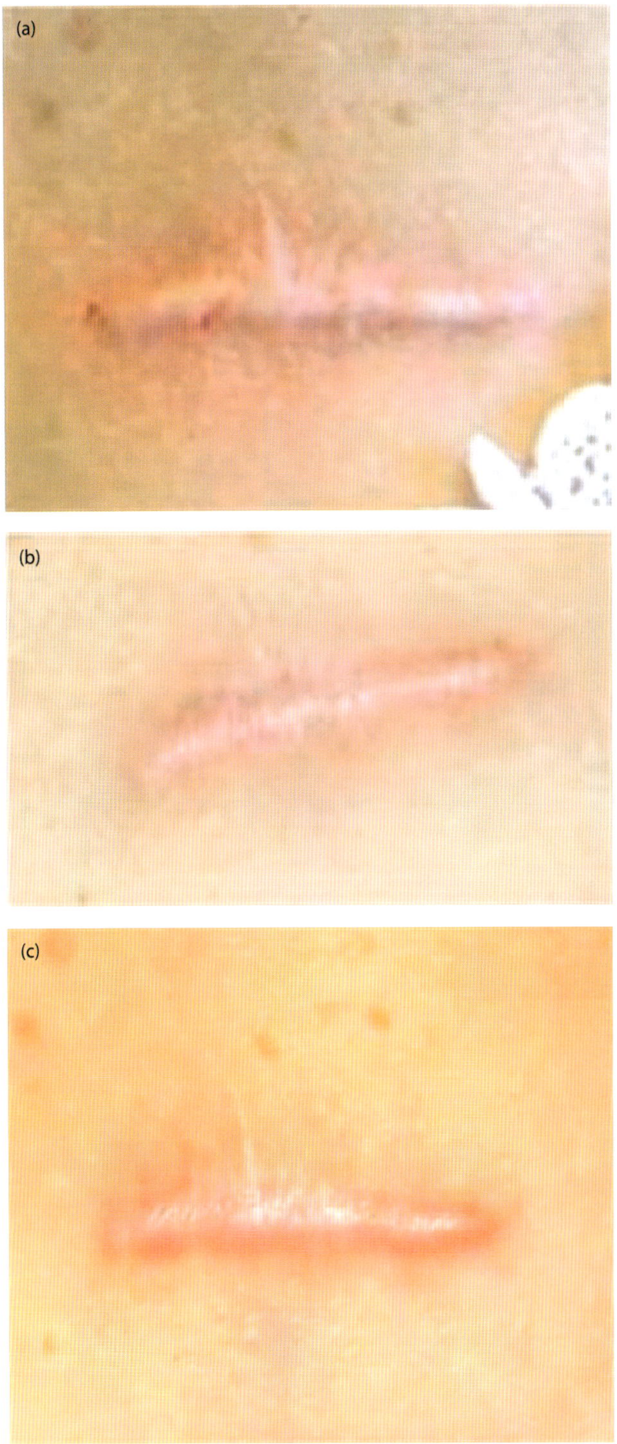

Figure 10.8 Pain in a hypertrophic scar on the upper chest after breast biopsy resolved in response to intralesional injection of OnaBTX-A: (a) Week 0: 3 cm painful and hypersensitive hypertrophic scar with a volume of about 0.4 mL, 10 months after breast biopsy, injected with 20 units of OnaBTX-A at 1 mL/100 units, 30 ga 1 inch needle, into a total volume of about 0.5 mL of scar; (b) Week 8: 1 week after relapse of discomfort, 8 weeks after injection, repeat dose of 20 units of OnaBTX-A at 1 mL/100 units; (c) Week 12: 4 weeks after second dose, completely pain free.

Diffuse pain, loss of function, and autonomic dysfunction are three main criteria suggested for diagnosis. Successful use of BoNT-A for this entity has been reported.[58,59]

Over the past 5 years, the author (KCS) has treated a 41-year-old woman who had an 8-year history of severe, refractory RSDS rendering her right arm and leg useless since injuries in a motor vehicle accident. She also had post-traumatic headaches with muscle spasm pulling her head to the right. The headaches and muscle spasm were also treated with OnaBTX-A. Initially injections were exceptionally painful and anxiety provoking. Anxiety was reduced in subsequent injection sessions by pretreating this patient with 80 mg of oxprenolol (a very lipid-soluble beta blocker which crosses the blood–brain barrier quite well and attenuates the central effects of adrenaline) together with 4 mg of lorazepam, 1–2 hours before injection of OnaBTX-A. Over the past several years, fentanyl 100–150 mcg administered intravenously 10 minutes before the injection sessions has been very helpful to reduce both anxiety and pain. Gradual improvement in the hyperalgesic component of her RSDS has also contributed to improved tolerance of the BoNTA injections.

The patient characterized her pain as coming predominantly from bone, and deep injections close to bone using a 30-gauge 1-inch needle, were of particular benefit. Subcutaneous and intramuscular injections of OnaBTX-A (a total of 120–400 units per session, about once a month) into the areas of discomfort in the right hand and arm gave substantial pain relief (for which the patient was very grateful) and also normalized skin color and temperature in the right hand and forearm within several minutes, but after one year of treatments there has not been any improvement in her ability to use the right hand. Even though the right hand remains useless, it is less of an impediment. It should be noted that reduction in pain and sensitivity has allowed this patient to take part in a greater range of activities of daily living and to participate more fully and effectively in physiotherapy and in society, so there has been an overall improvement in general functional ability. Treatment of the involved areas in the right lower leg and foot were also helpful. At times, the total dose of OnaBTX-A for treatment of headache and for treatment of RSDS in the right arm and leg reached 1200 units per month. This was well tolerated. After about 4 years of treatment her headaches, neck spasm, and RSDS in the right arm and lower leg improved to the point where OnaBTX-A in those areas was stopped, and the dose of OnaBTX-A declined to about 400 units every 2–3 months to control her headaches, neck spasm and pain in the right shoulder.

This is consistent with the observations of Cordivari[45] et al., who noted that four out of four of their patients with dystonia-complex regional pain syndrome affecting the hand had pain relief after treatment with BoNT-A (AboBTX-A), but only one of the four had functional improvement.

There is less concern now than in the past about the risk that a patient such as this, who was treated with high doses of OnaBTX-A, will develop antibodies against the OnaBTX-A formulation of BoNT-A. Jankovic et al.[21] found that blocking antibodies were detected in 4 of 42 (9.5%) cervical dystonia patients treated only with the original OnaBTX-A, but in none of the 119 patients ($p < 0.004$) treated exclusively with the current OnaBTX-A which has been on the market since late 1997.

BoNT-A for Improvement of Upper Thoracic Posture and "BOTOX® 'Breast Lift'"

BoNT-A has a long history of being used to improve posture in a variety of conditions.[60,61] The position of the shoulders is determined largely by the balance of forces between the pectoralis minor and pectoralis major muscles (Figure 10.9), which tend to rotate the shoulders medially and to depress the shoulders and the opposing muscles of the back, for example, the rhomboids. The use of BOTOX® to improve upper thoracic posture and so improve the presentation of the female breast has been detailed in the previous edition of this textbook[62] by both the present author (KCS) and Dr. Francisco

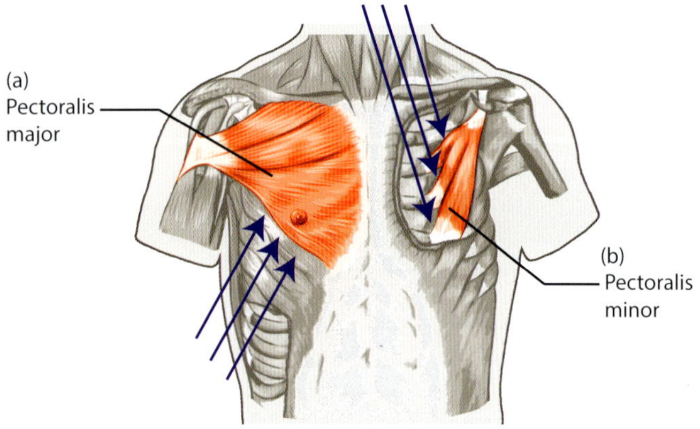

Figure 10.9 Typical injection sites for OnaBTX-A treatment of the pectoralis minor and pectoralis major muscles: (a) 15 units OnaBTX-A at each point, according to Francisco Perea-Atamoros; (b) 10 units OnaBTX-A at each point, according to Kevin C. Smith.

Perez-Atamoros, who also provides us with an update in this edition in Chapter 16.

This proposed mechanism of action has been criticized by Dr. Otto Wegelin (personal communication, April 2004), who argues:

1. The muscles (pectoralis minor and rhomboid minor) invoked to carry out the postural changes are far too small to do what is expected of them.
2. The muscles do not in fact rotate the shoulder but rather act primarily to stabilize the scapula—an entirely different function.
3. The muscles are not antagonistic in action, as are the frontalis and the orbicularis oculi, but rather synergistic.
4. There is no way to determine how much, if any, of the OnaBTX-A is actually acting on the pectoralis minor as the OnaBTX-A can diffuse widely in a three-dimensional plane unlike the forehead where there is the bony skull limiting diffusion.

Dr. Doris Hexsel (personal communication, July 2004), in a study of six women, was not able to obtain satisfactory results, and in two cases noted that the nipples hung lower.

Recently it has been reported that the combination of BoNT-A to relax muscles in the chest, when combined with a program of stretching to relax the chest muscles and exercises to strengthen muscles in the back, can produce a higher response rate and a greater duration of effect on upper thoracic posture than treatment with BoNT-A alone.[63–65]

Issues that remain to be resolved include optimization of patient selection, OnaBTX-A dosing, the placement of OnaBTX-A doses, the issue of placebo effect versus biomechanical effect, and elucidation of the mechanism of action.[66,67] T-2 weighted magnetic resonance imaging before and immediately after exercise is being evaluated as a technique to visualize and perhaps partially quantify the degree of flaccid paralysis induced by OnaBTX-A treatment.[68]

REFERENCES

1. Tsui JK, Eisen A, Mak E et al. A pilot study on the use of botulinum toxin in spasmodic torticollis. *Can J Neurol Sci* 1985;12(4):314–6.
2. https://www.ncbi.nlm.nih.gov/gquery/?term=botulinum+pain. Accessed January 13, 2016.
3. Smith K, Alam M. Botulinum toxin for pain relief and treatment of headache. In: Carruthers A, Carruthers J (eds) *Botulinum Toxin*, 2nd ed, Philadelphia, Elsevier; 2008, 93–104.
4. Smith KC, Goldberg D. Dermatologists can use botulinum toxin to treat headache. Point/counterpoint. *Practical Dermatology* 2004.
5. Finzi E, Rosenthal NE. Treatment of depression with onabotulinumtoxinA: A randomized, double-blind, placebo controlled trial. *J Psychiatr Res* 2014; 52:1–6.
6. Magid M, Reichenberg JS, Poth PE et al. Treatment of major depressive disorder using botulinum toxin A: A 24-week randomized, double-blind, placebo-controlled study. *J Clin Psychiatry* 2014; 75(8): 837–844.
7. Wollmer MA, de Boer C, Kalak N et al. Facing depression with botulinum toxin: A randomized controlled trial. *J Psychiatr Res* 2012; 46(5):574–581.
8. Reichenberg JS, Hauptman AJ, Robertson HT et al. Botulinum toxin for depression: Does patient appearance matter? *J Am Acad Dermatol* 2016; 74(1): 171–173.
9. Hennenlotter A, Dresel C, Castrop F et al. The link between facial feedback and neural activity within central circuitries of emotionenew insights from botulinum toxin-induced denervation of frown muscles. *Cereb Cortex* 2009; 19(3): 537–542.
10. Lewis MB. The positive and negative psychological potential of botulinum-toxin (Botox) injections. Abstract presented at: British Psychological Society Harrogate, North Yorkshire, En- gland, United Kingdom; April 9, 2013. Available from: URL: http://abstracts.bps.org.uk/abstracts/abstracts_home.cfm?&ResultsType=Abstracts&ResultSet_ID=9317&FormDisplayMode=view&frmShowSelected=true&localAction=details. Accessed January 5, 2016.
11. Allergan Reports Topline Phase II Data Supporting Advancement of BOTOX® (onabotulinumtoxinA) for the Treatment of Major Depressive Disorder (MDD). http://www.prnewswire.com/news-releases/allergan-reports-topline-phase-ii-data-supporting-advancement-of-botox-onabotulinumtoxina-for-the-treatment-of-major-depressive-disorder-mdd-300435486.html. Accessed April 9, 2017.
12. Van Beek AL, Lim PK, Gear AJ, Pritzker MR. Management of vasospastic disorders with botulinum toxin A. *Plast Reconstr Surg* 2007; 119(1): 217–26.
13. Stadlmaier E, Muller T, Hermann J, Graninger W. Raynaud's phenomenon: Treatment with botulinum toxin. *Ann Rheum Dis* 2005; 64(supple III): 275.
14. Sycha T, Graninger M, Auff E, Schnider P. Botulinum toxin in the treatment of Raynaud's phenomenon: A pilot study. *Eur J Clin Invest* 2004; 34(4): 312–3.
15. Kossintseva I, Barankin B. Improvement in both Raynaud's disease and hyperhidrosis in response to botulinum toxin type A treatment. *J Cutan Med Surg* 2008; 12(4): 189–93.
16. MacKenzie I, Burnstock G, Dolly JO. The effects of purified botulinum neurotoxin type A on cholinergic, adrenergic and non-adrenergic, atropine-resistant autonomic neuromuscular transmission. *Neuroscience* 1982; 7: 997–1006.
17. Morris JL, Jobling P, Gibbins IL. Differential inhibition by botulinum neurotoxin A of cotransmitters released from autonomic vasodilator neurons. *Am J Physiol Heart Circ Physiol* 2001; 281: H2124–H2132.
18. Morris JL, Jobling P, Gibbins IL. Botulinum neurotoxin A attenuates release of norepinephrine but not NPY from vasoconstrictor neurons. *Am J Physiol Heart Circ Physiol* 2002; 283(6): H2627–35.

19. Ansiaux R, Baudelet C, Cron GO et al. Botulinum toxin potentiates cancer radiotherapy and chemotherapy. *Clin Cancer Res* 2006; 12(4): 1276–83.
20. Matic DB, Lee TY, Wells RG, Gan BS. The effects of botulinum toxin type A on muscle blood perfusion and metabolism. *Plast Reconstr Surg* 2007; 120(7):1823–33.
21. Oskarsson E, Piehl Aulin K, Gustafsson BE, Pettersson K. Improved intramuscular blood flow and normalized metabolism in lateral epicondylitis after botulinum toxin treatment. *Scand J Med Sci Sports* 2008; 19: 323–328.
22. Cui M, Khanijou S, Rubino J, Aoki KR. Subcutaneous administration of botulinum toxin A reduces formalin-induced pain. *Pain* 2004; 107: 125–133.
23. Türk N, Ilhan S, Alp R, Sur H. Botulinum toxin and intractable trigeminal neuralgia. *Clin Neuropharmacol* 2005; 28(4): 161–162.
24. Aurora S. Botulinum toxin type A for the treatment of migraine. *Expert Opin Pharmacother* 2006; 7(8): 1085–95.
25. Welch MJ, Purkiss JR, Foster KA. Sensitivity of embryonic rat dorsal root ganglia neurons to Clostridium botulinum neurotoxins. *Toxicon* 2000; 38: 245–258.
26. Rapp DE, Turk KW, Bales GT, Coock SP. Botulinum toxin type A inhibits calcitonin gene-related peptide release from isolated rat bladder. *The Journal of Urology* 2006; 175: 1138–1142.
27. Durham PL, Cady R, Cady R. Regulation of calcitonin gene-related peptide secretion from trigeminal nerve cells by botulinum toxin type A: Implications for migraine therapy. *Headache* 2004; 44: 35–43.
28. Carlton SM, Hargett GL, Coggeshall RE. Localization and activation of glutamate receptors in unmyelinated axons of rat glabrous skin. *Neurosci Lett* 1995; 197(1): 25–8.
29. Wheeler-Aceto H, Porreca F, Cowan A. The rat paw formalin test: Comparison of noxious agents. *Pain* 1990; 40(2): 229–38.
30. Kreyden OP, Scheidegger EP. Anatomy of the sweat glands, pharmacology of botulinum toxin, and distinctive syndromes associated with hyperhidrosis. *Clin Dermatol* 2004; 22(1): 40–4.
31. Bansal C, Omlin KJ, Hayes CM, Rohrer TE. Novel cutaneous uses for botulinum toxin type A. *J Cosmet Dermatol* 2006; 5(3): 268–72.
32. Martos Díaz P, Bances del Castillo R, Mancha de la Plata M, Naval Gías L, Martínez Nieto C, Lee GY, Muñoz Guerra M. Clinical results in the management of Frey's syndrome with injections of Botulinum toxin. *Med Oral Patol Oral Cir Bucal* 2008; 13(4): E248–52.
33. Capaccio P, Torretta S, Osio M, Minorati D, Ottaviani F, Sambataro G, Nascimbene C, Pignataro L. Botulinum toxin therapy: A tempting tool in the management of salivary secretory disorders. *Am J Otolaryngol* 2008; 29(5): 333–8.
34. Laing TA, Laing ME, O'Sullivan ST. Botulinum toxin for treatment of glandular hypersecretory disorders. *J Plast Reconstr Aesthet Surg* 2008; 61(9): 1024–8.
35. Hill SE, Mortimer NJ, Hitchcock B, Salmon PJ. Parotid fistula complicating surgical excision of a basal cell carcinoma: Successful treatment with botulinum toxin type A. *Dermatol Surg* 2007; 33(11): 1365–7.
36. Lim YC, Choi EC. Treatment of an acute salivary fistula after parotid surgery: Botulinum toxin type A injection as primary treatment. *Eur Arch Otorhinolaryngol* 2008; 265(2): 243–5.
37. Marchese-Ragona R, Marioni G, Restivo DA, Staffieri A. The role of botulinum toxin in postparotidectomy fistula treatment. A technical note. *Am J Otolaryngol* 2006; 27(3): 221–4.
38. Konrad H, Karamfilov T, Wollina U. Intracutaneous botulinum toxin A versus ablative therapy of Hailey-Hailey disease—a case report. *J Cosmet Laser Ther* 2001; 3(4): 181–4.
39. Koeyers WJ, Van Der Geer S, Krekels G. Botulinum toxin type A as an adjuvant treatment modality for extensive Hailey-Hailey disease. *J Dermatolog Treat* 2008; 19(4): 251–4.
40. Swartling C, Naver H, Lindberg M, Anveden I. Treatment of dyshidrotic hand dermatitis with intradermal botulinum toxin. *J Am Acad Dermatol* 2002; 47(5): 667–71.
41. Wollina U, Karamfilov T. Adjuvant botulinum toxin A in dyshidrotic hand eczema: A controlled prospective pilot study with left-right comparison. *J Eur Acad Dermatol Venereol* 2002; 16(1): 40–2.
42. Kontochristopoulos G, Gregoriou S, Agiasofitou E, Nikolakis G, Rigopoulos D, Katsambas A. Letter: Regression of relapsing dyshidrotic eczema after treatment of concomitant hyperhidrosis with botulinum toxin-A. *Dermatol Surg* 2007; 33(10): 1289–90.
43. Zanchi M, Favot F, Bizzarini M, Piai M, Donini M, Sedona P. Botulinum toxin type-A for the treatment of inverse psoriasis. *J Eur Acad Dermatol Venereol* 2008; 22(4): 431–6.
44. Sifaki MK, Krueger-Krasagakis S, Koutsopoulos A, Evangelou GI, Tosca AD. Botulinum toxin type A—treatment of a patient with multiple cutaneous piloleiomyomas. *Dermatology* 2009; 218(1): 44–7.
45. Weinfeld PK. Successful treatment of notalgia paresthetica with botulinum toxin type A. *Arch Dermatol* 2007; 143(8): 980–2.
46. Dong M, Yeh F, Tepp WH et al. SV2 is the protein receptor for botulinum neurotoxin A. *Science* 2006 Apr 28; 3125773: 592–6.
47. Hamdy S, Samir H, El-Sayed M et al. Botulinum toxin: Could it be an effective treatment for chronic tension-type headache? *J Headache Pain* 2009; 10: 27–34.
48. Mathew NT, Kailasam J, Meadors L. Predictors of response to botulinum toxin type A (BoNT-A) in chronic daily headache. *Headache* 2008; 4: 194–200.
49. Aurora SK, Gawel M, Brandes JL et al. Botulinum toxin type A prophylactic treatment of episodic migraine: A randomized, double-blind, placebo-controlled exploratory study. *Headache* 2007; 4: 486–99.
50. Blumenfeld A. Botulinum toxin type A as an effective prophylactic treatment in primary headache disorders. *Headache* 2003; 4: 853–60.
51. Klein AW. The therapeutic potential of botulinum toxin. *Dermatol Surg* 2004; 30(3): 452–5.
52. Aoki KR. Evidence for antinociceptive activity of botulinum toxin type A in pain management. *Headache* 2003; 43(Suppl 1): S9–15.
53. Carruthers A, Carruthers J, Cohen J. Dilution volume of botulinum toxin type A for the treatment of glabellar rhytides: Does it matter? *Dermatol Surg* 2007; 33: S97–104.
54. Crowe R, Parkhouse N, McGrouther D. Neuropeptide-containing nerves in painful hypertrophic human scar tissue. *Br J Dermatol* 1994; 130(4): 444–52.
55. Takeba Y, Suzuki N, Kaneko A et al. Evidence for neural regulation of inflammatory synovial cell functions by secreting calcitonin gene-related peptide and vasoactive intestinal peptide in patients with rheumatoid arthritis. *Arthritis Rheum* 1999; 42(11): 2418–29.
56. Hart DA, Reno C. Pregnancy alters the *in vitro* responsiveness of the rabbit medial collateral ligament to neuropeptides: Effect on mRNA levels for growth factors, cytokines, iNOS, COX-2, metalloproteinases and TIMPs. *Biochim Biophys Acta* 1998; 1408(1): 35–43.
57. Jorgensen C, Sany J. Modulation of the immune response by the neuro-endocrine axis in rheumatoid arthritis. *Clin Exp Rheumatol* 1994; 12(4): 435–41.

58. Cordivari C, Misra VP, Catania S et al. Treatment of dystonic clenched fist with botulinum toxin. *Mov Disord* 2001; 16(5): 907–13.
59. Saenz A, Avellanet M, Garreta R. Use of botulinum toxin type A on orthopedics: A case report. *Arch Phys Med Rehabil* 2003; 84(7): 1085–6.
60. Traba Lopez A, Esteban A. Botulinum toxin in motor disorders: Practical considerations with emphasis on interventional neurophysiology. *Neurophysiol Clin* 2001; 31(4): 220–9.
61. Gallien P, Nicolas B, Petrilli S et al. Role for botulinum toxin in back pain treatment in adults with cerebral palsy: Report of a case. *Joint Bone Spine* 2004; 71(1): 76–8.
62. Smith KC, Pérez-Atamoros F. Other dermatologic uses of botulinum toxin. In: Benedetto AV, (ed). *Botulinum Toxin in Clinical Dermatology*. London: Taylor and Francis; 2006, 219–236.
63. Lang AM. Considerations for the use of Botulinum toxin in pain management. *Case Management* 2006; 11: 279–282.
64. Finkelstein I, Katsis E. Botulinum toxin type A (BotoxR) improves chronic tension-type headache by altering biomechanics in the cervico-thoracic area: A case study. *Cephalalgia* 2005; 25: 1189–1205.
65. Vad VB, Donatelli RA, Joshi M, Lang AM, Sims V. *O.N.E.U.P. Cervical Thoracic & Lumbar Pain Syndromes Program*. Beth Israel Medical Center, Office of Continuing Medical Education, New York. Accessed January 2008.
66. Smith KC, Arndt KA. *Lifting with Neurotoxins in Non-Surgical Skin Tightening and Lifting*, Alam M, Dover J (eds). Elsevier, in press, 2008; 107–16.
67. Smith KC. BOTOX®, perhaps augmented by a program of physiotherapy, may improve upper thoracic posture and the appearance of a “breast lift.” In: Alam M (ed). *Body Rejuvenation*. Taylor and Francis, in press, 2008.
68. Smith KC, Ludwig D, Price T. Unpublished observations. August 2005.

11 Medicolegal considerations of cosmetic treatment with botulinum toxin injections

David J. Goldberg

Botulinum toxin injections have become one of the most popular cosmetic treatments throughout the world over the past decade. However, the recognition of the effects of this toxin has been known for over a century. It was Justinus Kerner, a German physician, who first studied the potent effects of botulinum toxins during the Napoleonic Wars, after a reported increase in food-poisoning deaths in persons eating sausages. After a series of experiments on animals and self, he hypothesized that the toxin was produced under anaerobic conditions, that it acted on the autonomic and motor nervous system, and that it was lethal in small doses.[1] The use of botulinum toxins, for modern day medical purposes, began in the 1960s, when Scott et al. investigated the therapeutic uses of this drug in humans suffering from strabismus and blepharospasm.[2–4] In the United States, the Food and Drug Administration (FDA) approved botulinum toxin type A (BoNT-A) for these conditions in 1989. In 2000, the FDA expanded the approved indications to include cervical dystonia. In 2002, FDA approved the use of BoNT-A for cosmetic uses.

Independent surveys by the American Society for Aesthetic Plastic Surgery and the American Society of Plastic Surgeons suggested that, in 2002, between 1.1 and 1.6 million patients in the United States received cosmetic injections with BoNT-A. In 2008, the number had increased to 2.5 million patients. By 2013, the number of patients treated by both physicians and their associated providers was over 4 million patients. According to the American Society for Dermatologic Surgery in 2013, 1.5 million patients received botulinum toxin injections from dermatologists, an almost 25% increase from the 1.2 million patients who had received such injections in 2011. Finally, the American Society for Plastic and Reconstructive Surgery noted in 2014 that more than 385,000 men had received botulinum toxin injections that year—a 310% increase from the previous 10 years. These numbers clearly are increasing yearly both in the United States and elsewhere throughout the world.[5] Although a very safe substance when used with appropriate dosing, BoNT-A injections can be associated with complications. Such complications may be associated with medicolegal considerations. This chapter will review the reported BoNT-A-associated complications and the legal impact these implications may have on the injecting physician. A wide variety of complications may occur. It should be noted though that the most common complication, that of patient dissatisfaction, may have nothing to do with actual physician technique.

Patient dissatisfaction can, and should be, of concern to physicians who perform BoNT-A injections. The disgruntled patient typically fails to return for further treatment or, less commonly, may assert negligence and sue for economic damages.

Why do some patients fail to return for BoNTA injections? There are few published studies evaluating patient satisfaction and retention in dermatology for cosmetic procedures. Only one study has ever explored why a high percentage of patients may not return for repeat botulinum toxin injections.[6] In the study, a private cosmetic dermatology practice reviewed the charts of all patients who had received BoNT-A injections over a 2-year period to determine the patient retention rate, defined as the percentage of patients who returned for BoNT-A treatment within 6 months after the initial injection.[6] In particular, patients who had discontinued BoNT-A treatment after a single session were surveyed to learn their reasons for termination.

Between November 2002 and October 2004, 361 patients received BoNT-A cosmetic treatments for the first time. The chart review revealed that 55% (198/361) of these patients returned for additional BoNT-A injections, but that 45% (163/361) discontinued BoNT-A treatment, although 67% (109/163) of these patients continued to receive other cosmetic procedures. A retention rate of 55% was not as high as expected.

The practice surveyed 50 patients who had discontinued BoNT-A treatments after an initial injection. The most common reasons cited were procedural cost, perceived lack of product longevity, patient failure to reschedule treatment, and clinical effect falling short of expectations. In short, most of the reasons given (except possibly cost) are seemingly directly related to poor patient–physician communication.[6]

To improve communication, the practice decided to institute a mandatory 2-week post-treatment office evaluation for new BoNT-A patients to determine treatment effect, to administer touch-ups if needed, and to address patient expectations and treatment-related concerns. Since initiating this mandatory follow-up, retention rate of BoNT-A patients in the practice increased from 55% to 67%.

Thankfully, BoNT-A dissatisfaction leading to discontinuation of BoNT-A injections does not usually have associated medicolegal considerations. However, some patients dissatisfied with BoNT-A may actually have BoNT-A-induced associated complications. A review of BoNT-A adverse reactions occurring after treatments for medical and not cosmetic purposes reported 28 deaths and 17 seizures among 406 reports of serious adverse events.[7] All of these patients treated for their medical conditions received significantly higher dosages of BoNT-A than is commonly used for cosmetic treatments. Among the 28 deaths, 6 were attributed to respiratory arrest, 5 to myocardial infarction, 3 to cerebrovascular accident, 2 to pulmonary embolism, 2 to pneumonia (1 known to be aspiration pneumonia), 5 to other known causes, and 5 to unknown causes of death. Death occurred a median of 3 days after BoNT-A injection (range: <1 hour–120 days). The median age of BoNT-A recipients who died was 44 years (range: 3–91 years). Of the 28 patients who died, 26 had underlying systemic diseases with neuromuscular and/or respiratory issues leading to an elevated risk of mortality, in addition to the symptoms for which they received BoNTA. The possibility of a causal role for underlying diseases made it difficult to evaluate the role of BoNT-A in the fatalities. It would seem, based on these facts, that warning patients of the risk of seizures and death after BoNT-A used for cosmetic procedures is not legally required.

The more serious reported events associated with OnaBTX-A include dysphasia, muscle weakness, allergic reactions, and flu-like symptoms.[7] These have all been extraordinarily rare reported events, and may not always be directly related to the BoNT-A injection, and probably are not reasonable risks to discuss with patients who are seeking facial cosmetic BoNT-A injections.

Among 995 reported cosmetic cases with a nonserious complication, lack of intended cosmetic effect was most commonly noted. Injection site reaction, ptosis, muscle weakness, and headaches were frequently reported complications.[7]

What should be clear is that there are some obvious contraindications to BoNT-A use for cosmetic purposes. These would include prior allergic reaction, injection into areas of infection or inflammation, pregnancy (safety for use during pregnancy has not been established), or breastfeeding. Women who at the time they were injected were not aware they were pregnant thus far have had uneventful deliveries, and to date no teratogenicity has been attributed to botulinum toxin. Nonetheless, delay of injections would be the likely recommendation until pregnancy is complete and breastfeeding has ended.

Relative contraindications to BoNT-A treatment would include patients with diseases of the neuromuscular junction (e.g., myasthenia gravis) because of the underlying generalized muscle weakness seen with such diseases. Local weakness at injection sites would be expected in such patients. In addition, some medications decrease neuromuscular transmission and generally should be avoided in patients treated with botulinum toxin. These include aminoglycosides, penicillamine, quinine, and calcium channel blockers.[8]

The most common reactions to botulinum toxin injections are generally mild and transient and they are discussed in detail in their respective chapters on injection techniques (Chapters 13, 14, 15). Untoward sequelae commonly caused by a percutaneous injection include pain, edema, erythema, ecchymosis, headache, and hypesthesia. These also are generally mild and transient. The most common meaningful adverse effect is unwanted weakness in nontargeted muscles. Fortunately, unwanted weakness caused by the action of the toxin usually resolves in several months and in some patients in a few weeks, depending on the site, strength of the injections, and the muscles made excessively weak.[8] More infrequently experienced reactions to BoNT-A injections include nausea, fatigue, malaise, flu-like symptoms, and rashes at sites distant from the injection sites (see Appendix 6).

Muscle weakness is the result of the desired toxin effect on injected musculature. This can be a desired goal in most and a problem with imagined or presumptive medical legal overtones for others. For example, patients who depend on emotive expression, such as actors and politicians, can be significantly negatively impacted by a potential reduction in expression. Excess weakness following frontalis injection may cause paralysis rather than weakening of the muscle. Patients may report that they appear mask-like and further, that their brow feels heavy. If brow ptosis occurs, a hooded appearance may be present, and occasionally vision may be partially obstructed. If the lateral fibers of the frontalis have not been injected appropriately, a quizzical appearance may result in which the lateral brow is pulled up while the central brow is lowered. This can be improved by simply injecting a small amount of toxin into the lateral frontalis fibers.

Since brow depressors are generally weakened when treating glabellar lines, ptosis of the upper eyelid can occasionally result following improper injection technique in this region. This may occur as late as 2 weeks after injection. Ptosis is caused by migration of toxin through the orbital septum weakening the levator palpebrae superioris. It has been suggested that patients remain in an upright position for 3–4 hours following injection to lessen the risk of eyelid ptosis. There is, however, no scientific data to support this notion and this author no longer provides such advice to his patients.[9] Active contraction of the muscles under treatment may increase the uptake of toxin and decrease its diffusion. Ptosis can be treated with apraclonidine 0.5% eye drops. Apraclonidine is an alpha2-adrenergic agonist, which causes Müller's muscle to contract. It should be noted that apraclonidine is contraindicated in patients with documented hypersensitivity. Phenylephrine 2.5% can be used when apraclonidine is not available. Phenylephrine is contraindicated in patients with narrow-angle glaucoma and in patients with aneurysms.

Weakness of the lower eyelid or lateral rectus can occur following injection of the lateral orbicularis oculi. If severe lower lid weakness occurs, an exposure keratitis may result. If the lateral rectus is weakened, diplopia results. Treatment is symptomatic. This complication is best avoided by injecting at least 1 cm lateral to the lateral canthus and above the zygomatic arch.

Injection of platysma muscles can result in dysphagia from diffusion of toxin into muscles of deglutition. When this occurs, it usually lasts only a few days or weeks. Some patients may require soft foods. Although a swallowing weakness does not necessarily herald systemic toxicity, if it is severe, patients may be at theoretical risk of aspiration.

Some patients experience neck weakness after botulinum toxin injections into the neck. This may be especially noticeable when attempting to raise the head from a supine position. This is thought to occur from a weakening of the sternocleidomastoid muscles, either from direct injection or diffusion. This rare complication, anecdotally, appears to be more common in women with long, thin necks.

Generally, in the United States reasonable risks must be detailed to the prospective patient. Thirty-six serious adverse events and no deaths were reported to the FDA between 1989 and 2003 when related to the cosmetic use of neuromodulators. More than one-third were related to the legal off-label use of the drug. Non-serious adverse events included injection site reactions, lack of intended effect, ptosis, muscle weakness, and headache.[7] Any discussion of complications induced by botulinum toxin injections raises the issue of what is required in an informed consent.[10] What is a reasonable risk may be open to discussion. It represents the "standard of care." The duty of a physician using botulinum toxin is to use botulinum toxin in accordance with the standard of care. The standard of care is somewhat simplistically defined as "what would a reasonable physician do if in an identical situation with an identical patient." Although the elements of a cause of action in negligence are derived from formal legal textbooks, the standard of care is not necessarily derived from some well-known textbook.[11] It is also not articulated by any judge. The standard of care is defined by some, as whatever an expert witness says it is in the confines of a courtroom, and what a jury will believe. In a case against any cosmetic physician, the specialist must have the knowledge and skill ordinarily possessed by a specialist in that field, and has used the care and skill ordinarily possessed by a specialist in that particular field of specialty in the same or similar locality under similar circumstances. A dermatologist, plastic surgeon, otolaryngologist, internist, or aesthetic medicine physician will all be held to an equal standard. A failure to fulfil such a duty may lead to loss of a lawsuit by the physician. If the jury accepts the suggestion that the doctor mismanaged the case and that the negligence led to damages to the patient, then the physician will be liable. In the case of botulinum toxin injections, mistreatment may lead to both damages and physician liability. Conversely, if the jury believes an expert who testifies for the defendant doctor, then the standard of care, in that particular case, has been met. In this view, the standard of care is a pragmatic concept, decided case by case, and based on the testimony of an expert physician. The physician injecting botulinum toxin is expected to do this in the manner of a reasonable physician. A physician needs to perform a procedure in a manner that is considered by an objective standard as reasonable. For example, if a physician chooses to use a dilution of BoNT-A that is not in accordance with the manufacturer's suggested dilution instructions, but works well and gives optimal results, then this dilution would be considered reasonable and would not lead to loss of a medical malpractice lawsuit.

It is important to note that where there are two or more recognized approaches to injecting botulinum toxins, a physician does not fall below the standard of care by using any of the acceptable methods even if one method turns out to be less effective than another method. Finally, in many jurisdictions, an unfavorable result due to an "error in judgment" by a physician is not in and of itself a violation of the standard of care if the physician acted appropriately prior to exercising his professional judgment.

Evidence of the standard of care in a specific malpractice case includes laws, regulations, and guidelines for practice, which represent a consensus among professionals on a topic involving diagnosis or treatment, and the medical literature including peer-reviewed articles and authoritative texts. In addition, obviously, the view of an expert is crucial. Although the standard of care may vary from state to state in the United States, it is typically defined as a national standard by and for physicians.[12]

Most commonly for litigation purposes, as described above, expert witnesses articulate, in court, the standard of care. The basis of the expert witness testimony, and therefore the origin of the standard of care, is grounded in the following:

1. The witness's personal practice
2. The practice of others that he has observed in his experience
3. Medical literature in recognized publications
4. Statutes and/or legislative rules
5. Courses where the subject is discussed and taught in a well-defined manner

The standard of care is the way in which the majority of the physicians in a similar medical community would practice. If, in fact, the expert personally does not practice like the majority of other physicians, then the expert will have a difficult time explaining why the majority of the medical community does not practice according to his or her ways.[13]

It would seem then that in the perfect world, the standard of care in every case would be a clearly definable level of care agreed on by all physicians and patients. Unfortunately, in the typical situation the standard of care is an ephemeral concept resulting from differences and inconsistencies among the medical profession, the legal system, and the public.

At one polar extreme, the medical profession is dominant in determining the standard of care in the practice of medicine. In such a situation, recommendations, guidelines, and policies regarding varying treatment modalities for different clinical situations published by nationally recognized boards, societies, and commissions establish the appropriate standard of care. Even in some of these cases, however, factual disputes may arise because more than one such organization will publish conflicting standards concerning the same medical condition. Adding to the confusion, local societies may publish their own rules applicable to a particular claim of malpractice.

Thus, in most situations the standard of care is neither clearly definable nor consistently defined. It is a legal fiction to suggest that a generally accepted standard of care exists for any area of practice. At best, there are parameters within which experts will testify. The cosmetic physician's best defense that he is acting in accordance with the standard of care is to document appropriate risk assessment of the patient, provide appropriate medical record documentation, appropriate informed consent, and finally to utilize appropriate diagnostic and treatment approaches.[14]

American physicians have in recent years put forth substantial efforts toward standard setting, and specifying treatment approaches to various conditions. Clinical practice guidelines have been developed by specialty societies such as the American Academy of Dermatology, the American Society for Dermatologic Surgery, and the American Society of Aesthetic Plastic Surgery. The Institute of Medicine has defined such clinical guidelines as "systematically developed statements to assist practitioner and patient decisions about appropriate health care for specific clinical circumstances." Such guidelines represent standardized specifications for performing a procedure or managing a particular clinical problem.

Clinical guidelines raise thorny legal issues.[12] They have the potential of offering an authoritative and settled statement of what the standard of care should be for a given skin condition. A court would have several options when such guidelines are offered as evidence. Such a guideline might be evidence of the customary practice in the medical profession. A doctor acting in accordance with the guidelines would be shielded from liability to the same extent as one who can establish that he or she followed professional customs. The guidelines could play the role of an authoritative expert witness or a well-accepted review article. Using guidelines as evidence of professional custom, however, is problematic if they are ahead of prevailing medical practice.

Clinical guidelines have already had an effect on settlement, according to surveys of malpractice lawyers. A widely accepted clinical standard may be presumptive evidence of due care, but expert testimony will still be required to introduce the standard of care and establish its sources and its relevancy.

Professional societies often attach disclaimers to their guidelines, thereby undercutting their defensive use in litigation. The American Medical Association, for example, calls its guidelines "parameters" instead of protocols intended to significantly impact on physician discretion. The AMA further suggests that all such guidelines contain disclaimers stating that they are not intended to displace physician discretion. Such guidelines, in these situations, could not be treated as conclusive.

Plaintiffs usually will use their own expert witness, as opposed to the physician's expert, to define the standard of care. Although such a plaintiff's expert may also refer to clinical practice guidelines, the physician's negligence can be established in other ways as well. These methods include (1) examination of the physician defendant's expert witness, (2) an admission by the defendant that he or she was negligent, (3) testimony by the plaintiff, in a rare case where he or she is a medical expert qualified to evaluate the allegedly negligent physician's conduct, and (4) common knowledge in situations where a layperson could understand the negligence without the assistance of an expert.

It is clear then that although complications may occur following botulinum toxin injections, the plaintiff, to win his or her negligence cause of action against an aesthetic physician, must establish that his or her physician had a duty of reasonable care in treating him or her and had in fact breached that duty. That breach if proven, would then lead to some form of damages. A mere inconvenience to the plaintiff, even in the setting of a physician's breach, will usually not lead to physician liability in a cause of action for negligence. In general, most botulinum toxin induced complications are temporary and nothing more than an inconvenience. However, in those rare situations where a patient was not warned of a potential complication and the ensuing complication led to damages (such as the inability to work), there may be legal implications from the botulinum toxin induced complication.

In the United States, thankfully, lawsuits brought against physicians for negligent use of BoNT-A are quite rare. It is because the effects of BoNT-A wear off long before a court trial would begin. We discuss two examples of such lawsuits. In one case, a television anchorwoman was given BoNT-A in her frontalis region. Because of negligent technique, her eyebrows were lifted in the so-called mephisto pattern. Even though the deformity was treated to correction some weeks after the injection, she missed out on 2 weeks of work with its economic impact and associated embarrassment. She sued her physician. Although the case never went to trial, she settled for economic damages. Similarly, a musician working in a jazz band had

BoNT-A injected in his lip and for almost 1 month was unable to successfully blow into his musical instrument. As in the previous case, he settled for monies after bringing a lawsuit because of economic damages ensuing from his inability to play his instrument. A similar case occurred in which a patient claimed dysphagia after injections of BoNT-A into her neck. In all cases, the plaintiffs contended they were never warned that this complication might happen—clearly a breach in the standard of care.

BoNT-A injections into either the forehead or upper lip would be considered off-label since the FDA labeling (FDA-approval process) is for glabellar folds and lateral canthal folds only. In contrast to some countries in Europe where the physician use of a drug off-label is restricted, the FDA has traditionally encouraged off-label drug use by U.S. physicians and looks at this as a way of further developing medical research and care in the United States. However, the use of any drug (including BoNT-A) for off-label purposes can lead to problems for the physician. In one case brought to trial in the United States, a dermatologist was using OnaBTX-A off label for the treatment of headaches. The plaintiff subsequently developed a disabling illness and contended that it was caused by the off-label use of the OnaBTX-A by a physician who would not in general be treating headaches. Although the dermatologist, at trial, was found not to be culpable, the case is an example of what can happen when products are used off label. Some physicians are concerned that there will be increasing restrictions for off-label drug use. This has yet to be decided.[15]

Several years ago, the FDA mandated a "black box warning" for manufacturers selling botulinum toxins in the United States. Such mandatory information, must be provided with every vial of sold botulinum toxin. The warning contains the following:

- Read this information this time and every time you get botulinum toxin.
- Share this information with your family and caregivers.
- Problems with swallowing, speaking, or breathing may occur.
- These problems may occur weeks after the injections.
- Swallowing problems may require a feeding tube.
- Muscle weakness may occur all over the body.
- Loss over bladder control may occur.
- Death can happen.
- These problems could make it unsafe for you to drive a car or do other dangerous activities.
- This medication guide has been approved by the FDA.

Although it is clear that such a warning must be contained within the manufacturers' packaging, the obvious question remains. Is it necessary to warn patients of dire complications that have never been reported with the cosmetic use of neuromodulators product? Most clinicians are convinced that a warning would preclude patients from seeking elective cosmetic treatment. Unfortunately, there is no easy legal answer to the question. What can be advised is a practical approach of mentioning the "black box" warning in the consent and encouraging discussion with patients regarding the issue. It was hoped that a coalition of cosmetic dermatology, plastic surgery, and oculoplastic surgical societies would convince the FDA to reverse this warning. This has yet to occur.

Finally, it should be noted that one rare serious adverse event following the cosmetic use of BoNT-A has been wrongly associated with the FDA-approved product (BOTOX®; OnaBTX-A).[16] In a 2004 case, a non-dermatologist, non-core physician administered a high dose of unregulated and unlicensed research-grade BoNT-A to himself and three others to treat wrinkles.[16]). All developed respiratory paralysis but eventually recovered; the physician's license to practice medicine was suspended. Given that this became a well-publicized media case, it once again begs the question whether respiratory collapse needs to be included as a possible adverse event in the cosmetic use of BoNT-A. Certainly, this serious adverse event, if it were to occur, would result from a breach of physician duty and would be grounds for a lawsuit claiming major economic damages. However, any reasonable cosmetic dermatologist recognizes that this situation was unique to this case. The possibility of respiratory paralysis is virtually nonexistent when licensed FDA-approved BoNT-A is used in established doses for cosmetic purposes. Therefore, this adverse event need not be included on the consent form.

This case also highlights the need for physicians to be cognizant of "bootlegged" BoNT-A. Sellers of these products claim that they provide similar results when compared to licensed BoNT-A, but at a substantially reduced cost. Use of these products is a breach of the physician's professional duty to provide care. In addition to a potential lawsuit by a dissatisfied patient, other adverse outcomes include medical license suspension or revocation in one's state, and federal consequences.

CONCLUSION

In 1959, Lammana referred to botulinum toxin as "the most poisonous poison."[17] Written long before the notion of the aesthetic use of botulinum neurotoxins was conceived and its safety well established, Lammana's opinion of BoNT-A today could be used as ammunition by aggressive lawyers and their dissatisfied clients. Also, given the high rate of medical malpractice in the United States, physicians performing cosmetic dermatologic procedures are advised to institute certain measures when treating patients to reduce the likelihood of patient dissatisfaction and potential litigation. These include establishing a good rapport with their patients; prescreening patients prior to performing procedures, not only for obvious contraindications to treatment but also for any "warning signs" that might indicate the patient is looking for something that may not satisfy him or her; using appropriate consent forms that outline reasonable risks (see Appendix 5); and taking action to correct any potential adverse outcomes, should they occur. These steps are part of standard medical care and should be performed at all times. Understanding the medicolegal considerations of the cosmetic treatment with botulinum toxin injections remains an important part of everyday cosmetic practice.

REFERENCES

1. Erbguth F. Botulinum toxin, a historical note. *Lancet* 1998; 351: 1280.
2. Scott AB, Rosenbaum A, Collins CC. Pharmacological weakening of extraocular muscles. *Invest Ophthalmol Vis Sci* 1973; 12: 924–7.
3. Scott AB, Suzuki D. Systemic toxicity of botulinum toxin by intramuscular injection in the monkey. *Mov Disord* 1988; 3: 333–5.
4. Scott AB. Botulinum toxin injection of eye muscle to correct strabismus. *Trans Am Ophthalmol Soc* 1981; 79: 734–70.
5. American Society of Plastic Surgeons. Available at http://www.plasticsurgery.org/Patients_and_Consumers/Procedures/Cosmetic_Procedures/Botulinum_Toxin.html.
6. White L, Tanzi EL, Alster TS. Improving patient retention after botulinum toxin type A treatment. *Dermatol Surg* 2006; 32: 212–15.
7. Coté TR, Mohan AK, Polder JA, Walton MK, Braun M. Botulinum toxin type A injections: Adverse events reported to the US Food and Drug Administration in therapeutic and cosmetic cases. *JAAD* 2005; 53: 407–15.
8. Glogau RG. Review of the use of botulinum toxin for hyperhidrosis and cosmetic purposes. *Clin J Pain* 2002; 18(Suppl); S191–7.
9. Gart MS, Gutkowski KA. Aesthetic uses of neuromodulators: Current uses and future directions. *Plast Reconstr Surg* 2015; 55(Suppl): 62–9.

10. Gershon SK, Wise RP, Braun MM. Adverse events reported with cosmetic use of botulinum toxin A. *Pharmacoepidemiol Drug Saf* 2001; 10(Suppl): S135–6.
11. Furrow BF, Greaney TL, Johnson SH, Jost TS, Schwartz RL. *Liability in Health Care Law*, 5th ed. St. Paul, MN: West Publishing; 2004.
12. Hyams AL, Shapiro DW, Brennan TA. Medical practice guidelines in malpractice litigation: An early retrospective. *J Health Policy Law* 1996; 21: 289.
13. *Lamont v Brookwood Health Service, Inc.*, 446 So.2d 1018 (Ala.1983).
14. *Gannon v Elliot*, 19 Cal. App. 4th 1 1993.
15. Botox lawsuit is raising eyebrows. *NY Times*, April 4, 2004.
16. Jesitus J. Bogus botox sounds wake-up call. *Dermatology Times*, February 1, 2005. Available at: http://www.dermatologytimes.com/dermatologytimes/article/articleDetail.jsp?id=146023.
17. Lamanna C. The most poisonous poison. *Science* 1959; 130: 763–72.

APPENDIX 1 Comparison of different consensus reports of botulinum toxin dosing in different Western countries

Alisa A. Sharova

It is generally accepted that the different approved botulinum toxins (BoNTs) in use today are not identical, and neither are their treatment dosages completely interchangeable. In April 2009, the United States (U.S.) FDA assigned nonproprietary, generic-like names to each of the BoNTs, once again emphasizing their uniqueness and lack of full equivalency. BOTOX® was named onabotulinumtoxinA (OnaBTX-A), Dysport®—abobotulinumtoxinA (AboBTX-A) and Xeomin®—incobotulinumtoxinA (IncoBTX-A).

We compared the national and international consensus reports and recommendations on the use of AboBTX-A, OnaBTX-A and IncoBTX-A in the U.S., Russia, and Europe.[1–12] The complexity of this analysis is the lack of consensus on the use of all toxins in different countries, as well as the absence of a unified consensus design.

DOSE RATIO ANALYSIS

Results of the dose ratio comparisons of the approved BoNT-As are presented in Table A1.1. This analysis is also associated with certain difficulties, but we compared the ratios of OnaBTX-A versus AboBTX-A dosages in the U.S.; and IncoBTX-A versus AboBTX-A dosages in Russia and those of international consensus reports.

The most appropriate way to record our results would be to compare median dose values, that is, the most commonly used doses approved in the different countries included in this study. It is not always the same as the arithmetic mean value for a particular aesthetic treatment zone. However, the median doses were not always available in the different consensus reports.

Therefore, in cases where the median dose was not available, we used an arithmetic mean value of a dose range for comparison.

Results regarding dose ratios for OnaBTX-A:AboBTX-A and IncoBTX-A:AboBTX-A showed that in most cases there was both an increase and a decrease of the conventionally recognized ratio of 1:2.5.

According to U.S. recommendations, in five out of nine aesthetic areas OnaBTX-A:AboBTX-A ratio was above 1:2.5, and in the three areas it was lower.

Thus, the exact ratio of average dose 1:2.5 for OnaBTX-A:AboBTX-A (or very close to it) is true only for "crow's feet" and for the glabella. In the U.S. consensus reports, the ratio for OnaBTX-A:AboBTX-A (1:2.6) slightly differs for glabella only due to the fact that the average dose of AboBTX-A recommended for the treatment of this area is slightly higher (52.5 U) than in other countries (50 U).

In Russian consensus reports IncoBTX-A:AboBTX-A ratio is above 1:2.5 only for the treatment of the chin area (1:3.3); it is exactly 1:2.5 for the treatment of three zones (glabella, bunny lines, and depressor anguli oris [DAO]); and for the other five areas it is below 1:2.5. In the international consensus reports, IncoBTX-A:AboBTX-A dose ratio of 1:2.5 is true only for the glabellar out of the eight aesthetic zones considered, and it is above this value in the forehead area (1:3.5) and below in six other zones.

In all consensus reports, the dose ratio of OnaBTX-A or IncoBTX-A to AboBTX-A is 1:2.5 or below only for three aesthetic areas: crow's feet, DAO, and neck (platysmal) bands.

The dose ratio for IncoBTX-A and AboBTX-A for cervico-facial contour correction ("Nefertiti lift") is paradoxical. It is equal to 1:0.75 in the Russian and 1:0.9 in international consensus reports. Therefore, the average value of dose ratios for OnaBTX-A:AboBTX-A is 1:2.8, and for IncoBTX-A:AboBTX-A, it is 1:1.9.

COMPARATIVE ANALYSIS OF THE DIFFERENT RECOMMENDED DOSES OF THE DIFFERENT BoNT-As

The recommendations for each BoNT-A adopted in different countries are presented in Table A1.2. Recommendations regarding the number of injection points for the different BoNT-As are generally similar in all the consensus reports studied.

COMPARATIVE ANALYSIS OF THE RECOMMENDATIONS ON THE USE OF OnaBTX-A

Analysis of the recommendations on the use of OnaBTX-A was based on the published consensus reports from the U.S., Germany, and France[1–5] (Table A1.3). The most complete recommendations regarding the number of areas to treat with OnaBTX-A were presented in the German consensus report. It contains an expert opinion on the use of OnaBTX-A for the correction of wrinkles of the lower eyelid, eyebrow position, the zygomatic muscles, and the facial portion of the platysma ("Nefertiti lift").

In general, the recommendations regarding injection points and the doses of OnaBTX-A in the analyzed consensus reports are largely similar. The widest range of doses is presented in the German consensus.[3] This is because it contains opinions of 13 experts, and the average single recommendation is not presented. In Germany, higher doses are recommended for the treatment of glabella wrinkles and platysma bands, and in the United States, more wide dose ranges with high maximum doses are proposed for DAO correction.

There are conspicuous differences in the recommendations for the correction of perioral wrinkles in different countries. In the French consensus report it is recommended to correct first only the wrinkles of the upper lip. The lower lip wrinkles, if needed, are treated separately, during an additional visit. The U.S. and German consensus reports, on the contrary, propose to inject OnaBTX-A into the upper and lower lips during one session, starting with one point of injection in each of the four lip quadrants.

COMPARATIVE ANALYSIS OF THE RECOMMENDATIONS ON THE USE OF IncoBTX-A

Russian and international dose recommendations for the treatment of individual aesthetic facial zones are shown in Table A1.4.[10,1] The table shows that in the upper third of the face, the recommended doses are very similar. International guidelines only allow higher doses to correct the "crow's feet" (up to 30 U on each side) and the glabella (up to 50 U), while the Russian consensus recommends limiting the dose at 12 and 20 U, respectively.

The most significant difference in dosage used in the lower third of the face is related to the DAO correction. In the Russian consensus, the dose for one side of the face is 1.5–4 U, while international consensus suggests using 1–7.5 U of IncoBTX-A for each DAO.

Table A1.1 Dose Equivalence

Treatment zone	OnaBTX-A:AboBTX-A (U.S.)		IncoBTX-A:AboBTX-A (Russia)		IncoBTX-A: AboBTX-A (International)	
Frontal lines	10.5:30	1:2.8	15:20	1:1.3	10:35	1:3.5
Glabella	20:52.5	**1:2.6**	20:50	**1:2.5**	20:50	**1:2.5**
Crow's feet	10:25	**1:2.5**	12:20	1:1.7	20:22.5	1:1.1
Bunny lines	1.75:11	1:6.3	3:7.5	**1:2.5**	No	No
Perioral area[a]	4.5:15	1:3.3	5:9	1:1.8	5:10	1:2
Nasal tip	3:5	1:1.7	No	No	No	No
DAO	4.25:8	1:1.9	3:7.5	**1:2.5**	4.3:7.5	1:1.7
Nefertiti lift	No	No	20:15	1:0.75	15:13	1:0.9
Chin (total)	5:15	1:3	6:20	1:3.3	7:15	1:2.1
Neck (platysmal bands) (total)	50:75	1:1.5	55:70	1:1.3	45:70	1:1.5
Average		**1:2.8**		**1:1.9**		**1:1.9**

Note: No = data are not included in the consensus.
[a] The number of injection points for the correction of the perioral region in the U.S. consensuses is indicated for the upper and lower lips. In Russian and International consensuses it is indicated only for the upper lip.

Table A1.2 Recommendations on the Number of Injection Points for the Different BoNT-As

	OnaBTX-A			IncoBTX-A		AboBTX-A		
Treatment zone	**Germany[3]**	**France[1,2]**	**U.S.[4,5]**	**Russia[10]**	**International[11]**	**Russia[9]**	**International[6,7]**	**U.S.[8]**
Frontal lines	4–8	2–8	4–8/4–8	2–8	4–10	2–12	4–6	6
Glabella	5–7	2–5	5–7/5–7	5–6	5–7	3–5	5	3–5
Crow's feet	3–5	2–5	2–5/2–5	3–4	2–5	3–6	3	3–4
Lower eyelid	1–2	1–2	No/No	No	No	1–2	1–2	1
Bunny lines	2	1	No/1	1	No	2–3	2	2
Perioral area[a]	8	2–4	2–6/2–6	4	2–6	4–6	4–6	6
Nasal tip	1	1	1/No	No	No	1	1	1
DAO	1	1	No/1	1	1	1	1	1
Chin (total)	2	2	1–2/1–2	2	1–2	2	2	1–2
Nefertiti lift	No	No	No	2–3	3	2–5	2–4	No

Note: No = data are not included in the consensus.
[a] The number of injection points for the correction of the perioral region in the U.S. and German consensuses are indicated for the upper and lower lips. In the French consensus, it is indicated only for the upper lip.

Table A1.3 Analysis of the Dose Range/Median Dose (U) Range for OnaBTX-A (Doses Indicated are for One Side of the Face Only)

Treatment Zone	Germany[3]	France[1,2]	U.S.[4,5]
Frontal lines	6–24/10–15	10–20	6–15 6–15
Glabella	10–50/22	5–30/20	10–30/20 10–30/20
Crow's feet	8–15/12	6–16	5–15 5–15
Lower eyelid	0.5–2/2	1–2	No/No
Bunny lines	2–5/2	2–4	No 1–2.5
Perioral area[a]	4–8/8	2–4	4–5 4–5
Nasal tip	1–8/3	2–4	3/No
DAO	2	1–2	No 1–7.5
Chin	4–10/6	6–10	4–10/5 4–10
Neck (platysmal bands) (total)	60–80/60	Max. 50	40–60 40–60

[a] The number of injection points for the correction of the perioral region in the U.S. and German consensuses are indicated for the upper and lower lips. In the French consensus, it is indicated only for the upper lip.

Table A1.4 Analysis of the Dose Range/Median Dose (U) for IncoBTX-A (The Dose is Indicated for One Side of the Face Only)

Treatment zone	Russia[10]	International[11,12]
Frontal lines	10–20/15	5–15
Glabella	20	10–50/20
Crow's feet	12	10–30
Bunny lines	2–4	No
Perioral area (only upper lip)	4–6	4–6
DAO	1.5–4/3	1–7.5
Chin (total)	2–8/6	4–10
Nefertiti lift	20	15
Neck (platysmal bands) (total)	50–60	30–60

However, the Russian recommended doses compared to the international ones point to higher doses for the correction of cervico-facial contours ("Nefertiti lift"). As a result, the total dosage for the cervico-facial contour correction (DAO + platysma) becomes roughly the same in both of the analyzed consensus reports.

COMPARATIVE ANALYSIS OF THE RECOMMENDATIONS ON THE USE OF AboBTX-A

Analysis of the AboBTX-A dosages was based on the consensus reports adopted by the United States, Russia, and those of the

Table A1.5 Analysis of the Dose Range/Median Dose for AboBTX-A (The Dose Indicated is for One Side of the Face Only)

Treatment Zone	Russia[9]	International[6,7]	U.S.[8]
Frontal lines	10–30/20	20–60/30–40	15–75/30
Glabella	30–70/50	30–70/50	30–70/52.5
Crow's feet	10–25 /20	15–30	12.5–35/25
Lower eyelid	2–7.5	2.5	1.5–10/5
Bunny lines	5–10	5–10	2.5–20/11
Perioral area[a]	4–12/8–10	4–12/10	4.5–30/15
Nasal tip	10–20	10	3–20/5
DAO	5–10/7.5	5–10	3–12.5/8
Nefertiti lift	10–20	10–16	No
Chin (total)	10–30/20	10–20	9–25/15
Neck (platysmal bands) (total)	60–80	Max.100	40–150/75

[a] The number of injection points for the correction of the perioral region in the U.S. consensus is indicated for the upper and lower lips.

international consensus (Table A1.5).[6–9] The widest range of doses for almost all areas of the face is found in the U.S. consensus reports. Comparison of the consensuses shows that Russian experts prefer to use lower doses of AboBTX-A for forehead and "crow's feet" correction and slightly higher doses for nasal tip and chin correction.

The median dose of 5 U is provided in the U.S. consensus for correction of the lower eyelid. It does not differ from the dose proposed by Russian and international consensuses. However, in the Russian and international consensuses it is recommended not to administer at one point more than 2.5 U of AboBTX-A, so the dose is divided between two points. In the U.S. consensus only one injection point is indicated in the lower eyelid, that is, it is more than twice as high a dose at a single point of injection.

The U.S. consensus also recommends a higher dosage to correct perioral wrinkles, mainly due to the inclusion of not only the upper but also the lower lip.

CONCLUSION

A comparison of the consensus reports of the various countries on the use of the different approved BoNT-As shows that despite numerous studies, the exact dose ratio of OnaBTX-A, IncoBTX-A, and AboBTX-A doses is still a questionable issue. The comparative analyses of the available consensus reports suggest that BoNT-A equivalence coefficients for different muscles can vary significantly. This once again proves that each BoNT-A is unique, and simple dose extrapolation is absolutely *not* acceptable and should be avoided.

REFERENCES

1. Raspaldo H, Baspeyras M, Bellity P. et al. Upper- and mid-face anti-aging treatment and prevention using onabotulinumtoxin A: The 2010 multidisciplinary French consensus—part 1. *J Cosmet Dermatol* 2011; 10: 36–50.
2. Raspaldo H, Baspeyras M, Gassia V. et al. Upper- and mid-face anti-aging treatment and prevention using onabotulinumtoxin A: The 2010 multidisciplinary French consensus—part 2. *J Cosmet Dermatol* 2011; 10(2): 131–49.
3. Philipp-Dormston WG, Bergfeld D, Sommer B, and the Onabotulinumtoxin Consensus Group. Consensus recommendations on the use of onabotulinumtoxin A in aesthetic medicine. *JDDG* 2012; 11(Suppl. 1): 1–41.
4. Carruthers JDA, Glogau RG, Blitzer A, and the Facial Aesthetics Consensus Group Faculty. Advances in facial rejuvenation: Botulinum toxin type A, hyaluronic acid dermal fillers, and combination therapies–consensus recommendations. *Plast Reconstr Surg* 2008; 121(5 Suppl): 5S–30S.
5. Kane M, Donofrio L, Ascher B et al. Expanding the use of neurotoxins in facial aesthetics: A consensus panel's assessment and recommendations. *J Drugs Dermatol* 2010; 9(1 Suppl): s7–22; quiz s23–5.
6. Ascher B, Talarico S, Cassuto D et al. International consensus recommendations on the aesthetic usage of botulinum toxin type A (Speywood Unit)—Part I: Upper facial wrinkles. *J Eur Acad Dermatol Venereol* 2010; 24(11): 1278–84.
7. Ascher B, Talarico S, Cassuto D et al. International consensus recommendations on the aesthetic usage of botulinum toxin type A (Speywood Unit)—Part II: Wrinkles on the middle and lower face, neck and chest. *J Eur Acad Dermatol Venereol* 2010; 24(11): 1285–95.
8. Maas C, Kane MA, Bucay VW et al. Current aesthetic use of AbobotulinumtoxinA in clinical practice: An evidence-based consensus review. *Aesthet Surg J* 2012; 32(1 Suppl): 8S–29S.
9. Contemporary view of facial wrinkles therapy with Dysport. Consensus materials of International Expert Council with comments of Russian Expert Group. Publishing House *Cosmetic & Medicine*, 2014.
10. Yutskovskaya Y, Gubanova E, Khrustaleva I et al. IncobotulinumtoxinA in aesthetics: Russian multidisciplinary expert consensus recommendations. *Clin Cosmet Investig Dermatol* 2015; 8: 297–306.
11. Carruthers J, Fournier N, Kerscher M, Ruiz-Avila J, De Almeida RT, Kaeuper G. The convergence of medicine and neurotoxins: A focus on botulinum toxin type A and its application in aesthetic medicine—A global, evidence-based botulinum toxin consensus education initiative. Part II: Incorporating botulinum toxin into aesthetic clinical practice. *Dermatol Surg* 2013; 39: 510–25.
12. Prager W, Bee EK, Havermann I, Zschocke I. IncobotulinumtoxinA for the treatment of platysmal bands: A single-arm, prospective proof-of-concept clinical study. *Dermatol Surg* 2015; 41(Suppl 1): S88–92.

Index